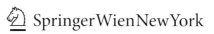

Bruno K. Podesser
David J. Chambers
(*Editors*)

New Solutions for the Heart

An Update in Advanced
Perioperative Protection

SpringerWienNewYork

Prof. Dr. Bruno K. Podesser
Department of Cardiac Surgery
Landesklinikum St. Pölten
Propst Führerstr. 4
3100 St. Pölten
Austria
bruno.podesser@meduniwien.ac.at

Dr. David J. Chambers
Cardiac Surgical Research
The Rayne Institute (King's College London)
St. Thomas Hospital
Westminster Bridge Road
London SE1 7EH
United Kingdom
david.chambers@kcl.ac.uk

This work is subject to copyright.
All rights are reserved, whether the whole or part of the material is concerned, specifically those of translation, reprinting, re-use of illustrations, broadcasting, reproduction by photocopying machines or similar means, and storage in data banks.

Product Liability: The publisher can give no guarantee for all the information contained in this book. The use of registered names, trademarks, etc. in this publication does not imply, even in the absence of a specific statement, that such names are exempt from the relevant protective laws and regulations and therefore free for general use.

© 2011 Springer-Verlag/Wien
Printed in Germany

SpringerWienNewYork is a part of Springer Science+Business Media
springer.at

Typesetting: SPI, Pondicherry, India

Printed on acid-free and chlorine-free bleached paper
SPIN: 80011542

With 39 Figures

Library of Congress Control Number: 2010937109

ISBN 978-3-211-85547-8   e-ISBN 978-3-211-85548-5
DOI 10.1007/978-3-211-85548-5
SpringerWienNewYork

Foreword (by Lawrence H. Cohn)

This interesting volume on advanced perioperative protection during cardiac surgery is an excellent compilation of past, present and future science of this very important and fundamental topic for every cardiac surgeon.

The Editors, Dr. Chambers and Podesser have assembled an all-star cast of excellent clinicians and scientists, experts in the general fields of basic cardiac research, cardioplegia research and clinical outcomes research. After an initial excellent historical chapter the various authors present much of the basic science of myocyte physiology, myocardial protection, subjects that have not been well understood. These basic concepts have been summarized beautifully in this book for clinicians and basic science investigators alike.

The next section discusses much of what is currently known about the clinical and physiological effect of cardioplegia on the beating and arrested heart, the optimal protection for the transplanted heart, specific recommendations for right heart protection and a variety of modalities to achieve optimal protection in these situations.

Finally, there are several chapters about the potential future of improved protective cardiac strategies during surgery for an increasing number of patients, particularly the elderly, who will require cardiac surgery over the next decades. The authors have done an excellent job in putting together the best of science and clinical practice of a subject which is critical to successful cardiac surgery and which was put into effect only 30 years ago with the institution of hyperkalemic cardioplegia. Cardioplegia has become a scientific and clinical requirement for excellence in heart surgery.

The results in heart surgery are superb today compared with yesterday and a book like this is very important to stimulate even better results as we operate on more and more elderly patients and patients in extreme heart failure. The editors are to be congratulated on a superb job of getting the best and the brightest authors and investigators in the area of myocardial protection and insisting that we not stand on our laurels, but look to even better physiologic and clinical pathologic correlations for the best protection of hearts during open heart surgery.

Department of Cardiac Surgery Lawrence H. Cohn
The Brigham & Women's Hospital
Harvard Medical School
Boston, MA, USA

Foreword (by Ernst Wolner)

Myocardial protection has been an integral part of cardiac surgery for the last 40 years after cardiac surgeons have realized in the early days that operations without protection of the heart lead to complications and fatalities. However, the story is not over yet. New challenges are waiting for surgeons and scientists. On the one hand, our surgical population is changing and we are today operating on older patients with often multiple co-morbidities; on the other hand, we are performing more complex operations than ever before.

The current book, edited by Podesser and Chambers, gives an excellent overview on the achievements in myocardial protection of the past, the current clinical strategies and the future direction of science in this important field of cardiac research. Both Dr. Podesser and Dr. Chambers have dedicated most of their experimental and clinical work during the last 25 years towards improvement of myocardial protection and helped us to understand basic concepts of ischemia and reperfusion in normal and failing hearts. The editors have assembled the "crème de la crème" of scientists around the world that work in this field of research. The result is a compendium of excellent contributions that cover the historic development of cardioplegic arrest. Then a systematic overview of the sites of injury, where injury happens, is presented. A special focus is placed on age and the possible influence of gender on myocardial protection strategies. Additionally, due to increasing clinical relevance, a spotlight is placed on protection of the right, the failing, and the transplanted heart. In the last section of the book, new approaches and technologies are discussed. The importance of the endothelium as the first line of injury and defense, followed by the effects of cardioplegia on the vascular system and the influence of radical scavengers are presented. Finally, alternative solutions to arrest the heart are discussed and new technologies to deliver cardioplegia and/or cell therapies, to improve perfusion of the explanted heart and to visualize cardioplegia are proposed to the reader.

I would like to congratulate all authors on their valuable contributions and, once again, the two editors for the tremendous work they have put into this book. The last comparable compendium is more than 15 years old. Therefore, this update in advanced perioperative protection is urgently needed. The results and strategies presented in this book will expand our knowledge on injury and protection of the heart and thereby can improve the outcome of our daily work. I think it is a valuable book for both cardiac surgeons and scientists.

Department of Cardiothoracic Surgery Ernst Wolner
Allgemeines Krankenhaus der Stadt Wien
Medizinische Universität Wien, Vienna, Austria

Preface

If I have seen a little further it is by standing on the shoulders of Giants.
Sir Isaac Newton (1643–1727), February 5, 1676, in a letter to Robert Hooke.

The mere formulation of a problem is far more essential than its solution, which may be merely a matter of mathematical or experimental skills. To raise new questions, new possibilities, to regard old problems from a new angle requires creative imagination and marks real advances in science.
Albert Einstein, (1879–1955)

Routine work can be accomplished easily and quickly by all who are willing to do so. However, almost everybody has to undergo a tiresome training to carefully and systematically reflect on complex processes.
Theodor Billroth, (1829–1894) "Über das Lehren und Lernen der medicinischen Wissenschaften an den Universitäten der Deutschen Nation" Vienna, 1876.

The idea for this book was conceived by Bruno Podesser in 2006, after realizing that there had been no comprehensive summary of myocardial protection during cardiac surgery since a book edited by HM Piper and CJ Preusse in 1993 (Ischemia-Reperfusion in Cardiac Surgery). It became more of a reality when I was invited to give a lecture at the Medical University, Vienna. Afterwards, we were chatting in a traditional Kaffeehaus in the old town of Vienna and I was persuaded (against my better judgement) to become part of the project as a Co-Editor (and author). This involved help in deciding a structure, and co-opting/persuading a number of eminent clinicians and scientists in the field of myocardial protection associated with cardiac surgery to write a chapter relevant to their expertise. It also became apparent that there was an expectation to write not one, but two, chapters (hence my reservations). Fortunately, the work involved in editing the other chapters was made relatively easy by the erudition of our authors.

That we have been successful in our endeavour can be seen within the book that has now been published. We hope this will be seen as a stepping-stone for continuing research in this field, and as an aid for the challenges that are before those of us involved in moving cardiac surgery forward as a modern and exciting specialty in medicine.

The quotes above encapsulate how we feel about our Authors and about how we hope that the book will be viewed. If it could act as a basis for future studies and stimulate more research in this field, we would be pleased with the achievement and consider the work involved worthwhile. The quest for new "solutions" to optimize protection in all aspects of cardiac surgery is a worthy goal, and one that is done primarily to benefit the patients who have to undergo such surgery.

We thank all the authors involved in this project, for agreeing to write for us and for the time and effort they have devoted to bringing the project to fruition. We appreciate that without their efforts this would not have been possible. Finally, we thank our families for putting up with the time spent away from home whilst working to finalize the end result.

Vienna and St. Pölten, Austria Bruno K. Podesser
London, UK David J. Chambers
May 2010

Contents

Contributors xiii

Part I Introduction

1 The Changing Population: The Surgeon's Challenge 3
Bruno K. Podesser

Part II Fundamentals

2 Fundamentals of the Past: Cardioplegia: The First Period Revisited 15
Sigurd Gunnes and Per Jynge

3 Sites of Injury: Myocyte 41
David J. Chambers

4 Sites of Injury: The Endothelium 57
Johann Wojta

Part III Special Focus

**5 Intraoperative Protection of the Myocardium: Effects
of Age and Gender** 73
James D. McCully and Sidney Levitsky

6 Protection of the Right Heart 93
Gábor Szabó

7 Protection of the Failing Heart 109
Bruno K. Podesser, Karola Trescher, and Wolfgang Dietl

8 Protection During Heart Transplantation 131
Allanah Barker and Stephen Large

Part IV   New Approaches and Technologies

9   The Endothelium As Target for Interventions 145
Seth Hallström and Bruno K. Podesser

10   Vascular Effects of Cardioplegic Arrest and Cardiopulmonary Bypass ... 167
Neel R. Sodha, Michael P. Robich, and Frank W. Sellke

11   Oxygen Radical Scavengers 179
Jack A.T.C. Parker and Uwe Mehlhorn

12   New Approaches to Cardioplegia: Alternatives to Hyperkalemia 199
David J. Chambers and Hazem B. Fallouh

13   Myocardial Protection via the Coronary Venous Route 221
Werner Mohl, Dejan Milasinovic, and Sarah Burki

14   Donor Heart Preservation by Continuous Perfusion 249
Andreas Zuckermann, Arezu Aliabadi, and Gernot Seebacher

15   Visualization of Cardioplegia Delivery 269
Lawrence S. Lee, Vakhtang Tchantchaleishvili, and Frederick Y. Chen

Author Index 283

Subject Index 285

About the Editors 287

Contributors

Arezu Aliabadi Department of Cardiac Surgery, Medical University of Vienna, Währinger Gürtel 18–20, 1090 Vienna, Austria

Allanah Barker Papworth Everard, Cambridge, CB3 8RE, UK

Sarah Burki Department of Cardiac Surgery, Medical University of Vienna, Währinger Gürtel 18–20, 1090 Vienna, Austria

David J. Chambers Cardiac Surgical Research/Cardiothoracic Surgery, The Rayne Institute (King's College London), Guy's & St. Thomas' NHS Foundation Trust, St. Thomas' Hospital, London, SE1 7EH, UK, david.chambers@kcl.ac.uk

Frederick Y. Chen Division of Cardiac Surgery, Brigham and Women's Hospital, Harvard Medical School, 75 Francis Street, Boston, MA 02115, USA, fchen@partners.org

Wolfgang Dietl Department of Cardiac Surgery, Landesklinikum St. Pölten, Propst Führerstr, 4,3100 St. Pölten, Austria, The Ludwig Boltzmann Cluster for Cardiovascular Research, Medical University of Vienna, Vienna, Austria

Hazem B. Fallouh Cardiac Surgical Research/Cardiothoracic Surgery, The Rayne Institute (King's College London), Guy's and St. Thomas' NHS Foundation Trust, St. Thomas' Hospital, London, SE1 7EH, UK

Sigurd Gunnes Department of Cardiothoracic Surgery, St. Olavs University Hospital, Trondheim, Norway; Department of Circulation and Medical Imaging, Norwegian University of Science and Technology, 7006 Trondheim, Norway, sigurd.gunnes@ntnu.no

Seth Hallström Institute of Physiological Chemistry, Center of Physiological Medicine, Medical University of Graz, Graz, Austria

Per Jynge Department of Medicine and Health Sciences, Linköping University, 58185 Linköping, Sweden, per.jynge@liu.se

Stephen Large Papworth Everard, Cambridge, CB3 8RE, UK, stephen.large@ papworth.nhs.uk

Lawrence S. Lee Division of Cardiac Surgery, Brigham and Women's Hospital, Harvard Medical School, 75 Francis Street, Boston, MA 02115, USA

Sidney Levitsky Division of Cardiothoracic Surgery, Beth Israel Deaconess Medical Center, Harvard Medical School, 110 Francis Street, Suite 2A, Boston, MA 02115, USA, slevitsk@bidmc.harvard.edu

James D. McCully Division of Cardiothoracic Surgery, Beth Israel Deaconess Medical Center, Harvard Medical School, 33 Brookline Avenue, DA-0734, Boston, MA 02115, USA, james_mccully@ hms.harvard.edu

Uwe Mehlhorn Department of Cardiothoracic and Vascular Surgery, University of Mainz, Mainz, Germany, uwe.mehlhorn@uni-mainz.de

Dejan Milasinovic Department of Cardiac Surgery, Medical University of Vienna, Währinger Gürtel 18–20, 1090 Vienna, Austria

Werner Mohl Department of Cardiac Surgery, Medical University of Vienna, Währinger Gürtel 18–20, 1090 Vienna, Austria, werner.mohl@meduniwien.ac.at

Jack A. T. C. Parker Department of Cardiothoracic and Vascular Surgery, University of Mainz, Mainz, Germany, jack.parker@ukmainz.de

Bruno K. Podesser Department of Cardiac Surgery, Landesklinikum St. Pölten, Propst Führerstr. 4, 3100, St. Pölten, Austria; The Ludwig Boltzmann Cluster for Cardiovascular Research, Medical University of Vienna, Vienna, Austria, bruno.podesser@meduniwien.ac.at

Michael P. Robich Beth Israel Deaconess Medical Center, Harvard Medical School, Boston, MA 02215, USA

Gernot Seebacher Department of Cardiac Surgery, Medical University of Vienna, Währinger Gürtel 18–20, 1090 Vienna, Austria

Frank W. Sellke Division of Cardiothoracic Surgery, Rhode Island Hospital and the Alpert Medical School of Brown University, APC 424, 593 Eddy Street, Providence, RI 02903, USA; Division of Cardiothoracic Surgery, Beth Israel Deaconess Medical Center, Harvard Medical School, Boston, MA 02215, USA, fsellke@lifespan.org

Neel R. Sodha Beth Israel Deaconess Medical Center, Harvard Medical School, Boston, MA 02215, USA

Gábor Szabó Abteilung Herzchirurgie, Chirurgische Universitätsklinik, Im Neuenheimer Feld 110, 69120 Heidelberg, Germany

Vakhtang Tchantchaleishvili Division of Cardiac Surgery, Brigham and Women's Hospital, Harvard Medical School, 75 Francis Street, Boston, MA 02115, USA

Karola Trescher Department of Cardiac Surgery, Landesklinikum St. Pölten, Propst Führerstr. 4,3100, St. Pölten, Austria; The Ludwig Boltzmann Cluster for Cardiovascular Research, Medical University of Vienna, Vienna, Austria

Johann Wojta Department of Internal Medicine, Allgemeines Krankenhaus der Stadt Wien, Medical University of Vienna, Währinger Gürtel 18–20, 1090 Vienna, Austria

Ernst Wolner Department of Cardiothoracic Surgery, Allgemeines Krankenhaus der Stadt Wien, Medical University of Vienna, Währinger Gürtel 18–20, 1090 Vienna, Austria

Andreas Zuckermann Department of Cardiac Surgery, Medical University of Vienna, Währinger Gürtel 18–20, 1090 Vienna, Austria, anandreas.zuckermann@meduniwien.ac.at

Part I
Introduction

The Changing Population: The Surgeon's Challenge

Bruno K. Podesser

Abbreviations

CABG   coronary artery bypass grafting
MI   myocardial infarction
avlg€   average logistic euro score

1.1 Historic Development and Current Trends in Cardiac Surgery

During the last 50 years cardiac surgery has developed from a sub-specialization of thoracic surgery to one of the most innovative and demanding fields in surgery. Whereas at the beginning palliative corrections of pediatric patients and adult valve patients have accounted for the majority of cases, today's cardiac surgical practice involves coronary artery bypass grafting, valve surgery, surgery of the large vessels, transplantation and pediatric surgery. In this book we will only focus on adult cardiac surgery.

During the last 20 years revascularization techniques have been refined and the majority of patients nowadays receives at least one arterial graft, for young individuals the advantages of two arterial grafts or an all-arterial concept is discussed (Navia et al. 2008). In valve surgery there has been a tremendous shift away from non-biological valve replacement towards biological prostheses and reconstructive techniques. For the first time ever, since 2004 the numbers of non-biological valves in the US are decreasing and those of biologic valves are increasing, because quality of life has become a major determinant in the selection of valve prostheses (Gammie et al. 2009). During the same

B.K. Podesser
Department of Cardiac Surgery, Landesklinikum St. Pölten, Propst Führerstr. 4, 3100 St. Pölten, Austria
The Ludwig Boltzmann Cluster for Cardiovascular Research, Medical University of Vienna, Austria
e-mail: bruno.podesser@meduniwien.ac.at

period the numbers of mitral valve reconstructions have reached an all-time high, thereby guaranteeing again a higher quality of life and a longer life expectancy (Gammie et al. 2009). The results of the surgery of the large vessels have improved from refined cerebro- and spinal protection techniques as well as from the development of endovascular stenting of the aneurysmatic part of the aorta (Grabenwoger et al. 2003; Ehrlich et al. 2009; Eggebrecht et al. 2003). In cardiac transplantation, new immunosuppressive drugs such as tacrolimus have become important alternatives to cyclosporine not only as back-up drug but as primary regimen (Podesser et al. 2005; Zuckermann and Aliabadi 2009).

The widening of the spectrum of operations is mainly due to new technologies that have become available to cardiac surgeons. Besides the already mentioned valve sparing techniques, these technologies are approaches to minimize the tissue damage and/or to miniaturize the skin and chest incisions. Some of these techniques have already gained considerable acceptance in the surgical community such as off-pump coronary revascularization (Puskas et al. 2009), endovascular stenting of the aorta (Ehrlich et al. 2009) or minimal-invasive approaches in aortic and mitral valve surgery (Walther et al. 2009; Casselman et al. 2003). Others such as robotic cardiac surgery are under critical re-evaluation regarding their efficacy (Robicsek 2008).

1.2
The Rightward Shift of the Age Curve: Representative Examples for Major Procedures

In the developed world the major challenge for our health care systems in general and for cardiac surgery in particular is the increasing age of the population. Whereas the distribution of the different age groups in the general population used to have a pyramid-shape, this curve today has a bell-shape that will further progress. The increasing rightward shift of the age curve already has a major impact on our daily practice today but will become even more evident during the next years (Fig. 1).

In CABG, the average age of a patient at the time of operation during the early 1990s was 61 years (Seitelberger et al. 1991), today's average age in our department is 68 years, females are 70 years old. Similarly, the average mechanical aortic valve patient in the early

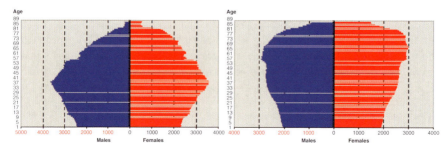

Fig. 1 Age distribution within the European Union: 2004 (*left panel*) and 2050 (*right panel*). *Source*: EuroCommerce 2006

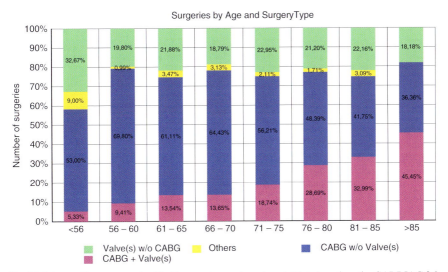

Fig. 2 Major cardiac surgery stratified by age in our department. Data based on the CARDIAC 2.0 software (STS data base form; S2 Engineering, Steyr, Austria) from the Department of Cardiac Surgery, Landesklinikum St. Pölten, Austria (n = 2347; 2007–2009); valves w/o CABG = aortic valves without CAGB; CABG + valves = CABG plus aortic valves; others = other major surgery such as mitral valve operations, aneurysms or dissections of the ascending aorta; CABG w/o Valves = CABG only

1980s was between 55 (Podesser et al. 1998) and 65 (Khan et al. 2001), the average biological aortic valve patient was 72 (Khan et al. 2001). Today's average age of aortic valve patients in our department is 72, if they receive an additional CABG they are 76 years old. In mitral surgery, patients were between 53 (Podesser et al. 1998) and 61 years (Moss et al. 2003). Today the average patient in our department who needs isolated mitral valve repair or replacement is 65, if they need additional CABG they are 71 years old. Finally, the average patient age in cardiac transplantation in the early 1990s was 43 years, today the patients are 49 years old (Aliabadi et al. 2007). Figure 2 summarizes the patients operated in our department between 2007 and 2009, stratified by age and major surgery groups.

1.3
Early Mortality in the 1990s and in 2010

In contrast to the rightward shift in age the postoperative outcome of these operations has been stable or even improved. In CABG perioperative mortality has remained at 3% between during the 1990s, as derived from the STS Data-base despite an observed increase in preoperative risk factors (Ferguson et al. 2002; Estafanous et al. 1998). When patients are operated with acute MI, hospital mortality is significantly higher: about 14% for patients during the first 24 h after MI, 8%, when operated between day 1 and 3, and 4%, when operated between day 4 and 15 post MI. Current mortality rates from our department

Table 1 Hospital mortality/30d mortality for major surgical procedures: early 1990s versus 2010

In%	CABG	CABG with acute MI	AV	AV and CABG	All MV repair	All MV replace	HTX (1y)
Early 1990s[a]	3	8	5	7	7.8	7.8	25
2010[b]	1.8	5.7	1.7	2.4	4	5	10
avlog€	4.1	8.9	7.0	8.7	7.3	9.4	n.a.

[a]Sources early 1990s: (Ferguson et al. 2002; Estafanous et al. 1998; Podesser et al. 1998; Marchand et al. 2001; Aliabadi et al. 2007)
[b]Data derived from CARDIAC 2.0 software (STS data base form; S2 Engineering, Steyr, Austria) from the Department of Cardiac Surgery, Landesklinikum St. Pölten, Austria (n = 2347; 2007–2009); HTX = heart transplant data with courtesy from Prof. Andreas Zuckermann, Medical University of Vienna, Austria; avlog€ = average logistic euro score

reflect exactly that trend. With an average logistic Euroscore (al€S) of 4.1 the overall 30-day mortality for CABG is 1.8%, for patients presenting with acute MI during the first 6 days average operative mortality is 5.7% (al€S 8.9).

In isolated aortic valve surgery operative mortalities during the late 1980s and early 1990s were around 5% (Podesser et al. 1998). Today, in our department the chance to die during the first 30 days after aortic valve replacement is 1.7% (al€S 7.0), if an additional CABG is performed, 30-day mortality is 2.4% (al€S 8.7). Mitral valve surgery in all databases has a higher risk than aortic valve surgery. Whereas Marchand reported for unselected isolated mitral valve surgery 7.8% (Marchand et al. 2001), today's chance to die during the first 30 days after unselected mitral valve replacement is 5% (al€S 9.4), during mitral valve repair is 4% (al€S 7.3). If an additional CABG is added, replacement has 7.7% (al€S 12.6) and repair 4.9% (al€S, 6.5) mortality in our own database. Finally, during cardiac transplantation 30-day mortality has nearly remained stable at 10% but one year survival increased from 75% in the early 1990s to 90% in 2010 (Aliabadi et al. 2007). Table 1 summarizes our own data and representative numbers from literature.

1.4
Why Could We Keep the Outcome Similar or Become Even Better?

In summary the data presented so far have shown us that in spite of an increasingly aging population with more and severer co-morbidities the outcome of our daily work has become better than ever before. What are possible reasons for that development?

1.4.1
Standardization of Procedures

Cardiac surgery is one of the areas in medicine with the highest degrees of standardization. One can visit an operation theater in North America, Europe or Asia and will find virtually the same operative techniques applied with similar or identical instruments performed. This is possible because (1) cardiac surgery is a very young domain that started out from a few centers or "schools" worldwide, (2) national cardiac surgery societies are small and dominated by three major associations in North America and Europe, whose scientific journals are also the most important media for research and technology transfer. (3) This point is more practical: the majority of operations are planned operations with well documented and prepared patients. Finally (4), cardiac surgery is a very conservative field similar to flying, because the surgeon is always at risk to loose a patient. Therefore new technologies take quite a long time to be accepted but if they get accepted, penetration rate is high.

1.4.2
Training

Hand in hand with standardization goes training. This incorporates both, the training of the young residents but also continuous education of surgeons in new technologies. Most universities and training hospitals have well documented training programs that have been developed in accordance with the national scientific associations under the guidance of the already mentioned supranational associations. Again, the annual meetings of these associations together with exchange programs and scholarships encourage the residents to move during their training. This standardizes knowledge and techniques and should become even more available in future. Also for advanced surgeons the annual meetings are a chance to develop their skills and update the knowledge during scientific sessions and techno-colleges. Besides, industry-driven technology and research transfer is an important source to gain new information and acquire technology.

1.4.3
Partners

The improved outcome data are also due to our partners in the operation theater and on the wards. Anesthetic regimens have changed dramatically during the last 15 years and a lot of our operations would not be possible without these changes. Here I would like to mention some of them without being complete. The importance of temperature control after cardiac surgery, and its effect on early outcome has been well-documented (Rajek et al. 1998; Pezawas et al. 2004). This simple target has made on-table extubation feasible and determined "shivering" as inacceptable side effect on the intensive care unit. The use of cervical peridural anesthesia (PDA) additionally to conventional inhalative regimens to block postoperative pain and consecutively improve respiratory capacity has become a valuable tool to reduce postoperative ventilation and ICU time and might be attractive in patients with COPD (Peterson et al. 2000). New drugs such as sevoflourane have been shown to have cardioprotective effects and have replaced in most operation theaters other forms of anesthesia (De Hert et al. 2004).

Similarly, in patients with severely reduced cardiac function levosimendan has become a valuable drug either for preoperative conditioning or acute intraoperative loading of these patients (Plöchl and Rajek 2004; Landoni et al. 2010). Similarly, the intraoperative guidance and quality control of transthoracic echocardiography has become a cornerstone of modern cardiac anesthesia and surgery.

But not only during the operation but also after it the demands have changed. Care and mobilization has been intensified so that the average patient is leaving the ICU and the hospital earlier. Nursing alone has been replaced by active and early mobilization by physiotherapists and nurses even in critically ill patients (O'Connor and Walsham 2009). Stroke patients undergo early neuro-rehabilitation thereby minimizing the long-term defects (Oden et al. 1998).

1.5
More Work To Do: What Is Next?

In my opinion, there is a lot of work ahead of us. This work is both, educational and conceptual and probably it will take major efforts, strength and energy to convince the surgical community and the surrounding. However, in order to make cardiac surgery fit for the next challenges the surgical community first has to identify these challenges. Only then we can address them for the sake of our patients.

1.5.1
Bi-Directional Education

Surgeons have to export their needs out of the surgical community to the gate-keeper, the cardiologists. We have to convince cardiologists that CABG has superior results in patients with three-vessel disease than PTCA and that CABG with good results is not feasible in patients that underwent "full metal jacket" revascularization by multiple coronary artery stents before. Patients have a right to be fully informed about their treatment options. Therefore all participating specialists should speak with the patients (Taggart 2009). Similarly, in patients with heart valve disease, timing is essential and determines the postoperative and long-term outcome. For example in mitral valve regurgitation, if left ventricular endsystolic dimension exceeds 45 mm, the chance to develop heart failure is dramatically increasing and can hardly be stopped or changed by operation (Wisenbaugh et al. 1994). There is an "optimal timing" for the operation and no chance that mitral regurgitation will disappear without operation- so why wait until the patient has additional pulmonary hypertension? The bottom line of these considerations is that we will not be able to keep the standards and the outcome if patient selection is not optimized. This can only be done in collaboration with the cardiologists, who have to realize that they don't loose a patient, if they refer him/her to surgery, but they gain one for long-term follow-up treatment.

Surgeons have to import new aspects and achievements into their daily routine. This means that we have to invite other specialists to help us in patient selection and preoperative preparation. Geriatricians have determined a new diagnosis in our increasingly older population: frailty. Frailty is characterized by vulnerability to acute stressors and is a consequence of decline in overall function and physiologic reserves (Singh et al. 2008). An estimated 7% of the US population older than 65 years and 30% of octogenarians are frail. The qualities to define frailty include mobility, strength, balance, motor processing, cognition, nutrition, endurance, and physical activity. Pathophysiologic pathways leading to frailty involve a multisystem cascade that includes neuroendocrine dysfunction with lower insulin-like growth factor and dehydroepiandrosterone sulfate and an altered inflammatory milieu with increased levels of C-reactive protein, interleukins, tumor necrosis factor alpha, and abnormal coagulation. Frailty predicts death and heralds the transition to disability in general populations (Singh et al. 2008). As our patients get older, we must consider the role of frailty. Simple "eye-bowling" is no longer enough to describe the preoperative status of our patients. Simplifications such as the stratification in "go-goes", "slow goes", and "no goes" can only be helpful, when an standardized institutional approach is chosen to assess and test these old candidates together with cardiologists, geriatricians, anesthesiologists, and physiotherapists.

1.5.2
New Concepts

The input mentioned before must lead also to new concepts that influence our daily work. The concept of myocardial protection is from the 1960s, with major innovations in the 1970s but has not changed in principle during the last 20 years (Bretschneider 1964; Hearse et al. 1975). In the meanwhile scientists and surgeons have realized that during cardiac surgery not only myocytes but also endothelial cells (Schölkens et al. 1987) and the cells of the conductance system are stressed. However, cardioplegic solutions were designed to protect myocytes and focused mainly on the ischemic period. Besides, myocardial protection was limited to intraoperative protection only and did not address the potential benefits of perioperative management (Podesser and Hallström 2007). We have shown convincing experimental evidence that pre- and intra-operative priming of the heart with endothelial-protective drugs can improve organ function and postischemic outcome (Podesser et al. 2002; Semsroth et al. 2005; Hallström et al. 2008).

It took surgeons a long time to realize that most cardioplegic solutions were developed and tested on healthy animal hearts. However, our patient's hearts are not healthy but have seriously altered coronary arteries, hypertension or are in failure. We therefore have started to use models of ischemic heart disease, heart failure, (Podesser et al. 2002), hypertension (Podesser et al. 2007), or the hostile environment of warm unprotected ischemia (Hallström et al. 2008) to test additives to currently used cardioplegic solutions or to study new solutions to arrest the heart (Trescher et al. 2009).

It is known that age influences the outcome in cardiac surgery and hearts of different ages have different needs. This is true for the very young and the very old heart. However, most cardioplegic solutions were tested experimentally on young adult hearts. Before the main interest was to study the differences in young hearts (Karck et al. 1995; Podesser et al. 1993). Recent experimental studies have shown considerable differences in old hearts during ischemia and reperfusion (McCully et al. 2007). These newly gained information might be interesting and influence our clinical work. Similarly, alternative solutions to arrest the heart that do not depend on hypopolarization but use beta-blocking agents are currently under evaluation and might change our clinical habits (Fallouh et al. 2010).

1.6
Summary

All in all, innovations are welcome from all sides and should involve preoperative diagnosis and treatment to address our patient's need and discover their weak spots such as heart failure, malnutrition, depression etc. Based on these findings the optimal and individualized treatment options during cardiac surgery and postoperative rehabilitation should be adopted. This book tries to address one segment of the puzzle and presents the latest developments and concepts in myocardial protection.

References

Aliabadi, A., S. Sandner, B. Bunzel, D. Dunkler, S. Mahr, M. Paireder, D. Zimpfer, S. Rödler, R. Herics, A. Rajek, G. Wieselthaler, M. Hülsmann, G. Wollenek, G. Weigel, U. Salzer-Muhar, E. Wolner, M. Grimm, and A. Zuckermann (2007) Recent trends in heart transplantation: the University of Vienna experience. Clin Transpl 81–97

Bretschneider, H.J. (1964) Survival time and recuperative time of the heart in normothermia and hypothermia. Verh Dtsch Ges Kreislaufforsch 30: 11–34

Casselman, F.P., S. Van Slycke, H. Dom, D.L. Lambrechts, Y. Vermeulen, H. Vanermen (2003) Endoscopic mitral valve repair: feasible, reproducible, and durable. J Thorac Cardiovasc Surg 125:273–282

De Hert, S.G., P.J. Van der Linden, S. Cromheecke, R. Meeus, A. Nelis, V. Van Reeth, P.W. ten Broecke, I.G. De Blier, B.A. Stockman, and I.E. Rodrigus (2004) Cardioprotective properties of sevoflurane in patients undergoing coronary surgery with cardiopulmonary bypass are related to the modalities of its administration. Anesthesiology 101: 299–310

Eggebrecht, H., D. Baumgart, A. Schmermund, C. von Birgelen, U. Herold, R. Wiesemes, J. Barkhausen, H. Jakob, and R. Erbel (2003) Endovascular stent-graft repair for penetrating atherosclerotic ulcer of the descending aorta. Am J Cardiol 91: 1150–1153

Ehrlich, M.P., H. Rousseau, R. Heijman, P. Piquet, J.P. Beregi, C.A. Nienaber, G. Sodeck, and R. Fattori (2009) Early outcome of endovascular treatment of acute traumatic aortic injuries: the talent thoracic retrospective registry. Ann Thorac Surg 88: 1258–1263

Estafanous, F.G., F.D. Loop, T.L. Higgins, S. Tekyi-Mensah, B.W. Lytle, D.M. Cosgrove, M. Roberts-Brown, and N.J. Starr (1998) Increased risk and decreased morbidity of coronary artery bypass grafting between 1986 and 1994. Ann Thorac Surg 65: 383–389

Fallouh, H.B., S.C. Bardswell, L.M. McLatchie, M.J. Shattock, D.J. Chambers, and J.C. Kentish (2010) Esmolol cardioplegia: the cellular mechanism of diastolic arrest. Cardiovasc Res 87: 552–560

Ferguson, T.B., B.G. Hammill, E.D. Peterson, E.R. DeLong, F.L. Grover, and S.T.S.N.D. Committee (2002) A decade of change-risk profiles and outcomes for isolated coronary artery bypass grafting procedures, 1990–1999: a report from the STS National Database Committee and the Duke Clinical Research Institute. Society of Thoracic Surgeons Ann Thorac Surg 73: 480–489; discussion 489–490

Gammie, J.S., S. Sheng, B.P. Griffith, E.D. Peterson, J.S. Rankin, S.M. O'Brien, and J.M. Brown (2009) Trends in mitral valve surgery in the United States: results from the Society of Thoracic Surgeons Adult Cardiac Surgery Database. Ann Thorac Surg 87: 1431–1437; discussion 1437–1439

Grabenwoger, M., T. Fleck, M. Czerny, D. Hutschala, M. Ehrlich, M. Schoder, J. Lammer, and E. Wolner (2003) Endovascular stent graft placement in patients with acute thoracic aortic syndromes. Eur J Cardiothorac Surg 23: 788–793; discussion 793

Hallström, S., M. Franz, H. Gasser, M. Vodrazka, S. Semsroth, U.M. Losert, M. Haisjackl, B.K. Podesser, and T. Malinski (2008) S-nitroso human serum albumin reduces ischaemia/reperfusion injury in the pig heart after unprotected warm ischaemia. Cardiovasc Res 77: 506–514

Hearse, D.J., D.A. Stewart, and M.V. Braimbridge (1975) The additive effects of potassium ions and hypothermia for the induction of elective cardiac arrest. Biochem Soc Trans 3: 417–420

Karck, M., G. Ziemer, M. Zoeller, S. Schulte, K.D. Juergens, H. Weisser, and A. Haverich (1995) Protection of the chronic hypoxic immature rat heart during global ischemia. Ann Thorac Surg 59: 699–706

Khan, S.S., A. Trento, M. DeRobertis, R.M. Kass, M. Sandhu, L.S. Czer, C. Blanche, S. Raissi, G.P. Fontana, W. Cheng, A. Chaux, and J.M. Matloff (2001) Twenty-year comparison of tissue and mechanical valve replacement. J Thorac Cardiovasc Surg 122: 257–269

Landoni, G., A. Mizzi, G. Biondi-Zoccai, G. Bruno, E. Bignami, L. Corno, M. Zambon, C. Gerli, and A. Zangrillo (2010) Reducing mortality in cardiac surgery with levosimendan: a meta-analysis of randomized controlled trials. J Cardiothorac Vasc Anesth 24: 51–57

Marchand, M.A., M.R. Aupart, R. Norton, I.R. Goldsmith, L.C. Pelletier, M. Pellerin, T. Dubiel, W. J. Daenen, P. Herijgers, F.P. Casselman, M.P. Holden, and T.E. David (2001) Fifteen-year experience with the mitral Carpentier-Edwards PERIMOUNT pericardial bioprosthesis. Ann Thorac Surg 71: S236–S239

McCully, J.D., A.J. Rousou, R.A. Parker, and S. Levitsky (2007) Age- and gender-related differences in mitochondrial oxygen consumption and calcium with cardioplegia and diazoxide. Ann Thorac Surg 83: 1102–1109

Moss, R.R., K.H. Humphries, M. Gao, C.R. Thompson, J.G. Abel, G. Fradet, and B.I. Munt (2003) Outcome of mitral valve repair or replacement: a comparison by propensity score analysis. Circulation 108(Suppl 1): 90–97

Navia, D., M. Vrancic, G. Vaccarino, F. Piccinini, H. Raich, S. Florit, and J. Thierer (2008) Total arterial off-pump coronary revascularization using bilateral internal thoracic arteries in triple-vessel disease: surgical technique and clinical outcomes. Ann Thorac Surg 86: 524–530

O'Connor, E.D., and J. Walsham (2009) Should we mobilise critically ill patients? A review Crit Care Resusc 11: 290–300

Oden, K.E., C.G. Kevorkian, and J.K. Levy (1998) Rehabilitation of the post-cardiac surgery stroke patient: analysis of cognitive and functional assessment. Arch Phys Med Rehabil 79: 67–71

Peterson, K.L., W.M. DeCampli, N.A. Pike, R.C. Robbins, and B.A. Reitz (2000) A report of two hundred twenty cases of regional anesthesia in pediatric cardiac surgery. Anesth Analg 90: 1014–1019

Pezawas, T., A. Rajek, M. Skolka, B. Schneider, and W. Plöchl (2004) Perspectives for core and skin surface temperature guided extubation in patients after normothermic cardiopulmonary bypass. Intensive Care Med 30: 1676–1680

Plöchl, W., and A. Rajek (2004) The use of the novel calcium sensitizer levosimendan in critically ill patients. Anaesth Intensive Care 32: 471–475

Podesser, B.K., and S. Hallström (2007) Nitric oxide homeostasis as a target for drug additives to cardioplegia. Br J Pharmacol 151: 930–940

Podesser, B.K., V. Hausleithner, R. Seitelberger, G. Wollenek, E. Wolner, and H. Steiert (1993) New developments in the isolated working heart: a comparison of neonatal, immature, and adult rabbits after sixty minutes of ischemia in respect to hemodynamic and biochemical parameters. J Pharmacol Toxicol Methods 30: 189–196

Podesser, B.K., G. Khuenl-Brady, E. Eigenbauer, S. Roedler, A. Schmiedberger, E. Wolner, and A. Moritz (1998) Long-term results of heart valve replacement with the Edwards Duromedics bileaflet prosthesis: a prospective ten-year clinical follow-up. J Thorac Cardiovasc Surg 115: 1121–1129

Podesser, B.K., J. Schirnhofer, O.Y. Bernecker, A. Kröner, M. Franz, S. Semsroth, B. Fellner, J. Neumüller, S. Hallström, and E. Wolner (2002) Optimizing ischemia/reperfusion in the failing rat heart–improved myocardial protection with acute ACE inhibition. Circulation 106: 1277–1283

Podesser, B.K., M. Rinaldi, N.A. Yona, L.A. Pulpón, J.P. Villemot, A. Haverich, D. Duveau, G. Brandrup-Wognsen, E. Gronda, A. Costard-Jäckle, M.G. Crespo-Leiro, C.S. Khazen, M. Viganó, J. Segovia, M.F. Mattei, W. Harringer, M. Treilhaud, K. Karason, M. Mangiavacchi, and G. Laufer (2005) Comparison of low and high initial tacrolimus dosing in primary heart transplant recipients: a prospective European multicenter study. Transplantation 79: 65–71

Podesser, B.K., M. Jain, S. Ngoy, C.S. Apstein, and F.R. Eberli (2007) Unveiling gender differences in demand ischemia: a study in a rat model of genetic hypertension. Eur J Cardiothorac Surg 31: 298–304

Puskas J.D., V.H. Thourani, P. Kilgo, W. Cooper, T. Vassiliades, J.D. Vega, C. Morris, E. Chen, B. J. Schmotzer, R.A. Guyton, and O.M. Lattouf (2009) Off-pump coronary artery bypass disproportionately benefits high-risk patients. Ann Thorac Surg 88: 1142–1147.

Rajek, A., R. Lenhardt, D.I. Sessler, A. Kurz, G. Laufer, R. Christensen, T. Matsukawa, and M. Hiesmayr (1998) Tissue heat content and distribution during and after cardiopulmonary bypass at 31 degrees C and 27 degrees C. Anesthesiology 88: 1511–1518

Robicsek F (2008) Robotic cardiac surgery: Time told!. J Thorac Cardiovasc Surg 135: 243–246

Schölkens, B.A., W. Linz, and Y.F. Han (1987) Heart and vascular wall as targets for tissue converting enzyme inhibition. Clin Exp Hypertens A 9: 427–433

Seitelberger, R., W. Zwölfer, S. Huber, S. Schwarzacher, T.M. Binder, F. Peschl, J. Spatt, C. Holzinger, B. Podesser, and P. Buxbaum (1991) Nifedipine reduces the incidence of myocardial infarction and transient ischemia in patients undergoing coronary bypass grafting. Circulation 83: 460–468

Semsroth, S., B. Fellner, K. Trescher, O.Y. Bernecker, L. Kalinowski, H. Gasser, S. Hallström, T. Malinski, and B.K. Podesser (2005) S-nitroso human serum albumin attenuates ischemia/reperfusion injury after cardioplegic arrest in isolated rabbit hearts. J Heart Lung Transplant 24: 2226–2234

Singh, M., K. Alexander, V.L. Roger, C.S. Rihal, H.E. Whitson, A. Lerman, A. Jahangir, and K.S. Nair (2008) Frailty and its potential relevance to cardiovascular care. Mayo Clin Proc 83: 1146–1153

Taggart, D.P. (2009) Coronary revascularization–2009: state of the art. Semin Thorac Cardiovasc Surg 21: 196–198

Trescher, K., M. Bauer, W. Dietl, S. Hallström, N. Wick, M. Wolfsberger, R. Ullrich, G. Jürgens, E. Wolner, and B.K. Podesser (2009) Improved myocardial protection in the failing heart by selective endothelin-A receptor blockade. J Thorac Cardiovasc Surg 137: 1005–1011

Walther, T., T. Dewey, M.A. Borger, J. Kempfert, A. Linke, R. Becht, V. Falk, G. Schuler, F.W. Mohr, M. Mack (2009) Transapical aortic valve implantation: Step by step. Ann Thorac Surg 87: 276–283

Wisenbaugh, T., D. Skudicky, and P. Sareli (1994) Prediction of outcome after valve replacement for rheumatic mitral regurgitation in the era of chordal preservation. Circulation 89: 191–197

Zuckermann, A.O., and A.Z. Aliabadi (2009) Calcineurin-inhibitor minimization protocols in heart transplantation. Transpl Int 22: 78–89

Part II
Fundamentals

Fundamentals of the Past: Cardioplegia: The First Period Revisited

2

Sigurd Gunnes and Per Jynge

2.1
Historical Overview

Techniques for controlling the heart during cardiopulmonary bypass (CPB) and aortic occlusion have occupied and still occupy a centre stage in cardiac surgical research. The first 25–30 years started with diverse attempts at cardiac arrest and subsequently at myocardial protection and, after initial failures, this became a successful period with development of concepts and techniques that still apply. The period thereafter is in the authors' opinion to a large extent characterized by continuous reassessment and refinement of principles and of consolidation of techniques. Notwithstanding, major new developments have taken place in molecular biology, physiology and pharmacology as well as in surgical practice. Within this context not only intraoperative but truly perioperative myocardial protection with improvements in diagnostic techniques, drug treatment, anesthesia and intensive care has come into focus and allowed cardiac surgery to take on more seriously ill patients. This chapter is written with the intention to provide insight in the thinking and problem solving during the early period until 1980–1985. It presents the history of what is well known as "cardioplegia" and thereafter presents some concepts and issues considered at the time. Only briefly are comments made that relate to current principles and practice.

2.1.1
Background and Definitions

When open heart surgery took off after the development of heart-lung machines (Gibbon 1954; Lillehei et al. 1956; Rygg and Kyvsgaard 1958), a partly unforeseen challenge was that

S. Gunnes
Department of Cardiothoracic Surgery, St. Olavs University Hospital, Trondheim, Norway
Department of Circulation and Medical Imaging, Norwegian University of Science and Technology, 7006 Trondheim, Norway
e-mail: sigurd.gunnes@ntnu.no

P. Jynge (✉)
Department of Medicine and Health Sciences, Linköping University, 58185 Linköping, Sweden
e-mail: per.jynge@liu.se

the unloaded heart on CPB continued to beat and had to be arrested in order to provide conditions for anatomic repair (Melrose 1980). Soon thereafter a further discovery was that surgical needs conflicted with myocardial demands. The needs of the surgeon include rapid induction, maintenance and easy reversal of cardiac arrest, a relaxed heart to allow for mobilization and traction, a preferably bloodless and unobscured field, and sufficient time for adequate correction of cardiac or coronary defects. A fulfillment ideally implies reversible induction of diastolic arrest, that coronary perfusion with blood may be avoided or minimized, and that periods of myocardial ischemia might be well tolerated.

Myocardial demands, on the other hand, requires that the cell machinery remains intact with rapid restoration of metabolism and function after cardiac arrest. An optimal procedure for the heart thus indicates that ischemia should preferably be avoided or that harmful effects induced by any inherent ischemia can be delayed and that a consequent reperfusion results in an uneventful recovery. In spite of all improvements made with time, the need-demand contradiction still represents a potential conflict in the everyday practice of cardiac surgery, not least when considering the state of the patient being operated upon.

Early techniques that were widely used to arrest and/or protect the heart were based on single or combined modalities such as:

- Hypothermia, systemic and/or supplied by topical cooling (Bigelow et al. 1950; Shumway et al. 1959; Swan 1973)
- Global ischemia with continuous or intermittent aortic occlusion (Cooley et al. 1962) and
- Aortic root or intracoronary perfusion with blood (Kay et al. 1958) and, when needed, electively induced ventricular fibrillation (Senning 1952).

Whereas these modalities alone or combined have survived up to the present day, during the 1970s they were mostly supplemented with or replaced by arresting the heart by "*cardioplegia*" based on chemical means (Bleese et al. 1978; Bretschneider et al. 1975; Follette et al. 1978a; Gay and Ebert 1973; Hearse et al. 1976a; Roe et al. 1977; Tyers et al. 1977). In general terms *cardioplegia* can be defined as a technique involving single or repeated injections, infusions or perfusions into the aortic root or into the coronary vasculature of a hypo- or normothermic solution (primarily) designed to arrest the heart (stricter sense) and (secondarily) also to protect the myocardium (wider sense) during aortic cross-clamping with global ischemia.

How the overall procedure of cardioplegia provided myocardial protection appeared as a very complex issue and many sophisticated explanations were forwarded. In more pragmatic terms, however, the salient properties of what was to become *cold chemical cardioplegia* could be divided into *three additive components* (Hearse et al. 1981a):

- *Chemical arrest* or the sparing of cell energy through rapid induction of arrest in diastole.
- *Hypothermia* or slowing the rate of cellular reactions thereby delaying energy decay and other deleterious processes during ischemia.
- *Additional protection* related to protective agents that prevent or reverse unfavourable ischemia-induced cellular changes.

Energy-sparing obtained by chemically induced diastolic arrest and by simultaneously added hypothermia at 20°C reduces myocardial oxygen demands (MVO_2) by almost 95%

and is therefore an obvious mutual factor explaining the efficacy of cold cardioplegic techniques. That hypothermia not only retards energy consumption but also degenerative cellular reactions during ischemia underpins its central role as the second component of cardioplegia (Bretschneider 1964; Hearse et al. 1976a). The third component may be more difficult to define, but, as was subsequently shown, the incorporation into coronary infusates of magnesium (Hölscher 1967; Hearse et al. 1976a), a buffering agent such as histidine (Bretschneider 1980; Preusse et al. 1979), and of metabolic substrates and of oxygen (Bleese et al. 1976; Bretschneider 1980; Follette et al. 1978a; Buckberg 1979) combats ischemia and adds further to the efficacy of cardioplegic procedures.

The early history of cardioplegia can be divided into three distinctly different phases with shifting opinions and practice: the birth and burial 1955–1960; the survival years 1960–1970; and the rediscovery and international acceptance during the 1970s. Each of these periods were dominated by eminent surgeons and scientists making their individual imprints upon the ongoing developments.

2.1.2
Birth and Burial

At the birth of open heart surgery the search for agents to stop the heart to improve conditions for surgical repair focused on a wide variety of pharmaceuticals (Lam et al. 1955; Melrose 1980) such as acetylcholine, muscle relaxants, antihistamines, and local anesthetics. Stimulated by Ringer's work (Ringer 1883) on the opposing effects of calcium and potassium upon the heart beat, Melrose and associates (Melrose et al. 1955) investigated the cardioplegic properties of potassium. After gaining experience in dogs they applied aortic root injections of potassium citrate for arrest of the human heart. The potassium citrate, maintained highly concentrated in glass vials prior to use, was dissolved in 30 ml batches of blood giving an injectate concentration in excess of 200 mM. The injection provided immediate cardiac arrest and conditions for short-lasting anatomic repair. Accordingly, Melrose's report in 1955 led to international recognition and adoption of his technique. In these very pioneering days of cardiac surgery bypass time was kept to an absolute minimum, ventricular fibrillation was feared and safe coronary perfusion techniques were yet to come. In this situation potential hazards of the Melrose solution were not easily detected. However, in 1959 it was reported (Helmsworth et al. 1959) that myocardial necrosis could always be found in dog hearts after potassium citrate arrest, and in 1960 this finding was confirmed by evidence in patients (McFarland et al. 1960). These two papers then led to the abandonment of chemically induced cardioplegia as it was now known. In retrospect, it is easy to forget how close Melrose came, in animal experiments, to establish a more rational use of potassium, and also that he was an early predecessor of modern blood cardioplegia.

2.1.3
Survival and Success

During the 1960s German scientists started research on cardioplegia and laid the basis for its future principles and general management. Hölscher observed the arresting and protective properties of magnesium and the local anesthetic procaine (Hölscher 1960, 1967) and proposed that the toxicity of the Melrose solution was due to citrate chelation of endogenous magnesium and calcium. Some years later, Kirsch (Kirsch et al. 1972) described the efficacy of injecting a highly concentrated solution of magnesium aspartate (161 mM) and procaine (11 mM) into the aortic root. The Kirsch *injection cardioplegia* combined with systemic hypothermia and topical cooling was introduced clinically in 1969 and gained popularity not least due to its simplicity.

2.1.3.1
Bretschneider and Söndergaard

The most influential German group of the 1960s, headed by Bretschneider, advocated hypothermia combined with very thorough myocardial equilibration by a single infusion of a cold (4°C) cardioplegic solution, ie *cold chemical cardioplegia* (Bretschneider 1964; Reidemeister et al. 1967; Nordbeck et al 1974; Bretschneider et al. 1975), this to be assisted by systemic hypothermia (15–20°C). Important observations mainly in ex vivo and in vivo dog hearts were:

- Energy-consuming ventricular fibrillation in hearts arrested by deep hypothermia without cardioplegia
- The considerable time required for complete equilibration of temperature between the coronary infusate and the myocardium during cooling
- The relationship between different forms of chemical arrest and myocardial oxygen demand
- The role of tissue ATP as a predictor of myocardial recovery from ischemia.

During the 1960s the Bretschneider group developed a number of "intracellular" solutions employing sodium plus calcium depletion for inducing a nondepolarized cardiac arrest thus minimizing transmembrane gradients of these ions at end of infusion and preferably also during subsequent ischemia. The solutions, as represented by no 3 in Table 1, were sodium-poor (5–12 mM) and calcium-free, included procaine (7.4–11.0 mM or finally zero), and contained almost normal or moderately elevated potassium (5–10 mM) and magnesium (1–9 mM).

Söndergaard in Denmark introduced the Bretschneider solution no. 3 into clinical use in 1964 and may be regarded as the surgical pioneer of modern cardioplegia. In 1975 he reported (Söndergaard et al. 1975) on 100 aortic valve operations with aortic occlusions of 80–120 min and with a low 6% mortality. Indirectly Søndergaard was also one of the early innovators of blood cardioplegia since the Bretschneider procedure advocated at the time involved two steps:

- Firstly, the infusion of a cold mixture of blood, glucose, mannitol and procaine in order to keep the heart oxygenated and rapidly arrested during the initial cooling phase; and
- Secondly, the infusion with myocardial equilibration of the cardioplegic solution itself.

In retrospect, it is fair to state that the total work by Bretschneider and associates remained underrated for an unfortunately long time. Contributing to this were the international neglect of cardioplegia in the 1960s and the apparent complexity of proposed principles and techniques.

Table 1 The composition of the Bretschneider (BR) and the St. Thomas' Hospital (STH) cardioplegic solutions

Component (mM)	BR no 3	BR-HTK	STH-1	STH-2
NaCl	12	18	144	120
NaHCO$_3$				10
KCL	10	10	20	16
MgCl$_2$	2	4	16	16
CaCl$_2$		0.02	2.2	1.2
Procaine–HCl	7.4		1	
Mannitol	239	33		
Histidine		180		
Histidine–HCl		18		
Tryptophan		2		
α-ketoglutarate		1		
pH	5.5–7.0	7.1 (25°C)	5.5–7.0	7.8
Osmolality (mOsm/Kg H$_2$O)	290 (320)	280 (302)	300–320	285–300

2.1.3.2
International Reawakening

During the 1970s the international interest in chemical arrest of the heart reawakened, and by the end of the decade the procedure of cold chemical cardioplegia had gained close to universal acclaim as the most useful approach to an adequate surgical and metabolic handling of the heart. In USA Gay, Levitsky, Roe, Tyers and Buckberg reassessed the use of potassium below 40 mM (Table 2) for inducing cardiac arrest (Gay and Ebert 1973; Levitsky 1977; Roe et al 1977; Tyers et al. 1977).

Whereas Buckberg initially advocated crystalloid solutions (Nelson et al. 1976), he (Follette et al. 1978a; Buckberg 1979) soon changed to blood as the vehicle for potassium induced cardioplegia (Table 3) and advocated intermittent perfusion with cold cardioplegic blood plus systemic hypothermia during aortic occlusion. Buckberg also proposed that the myocardium should be kept in a diastolic arrested state with warm cardioplegic blood during the initial reperfusion phase (Follette et al 1978b) and thereafter recommended warm blood cardioplegia during the induction phase (Rosenkranz et al 1986). Also the Buckberg group assessed quantitatively noncoronary collateral flow in the washout of cardioplegic solutions (Brazier et al 1975) and confirmed the necessity of repeated administration or *multi-dose cardioplegia* as also advocated by Engelmann et al. (1978).

In Germany Bleese and Döring (Bleese et al. 1976; Bleese et al. 1978) developed and applied clinically intermittent or nearly continuous perfusion with a cold oxygenated crystalloid cardioplegic solution (Table 2), this as an improvement upon their previous practice with the Kirsch injection technique. Also the Bretschneider group reassessed their formulations (Bretschneider 1980; Gebhard et al. 1983; Preusse et al. 1979, 1980; Preusse 1993) and while still keeping to sodium and calcium withdrawal for chemical arrest, they

Table 2 The composition of four different crystalloid cardioplegic solutions

Components (mM)	Hamburg	Tyers	Gay-Ebert	Roe
NaCl	25	88	38	27
NaHCO$_3$	25		10	
Na-acetate		27		
Na-gluconate		23		
KCl	5	20	40	20
KHCO$_3$		10		
MgCl$_2$		1.5		
Mg-aspartate	2			1.5
CaCl$_2$	0.5	0.5		
Procaine–HCl	4			
Glucose	10		277	278
Mannitol	200			
Hydroxyethyl starch	6%			
Special additives	Oxygen Methylprednisolone Gentamycin	Heparin		Tris
Osmolality (mOsm/Kg)	320	275	365	347
Oncotic pressure (mm Hg)	35 mm Hg			
Oxygen tension	>600 mm Hg			

Observe that the Hamburg and the Tyers solutions are based on a largely extracellular ionic matrix containing calcium and sodium whereas the Gay-Ebert and Roe solutions are formulated intracellularly with zero calcium and low to intermediate levels of sodium. The oxygenated Hamburg solution is applied for intermittent or subcontinuous perfusion whereas the other solutions are administered by infusion. All solutions are applied under hypothermic conditions

Table 3 Blood cardioplegia solution (Follette et al. 1978a)

Component	Concentration
Blood from CPB circuit	1,000 ml
KCl	26 mM
CPD* from standard blood storage bag	20 ml
Tris (0.3 M)	20 ml
Final cardioplegic solution	
K$^+$	30 mM
Ionized Ca^{2+}	0.30 mM
Hematocrit	20%
Osmolarity	355 mOsm/KgH$_2$O
pH	7.7

CPD citrate-phosphate-dextrose

filled the available osmolal gap with the amino acid histidine. This was based on the group's finding of interstitial (reflecting intracellular) pH as an important marker for survival as

ATP. The histidine/histidine–Cl buffer pair (180–18 mM) possesses an ideal temperature profile (Rahn et al. 1975) for preservation of optimal pH during hypothermia, and histidine may scavenge reactive oxygen species (ROS) like singlet oxygen and hydroxyl radicals (Kukreja et al. 1991). In the new solution procaine was omitted in favour of a rise in magnesium. With minor changes this latter formulation has survived to the current date, now in the form (Table 1) of the Bretschneider histidine-tryptophane-α-ketoglutarate (HTK) solution (Custodiol^{TM}, Dr. F. Köhler Chemie, Alsbach-Hähnlein, Germany).

2.1.3.3
British Rediscoveries

During the 1970s cardioplegia regained the interest of British scientists. In 1972 Proctor, working on design and performance of oxygenators for CPB, reported on his experience (Proctor 1972) in long term donor heart preservation. By applying continuous coronary perfusion with an oxygenated hypothermic (4°C) extracellular-type crystalloid solution containing procaine and colloids, dog hearts were kept alive for up to 4 days. However, the main forward drive in cardioplegia research was the group headed by Hearse and Braimbridge at St. Thomas' Hospital in London. Thus by applying isolated hearts from small animals, mainly rats, for screening of mechanisms and agents the group (Hearse et al. 1974, 1975, 1976a, b, 1978a, b) characterized individually and together multiple factors involved in cardiac arrest and in myocardial protective interventions during ischemia and reperfusion. These studies were accompanied by in-depth analyses into the very complex pathophysiology of myocardial ischemia and reperfusion. Principal findings from small animal hearts were confirmed in dogs on CPB (Rosenfeldt et al. 1980; Jynge et al. 1981). In conclusion the group emphasized pragmatically the importance of a careful approach to the formulation of coronary infusates. Thus they should preferably deviate as little as possible from the extracellular fluid they were to replace and they should be based on a close dose-response characterization of main ionic constituents like potassium and magnesium and of potential additives (Hearse et al. 1981c; Chambers and Braimbridge 1993).

A St. Thomas' Hospital solution no 1 (STH-1) with moderately elevated potassium (20 mM) and magnesium (16 mM) and a small additive of procaine (1 mM) in an *extracellular* ionic matrix was introduced clinically by Braimbridge in 1975 and he reported (Braimbridge et al. 1977) encouraging initial experience in 1977. Thus, a comparison of patients undergoing valve replacements using STH-1 and hypothermia (1975–1976) with his previous (1972–1975) practice of coronary perfusion with blood, demonstrated a substantial benefit. The obvious advantages of working in a bloodless field were also acknowledged.

Further preclinical studies (Jynge et al. 1978, 1981; Jynge 1980) confirmed the importance of maintaining near to normal extracellular concentrations of calcium and sodium avoiding major fluctuations in these key ions during and following coronary infusion of cardioplegic solutions. On the basis of the accumulated experience from ex vivo rat and in vivo dog studies an isosmolal St. Thomas' Hospital solution no 2 (STH-2) was formulated with moderate elevations of potassium (16 mM) and magnesium (16 mM) together with near to normal sodium (120 mM) and calcium (1.2 mM) and a minor content of bicarbonate (10 mM) for initial pH control. This purely ionic and crystalloid solution can, without constraints concerning its administration, be applied for single-dose or multi-dose cardioplegia depending on the duration of aortic occlusion and on the washout by noncoronary collateral blood flow. Commercially available STH-2 (Plegisol™, Hospira Inc., Lake Forest, Illinois, USA) and STH-1 made up by local hospital pharmacies are still in broad clinical use, mostly for its simplicity of application.

2.1.4
Status After 25 Years

At the end of the first 25 years with diverging opinions some main principles were acknowledged and already applied clinically with apparent success. The recommended cardioplegic solutions were largely crystalloid, whether based on an *intracellular* or "Bretschneider-like" ionic formulation or on an *extracellular* and "St. Thomas' Hospital-like" ionix matrix. Furthermore, *blood cardioplegia* with potassium-enriched and low-calcium containing blood was underway, especially in USA where Buckberg (Buckberg 1979) now predicted an end to the "cardioplegic controversy" concerning type of solution to use. The pro's and con's of hypothermia and the importance of avoiding a reperfusion injury were also recognized. The status at the time cannot be better presented than in the summing up by Kirklin (1979) at the first transatlantic workshop on cardioplegia held in New York in 1979: "The technique of cold cardioplegia has without question enormously improved surgical exposure and ease of operating during cardiac surgery. Properly done, it has severely reduced the incidence of myocardial necrosis, and thereby improved postoperative cardiac performance. It has thus made care of the patient in the early postoperative period much simpler than it was in earlier times. Most patients now convalesce easily, do not need special interventions, and are dismissed from hospital on the fifth or sixth day following the operation. We do not have proof that late myocardial failure will be reduced through the use of this technique, but it seems likely that this will be the case".

Kirklin further stated from a multifactorial analysis of risk factors and his team's clinical success that only one negative predictive factor was not improved by cold cardioplegia, namely preoperative myocardial failure with patients being NYHA functional classes III or IV. This statement from 1979 is appropriate to cite since we still, despite major later developments, are dealing with the problem of providing adequate protection to the failing heart, particularly in the elderly.

2.2
Concepts and Issues

The above, apparently successful, story from the first period of cardioplegia would not have been possible without major developments made in close collaboration between surgeons and basic scientists. Below five main concepts and issues have been selected for brief presentation as important lessons that had to be understood at the time.

2.2.1
Energy, Metabolism and Recovery from Ischemia

A most obvious key to myocardial protection was found in cell energetics and in the content and function of ATP. However, with mitochondrial respiration already discovered and the ATP producing proton circuit recently characterized (Mitchell 1966), still the diverse roles of ATP as the life-giving molecule and mechanisms of its transport and its translation to work were only partly known at the start of the 1970s. In cardioplegia and ischemia research two energy related concepts became subject to considerable debate: time and temperature limits for expected survival from surgical ischemia; and mechanisms and causes of ischemia-induced contracture.

2.2.1.1
Rescucitation Time

Bretschneider's main approach was to accept an uninterrupted long period of total ischemia which should be well tolerated by applying cold chemical cardioplegia (Bretschneider 1964; Reidemeister et al. 1967; Preusse 1993). He established an early focus of attention on conservation of cell energy and proposed that chemical arrest spared cell ATP stores, that hypothermia delayed ATP depletion and that an appropriate buffering system might provide anaerobic production of a minor, but important, amount of ATP. He also formulated the concept of *practical resuscitation time* or *t-ATP* as the time required for myocardial ATP to fall from about 6 mmol/g wet weight to 4 mmol/g wet weight. This level was shown to be critical for functional recovery from ischemia and rapid weaning from CPB. As shown from isolated dog hearts during total global ischemia at 25°C (Fig. 1), t-ATP increased from 60 min in control hearts to 200 min with the Bretschneider solution no 3 and further to 280 min with a high concentration of the extracellular histidine buffer in the HTK solution (Bretschneider et al. 1975; Bretschneider 1980).

In other experiments the Bretschneider group showed that the slower decay of tissue ATP by HTK was closely paralleled by a gradual consumption of cellular glycogen stores and a rise in tissue lactate (Nordbeck et al. 1974; Preusse et al. 1979; Gebhard et al. 1983). In later studies interstitial pH measurements showed that conservation of interstitial pH (critical limit 6.0), or more precisely avoidance of severe acidosis was instrumental for subsequent recovery of function (Preusse 1993).

Experiments by the Hearse group were in accordance with Bretschneider's findings on relationships between ATP conservation and cardiac function (Hearse et al. 1974). Thus, recovery of cardiac output in isolated working rat hearts depended greatly on the content of ATP at the end of ischemia: 12 μmol/g dry weight (50% of normal) formed a lower level for expectancy of any recovery; and above this level an almost linear correlation was found between ATP and cardiac output. Altogether, these studies by leading scientists documented the very crucial role of cellular ATP levels in the coupling between metabolism and function. In subsequent studies on how to provide anaerobic energy production during ischemia, the Hearse group showed that stimulation of glycolysis in zero flow conditions

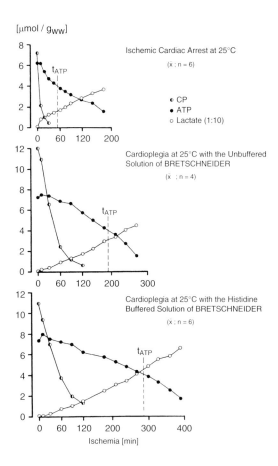

Fig. 1 *Myocardial content of ATP, creatine phosphate (CP) and lactate during ischemia.* Control hearts and hearts receiving initial perfusion with nonbuffered Bretschneider solution no 3 and buffered Bretschneider HTK solution. Results were obtained from isolated dog hearts kept ischemic at a myocardial temperature of 25°C. (Reproduced from Preusse 1993 by permission of Kluwer Academic Publishers)

was deleterious and hence glucose (Hearse et al. 1978b) or lactate (Hearse et al. 1978b) were not recommended as additives to the STH solutions.

2.2.1.2
The Stone Heart Challenge

In 1967 and 1969 the first reports appeared (Taber et al. 1967; Najafi et al. 1969) which documented transmural or subendocardial (Cooley et al. 1972) myocardial necrosis and low cardiac output after valve replacements. In 1972 Cooley, the proponent of normothermic ischemic arrest (Cooley et al. 1962), described the "*stone heart*" (Cooley et al. 1972); this was an irreversible contracture that occurred occasionally during and following nonprotected aortic occlusions, particularly in hypertrophied hearts. At the time this was taken up as a challenge for biochemists to become involved in surgical research (Katz and Tada 1972). Evidence that ATP depletion was the etiological factor behind stone heart formation was first provided by Hearse and associates in 1977 (Hearse et al 1977). Using isolated rat hearts with left ventricular pressure recordings and tissue ATP measurements at brief intervals, they showed that the onset of contracture (rise in resting tension) during ischemia started when ATP was reduced by approximately 50%, and that ATP-hydrolysis and contracture accelerated thereafter. The time to onset and also the extent of contracture could be delayed or diminished by interventions that reduced myocardial energy demands including potassium arrest, magnesium elevation, calcium antagonists and hypothermia. Conversely, metabolic poisoning had the opposite effect. From further experiments it was concluded that ischemic contracture was the result of ATP depletion forming rigor complexes between actin and myosin, that the onset of contracture was a purely ATP related event, and, that only the final extent of contracture was influenced by calcium-sensitive mechanisms. The stone heart paper contributed to our knowledge of the pathophysiology of ischemia and was of importance in turning surgeons towards new techniques for myocardial protection.

2.2.2
Hypothermia: The Second Component of Protection

2.2.2.1
Hypothermia on Its Own

In spite of more recent sceptical attitudes (Salerno 2007), hypothermia has followed cardiac surgery from the earliest until the most recent days. The first intracardiac operations with inflow occlusion and total circulatory arrest were undertaken with moderate hypothermia induced by body surface cooling (Bigelow et al. 1950). During this phase it was shown (Swan 1973) that systemic hypothermia slowed both heart rate and myocardial oxygen demands. Thus at 26°C oxygen consumption was reduced by 75% but at lower temperatures the rate of decline was less. Also below this level ventricular fibrillation was frequently observed. It was concluded that moderate hypothermia with a systemic temperature between 32°C and 29°C would reduce myocardial energy requirements substantially without imposing any hazard to cardiac function. Somewhat later, an "ice age" started with systemic hypothermia supplemented with topical cooling and use of saline slush (Shumway et al. 1959). Also intermittent ischemic arrest combined with systemic and topical hypothermia became a common technique.

In experimental studies of hypothermia as a separate modality for arrest and protection two particularly important observations were made. The first was that whereas heart rate fell almost linearly with temperature (Archie and Kirklin 1973), the force of each contraction increased (Coraboeuf and Weidmann 1954). The second was that myocardial oxygen consumption, although being gradually lowered together with temperature, actually increased when calculated for each heart beat (Archie and Kirklin 1973). On further cooling ventricular fibrillation also raised myocardial oxygen requirements. Accordingly, hypothermia, however effective in slowing basal metabolism, which accounts for 15–20% of normal myocardial oxygen demand (Braunwald 1969; Challoner 1968), was less efficient in reducing electromechanical activity accounting for the remaining 80–85%.

2.2.2.2
Hypothermia Plus Cardioplegia

The above problem was solved with the arrival of chemical arrest in diastole. Thus chemical cardioplegia reduces oxygen consumption from 6 to 8 ml/100g/min in the empty beating heart to 0.5–1.5 ml/100g/min at normothermia (Buckberg et al. 1977) and, when applied at 20°C or 15°C, a further reduction to 0.30 ml/100 g/min and 0.15 ml/100 g/min respectively can be expected (Preusse 1993). In line with this, hypothermia fulfils the role as the second component of myocardial protection by complementing the first, i.e., chemical arrest.

The efficacy of hypothermia is apparent from Fig. 2 showing the results from isolated working rat hearts protected by preischemic infusion of a cardioplegic solution (Hearse 1982). When temperature of cardioplegic infusion (2 min) and ischemia (60 min) was kept at 37°C, the hearts were unable to recover any cardiac output during normothermic reperfusion (15 min). In contrast, at or below 20°C the recovery was 90% or higher. An important observation at the time was that the dose-response curve of hypothermia was nonlinear with a marked inflection between 32°C and 24°C. The inflection was explained by lipid phase transitions in cell membranes (Inesi et al. 1973; Gordon et al. 1978) conferring an extra slowing of membrane embedded transporters and enzymes. An interpretation of the above rat heart study would be that cardioplegia with moderate hypothermia is safe for shortlasting aortic occlusions with temperature in the range of 24–28°C, but safer still when kept closer to 20°C.

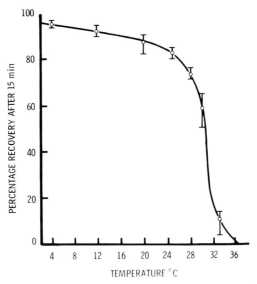

Fig. 2 *The second component of protection: hypothermia.* Isolated working rat hearts were subjected to 60 min of ischemia after receiving preischemic infusion of St. Thomas' Hospital solution no 1 enriched with ATP and creatine phosphate. Temperature of infusion and ischemia as indicated. Hearts were reperfused for 15 min with recording of aortic flow rate. Observe the sharp inflection between 33 and 24°C, and that below 20°C a full recovery is obtained. (Reproduced from Hearse 1982 by permission of Editrice CLUEB, Bologna)

2.2.2.3
Hypothermic Injury

Hypothermia induces a complex mixture of both beneficial and detrimental effects in homeothermic species (Hearse et al. 1981b) and optimal temperature levels for the entire body on CPB and for the arrested heart are still questioned. A particular issue that was heavily debated in the 1970s was the potential induction of a more advanced hypothermic injury with a major loss of protection. Careful reanalysis of a large number of studies (Hearse et al. 1981b) showed that hypothermic injury with loss of protective properties from a progressive decrease in myocardial temperature resulted when three main factors coincided: rapid and extensive cooling by coronary infusion or perfusion; use of noncardioplegic solutions; and presence of myocardial ischemia. The immediate consequence of the two first factors was cold shock induced release of calcium from sarcoplasmic reticulum (SR) (Endo 1977) accompanied by a slow reuptake into the SR (Katz and Repke 1967). Elevated intracellular calcium then activates energy-wasting and unfavourable cellular reactions. While these latter changes might be overcome by maintaining perfusion and energy production, the simultaneous presence of ischemia with further inhibition of metabolism acts to exacerbate cold-induced changes. Apparently, canine hearts were able to survive deep hypothermic perfusion for days (Proctor 1972) when the perfusion medium was formulated with an immediately arresting agent.

In essence, it seems that the immediate induction phase of cardioplegia is most important and adds a partial confirmation to the practice subsequently proposed by the Buckberg group (Buckberg 1979) with warm induction prior to cooling when using blood cardioplegia.

2.2.3
Calcium Control

2.2.3.1
Calcium Takes Centre Stage

In parallel with the history of cardioplegia major discoveries on cell calcium regulation saw the light of day. Important observations were made on the sarcolemmal sodium–calcium exchange (Langer 1977), on the SR for intracellular calcium storage-release (Ebashi and Lippman 1962; Katz and Repke 1967; Endo 1977), and on a new class of negative inotropic drugs and vasodilators with properties as antagonists of sarcolemmal slow calcium channels (Fleckenstein 1971). In addition, models of acute myocardial infarction in dog hearts demonstrated how cell calcium control might be at stake during ischemia and more so during reperfusion (Jennings et al. 1960; Jennings and Reimer 1979). Altogether, the growing acceptance of cell calcium as crucial in myocardial injury and protection had great impact upon the development of cardioplegia as an applied science. The accumulated knowledge at the end of the 1970s thus revealed multiple roles of calcium when formulating cardioplegic solutions and when applying them in combination with hypothermia for myocardial protection during aortic occlusion.

2.2.3.2
Cardioplegia and the Calcium Paradox

A controversial issue was the use of calcium-free coronary infusates and the possibility that an extensive calcium washout might induce a *calcium paradox*. Thus when calcium is reintroduced to a myocardium with a sarcolemma depleted of a critical high affinity fraction of calcium maintaining its integrity (Frank et al. 1977), cell calcium overload with contracture and membrane injury is immediate and massive (Zimmerman et al. 1967).

Some studies indicated that the calcium-free Bretschneider solutions might induce a calcium paradox (Jynge et al. 1977; Jynge et al. 1978; Jynge 1982; Ruigrok et al 1983) as indicated in Fig. 3. However, these solutions were apparently safe since they were sodium-poor and applied under deep hypothermia (Jynge 1980; Gebhard et al. 1983; Jynge 1983) which seemed to stabilize the sarcolemma against removal of a critical fraction of calcium. Furthermore, in the clinical situation with aortic occlusion noncoronary collateral flow is likely to ensure the presence of at least some calcium in the sarcolemma. When studying different formulations and situations in isolated rat hearts (Jynge 1983), trace calcium (25 µM), magnesium elevation, low sodium and simultaneous hypothermia during calcium-free perfusion prevented or delayed the paradox. Conversely, normal sodium, elevated potassium, calcium-binding anions like phosphate and citrate, ischemia and a warm heart were provocative factors.

In retrospect, the myocardial injuries inflicted by the Melrose solution (Melrose 1980) might be interpreted as the consequences of citrate induction of a calcium paradox. It is of interest to note that the most recent version of the Bretschneider HTK solutions (Custodiol) is formulated with a minor calcium additive (20 µM).

2.2.3.3
Ionic Interactions and Calcium Control

As already indicated, the relationship between calcium and sodium was shown to be essential for optimal formulation of cardioplegic solutions. Thus in the bidirectional sodium–calcium exchange of the sarcolemma three sodium ions are exchanged with one calcium ion for calcium influx (during depolarization) and efflux (during repolarization). A practical consequence is that lowering of extracellular sodium during coronary infusion of a sodium-poor cardioplegic solution has to be matched by a far more extensive reduction in extracellular calcium in order to induce diastolic arrest. Thus, the window for incorporating calcium in the Bretschneider solution No. 3 was marginal in normothermic rat hearts (Fig. 3) (Jynge 1982) and below 50 µM in hypothermic dog hearts (Gebhard et al. 1983). In addition it was found that myocardial equilibration with this sodium-poor and calcium-free solution might go through intermediate stages due to sodium–calcium interactions prior to achieving the lowest oxygen requirement.

According to recommendations the Bretschneider HTK solution has to be infused in a single-dose manner over 6–8 min requiring a volume of 2–3 L in adult patients. Most intriguingly, experiments in hypothermic ischemic dog hearts (Warnecke et al. 1981) documented that electromechanical reactivation required less washout of cardioplegic

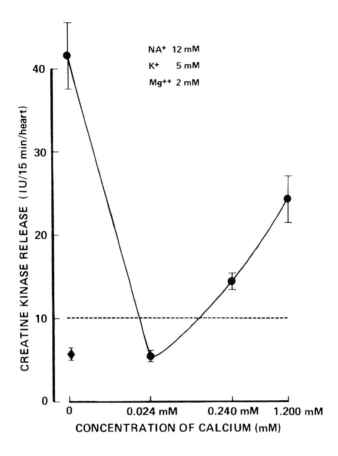

Fig. 3 *Sodium-poor coronary infusates and optimal calcium.* The accumulated creatine kinase (CK) release during reperfusion (15 min) after ischemia (30 min) in isolated normothermic rat hearts is shown. Hearts (●) received preischemic infusion for 2 min (8 ml) of Bretschneider solution no 3 devoid of or supplemented with calcium. Hearts (♦) receiving preischemic infusion over 2 min with less voume (4 ml) of Bretschneider solution devoid of calcium. The dotted line shows the level of CK release on reperfusion of control hearts. (Reproduced from Jynge 1982 by permission of Editrice CLUEB, Bologna)

solution after arrest with the HTK solution than with the STH-2 solution. As a consequence of gradual noncoronary collateral inflow of blood, myocardial protection with the otherwise superior BR-HTK was reduced but slightly improved with STH-2. It is difficult to explain these differences except by differences in reequlibration patterns with the extracellular ionic environment of inflowing blood. The STH-2 solutions containing near to normal sodium showed a broad calcium window in ischemic rat hearts (Yamamoto et al. 1984) with concentrations optimal for postischemic recovery in the range 0.6–1.2 mM. Furthermore, the tolerance to preischemic sodium depletion in the presence of normal calcium was also considerable (Jynge 1982) as documented by postischemic CK release in rat hearts (Fig. 4). Intriguingly, elevated potassium (16 mM) was more sensitive to sodium reduction than

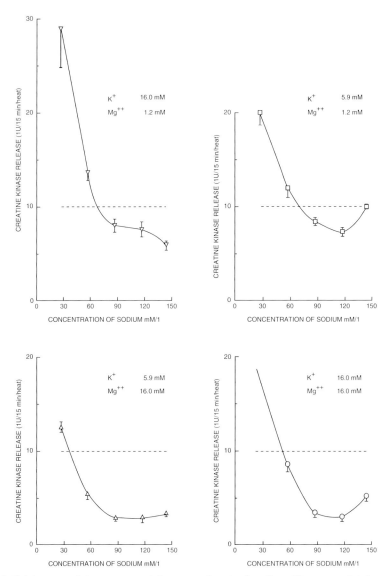

Fig. 4 *Calcium-containing coronary infusates and optimal sodium.* The accumulated creatine kinase (CK) release during reperfusion (15 min) after ischemia (30 min) in isolated normothermic rat hearts is shown. Hearts received preischemic infusion (2 min and 8 ml) of solutions with a fixed concentration of calcium (1.2 mM) but different concentrations of sodium (30–150 mM). Sodium chloride was substituted with mannitol. Substitution with choline chloride revealed similar results. The *dotted line* shows the level of CK release on reperfusion of control hearts. (Reproduced from Jynge 1982 by permission of Editrice CLUEB, Bologna)

elevated magnesium (16 mM) whereas the combined elevations revealed an intermediate sodium sensitivity with an optimal level of 90–120 mM. These results contributed to the formulation of the STH-2.

Altogether, it appeared that the main advantages with an extracellular type ionic formulation as applied in the crystalloid STH-2 solution, as well as in composite blood cardioplegia solutions, were less complex equilibration with the extracellular ionic environment and less rigorous infusion requirements except for multi-dose administration to counteract washout by noncoronary inflow of blood. Conversely, the major and outweighing advantage with intracellular solutions as exemplified by Bretschneider HTK was the large osmolal space available for inclusion of a high concentration of the beneficial histidine buffer.

2.2.4
Reperfusion

In 1960 Danforth and Bing reported detailed metabolic studies (Danforth et al 1960) on glycolytic fluxes during global myocardial ischemia and reperfusion while the Jennings' group (Jennings et al. 1960) simultaneously described functional and structural consequences associated with reperfusion in regional ischemia. In an anticipated reversal to normal conditions after aortic cross-clamping three phases of reperfusion were then identified (Hearse 1982). During the initial seconds to minutes of reperfusion the return of oxygen causes an immediate resumption of oxidative metabolism and reactivation of electromechanical function. The second phase, occurring over the next few minutes, leads to the reversal of ischemia-induced cell swelling and restoration of normal patterns of ion regulation and of metabolites and cofactors. The third phase requiring hours to days involves the repair of damaged organelles like mitochondria and cell membranes and the restoration of normal metabolic pathways including de novo synthesis of adenine nucleotides.

In surgical practice it was soon discovered that securing the myocardial transition from an almost hibernating to a fully working state is a complex process. Thus reperfusion pressure had preferably to be lowered to prevent edema formation (Engelman et al. 1978; Lindal et al. 1995), ventricular fibrillation had to be rapidly converted (Buckberg 1977) and residual air within heart chambers and coronary arteries had to be taken care of (Goldfarb and Bahnson 1963). A further obstacle to circumvent was the "no reflow" phenomenon (Leaf 1973; Brachfeld 1974; Fabiani 1976) induced by swelling of endothelial cells with venular trapping of neutrophils attracted by inflammation and compounded by the compressive forces of contracture and cellular plus interstitial edema. This fitted well with both earlier (Jennings et al. 1960) and later (Jennings and Reimer 1979) observations from the Jennings' group of specific reperfusion injuries that were initiated on return of blood and oxygen to a previously ischemic myocardium. It was also shown that reperfusion injury might express itself in reperfusion arrhythmias, in prolonged myocardial recovery with metabolic and contractile dysfunction (later to become known as "stunning"), and in an accelerated necrosis in tissue already doomed by ischemia. However, the fourth entity of a lethal reperfusion injury potentially amenable to therapeutic interventions (Hausenloy and Yellon 2008) was not yet recognized, as were neither preconditioning (Murry et al. 1986) nor postconditioning (Zhao et al. 2003) both potent endogenous syndromes in prevention or amelioration of reperfusion injuries.

When shedding light upon basic mechanisms the Hearse group compared three "re-admission" syndromes of relevance for events taking place on a cellular level during postischemic reperfusion (Hearse et al. 1979). In studies in isolated rat hearts myocardial creatine kinase (CK) release to the asanguineous perfusion medium was rapid with a maximum within 2 min of readmission. Three levels of peak CK release were observed: far the highest on readmission of calcium after calcium-free perfusion (>400 IU/min/g dry wt.); intermediate on reoxygenation after hypoxia (>50 IU/min/g dry wt.); and the lowest (~10 IU/min/g dry wt.) during reperfusion with oxygenated and calcium-containing medium after severe ischemia. In the readmission syndromes both calcium and reactive oxygen species (ROS) were identified as main culprits inducing immediate contracture and severe mechanical stress to injured cell and mitochondrial membranes with cell death and a graded CK release as the end result. In retrospect, it is of interest to note that the two factors, initial calcium overload and initial ROS release, together activate mitochondrial permeability transition pores and lethal reperfusion injury which may be inhibited or ameliorated by postconditioning procedures and drugs (Hausenloy and Yellon 2008).

Attempts to utilise antioxidants, whether pure scavengers or catalytic agents, were in their infancy at the start of the 1980s, but already some interest was on using key antioxidant enzymes (Fridovich 1974) like superoxide dismutase (SOD) and catalase (CAT). Thus, in 1982 Shlafer found that supplementation of SOD plus CAT to a cardioplegic solution gave superior protection during hypothermic ischemia than afforded by the solution itself and concluded that cytotoxic ROS contributed to a separate reperfusion injury (Shlafer et al. 1982). These findings were later both confirmed (Gardner et al. 1983; Ambrosio et al. 1987; Ytrehus et al. 1987) and negated (Gallagher et al. 1986; Uraizee et al. 1987) by other investigators. Apparently, shortcomings of native SOD or CAT enzymes, not least by being macromolecules, can be overcome by applying synthetic small molecular mimetics that are more likely to enter target cells and act intracellularly. Accordingly, more recent studies have shown that salen mangenese complexes (Tanguy et al. 1996) and manganese-dipyridoxyl dietethylene diamide (Karlsson et al. 2001) were effective in reducing reperfusion arrhythmias and myocardial infarct size.

2.2.5
Blood as Cardioplegic Vehicle

At the end of the 1970s influential new ideas came from protagonists of blood cardioplegia (Buckberg 1979; Barner et al. 1979). Thus Buckberg (as the foremost protagonist) claimed to have found a solution to discrepancies between different crystalloid "schools" of thought and practice. Based on the early experience of Melrose (Melrose et al. 1955) he proposed the use of blood as vehicle for an extracellular type, elevated-potassium and reduced-calcium based cardioplegia (Table 3). A number of apparent advantages were proposed, such as regular intermittent administrations to maintain aerobic metabolism, buffering by blood at an optimal pH, potential scavenging of ROS by blood constituents, and oncotic prevention of cell swelling and improvement in capillary distribution.

In a pioneering study published in 1978 Follette et al. (1978b) compared the efficacy of three protective procedures in dogs on CPB: continuous normothermic perfusion in the

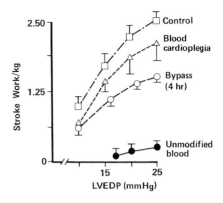

Fig. 5 *Blood cardioplegia and myocardial protection in dogs.* Stroke work during progressive volume loading after continuous normothermic perfusion (bypass) and hypothermic ischemia with unmodified blood or blood cardioplegia. For detailse, see text. (Reproduced from Follette et al. 1978a by permission of the American Heart Association, New York)

empty beating heart (continuous bypass); hypothermic ischemia with multidose infusion of cold (22°C) blood (unmodified blood); and hypothermic ischemia with multidose administration of cold (22°C) cardioplegic blood (blood cardioplegia). Infusions were given at 20 min intervals during 120 min of ischemia and before aortic declamping. As shown in Fig. 5, the recovery of stroke work, after 30 min of reperfusion, following cardioplegia was improved compared to continuous bypass and not significantly reduced below control values. However, the unmodified blood group of hearts hardly recovered any function at all. Myocardial ATP and creatine phosphate were well maintained with continuous bypass and intermittent ischemia with multi-dose blood cardioplegia but fell by 45% with unmodified blood. Clearly this study demonstrated the efficacy of blood cardioplegia, but for eventual comparison it lacked a control group with crystalloid cardioplegia. In retrospect, however, it is to be noted that in high risk patients undergoing CABG (Ibrahim et al. 1999) significantly enhanced myocardial protection with positive effects upon arrhythmias, recovery of function and myocardial high energy phosphates was provided with blood-based compared to crystalloid-based St. Thomas' Hospital solution (STH-1).

A particular question at the time was the efficacy of cold blood as a vehicle for oxygen delivery. Thus impairment of capillary flow by sludging of erythrocytes was partly feared. Another concern was that blood oxygen delivery might prove ineffective due to enhancement of oxygen–haemoglobin affinity by hypothermia and a high pH. As seen in Fig. 6 from Follette's initial study (Follette et al. 1978a) myocardial oxygen uptake in dog hearts receiving intermittent infusions with unmodified cold blood was 1.8 ml O_2/min/100 g while hearts arrested by blood cardioplegia consumed only 0.75 mlO_2/min/100 g. This approximate 2.5 fold higher value in hearts arrested solely by cold most probably resulted from a higher wall tension and ventricular fibrillation but might also be attributed to a lower pH of the infusate releasing more oxygen from haemoglobin. While these results undoubtedly showed that oxygen was released from cold blood, some might also have come from that physiologically dissolved in plasma. By undertaking oxygen debt calculations of the data presented it seemed likely that oxygen delivery might have had two almost equally important sources. In the search for other salient effects, it was later shown that the high buffering capacity with the histidine-imidazole-bicarbonate system of erythrocytes and the

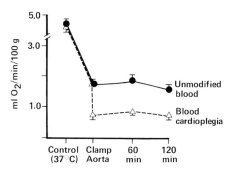

Fig. 6 *Blood cardioplegia and myocardial oxygen consumption in dogs.* Observe the higher oxygen uptake in hearts receiving unmodified cold blood during prolonged aortic clamping than in hearts receiving cold cardioplegic blood. For details-see text. (Reproduced from Follette et al. 1978a by permission of the American Heart Association, New York)

high content of scavenger and catalytic antioxidants (Illes et al. 1989a, b) were important contributing factors behind the efficacy of blood cardioplegia.

A convincing aspect of blood cardioplegia procedures has been optimal reanimation of hearts following aortic occlusion thus bridging the gap between ischemic and normal metabolism. Evidence was soon provided (Follette et al. 1978b; Kirklin 1990) that postischemic recovery of function could be improved considerably through keeping the heart arrested by perfusion with warm cardioplegic blood for the first few minutes after ischemia but before aortic declamping. This diverts energy production away from early reactivation of ionic pumps and towards early cellular repair. In parallel, unfavourable resumption of contractile function with mechanical stress upon weakened cell membranes is avoided in this critical phase. A further benefit of warm cardioplegic blood reperfusion beside that of electromechanical unloading, acid buffering and antioxidant effects, was the observation that addition (Lazar et al. 1980a) of amino acid substrates like glutamate and aspartate enhanced the recovery of metabolism.

The overall progress in reperfusion strategy (Buckberg 1995) was further extended by applying an extra period of warm blood cardioplegic perfusion (secondary cardioplegia) in failing hearts (Lazar et al. 1980b), to improve metabolism and function prior to weaning from CPB. The experience from reperfusion with warm cardioplegic blood was in 1983 (Rosenkranz et al. 1986) logically transferred to the introduction side of cardiac operations. The new concept of warm cardioplegic induction was based on the realization that in ischemic and energy-depleted hearts the induction of cardioplegia in reality represents an essentially first phase of reperfusion, and that a potential activation of cellular defence might improve myocardial tolerance to the forthcoming ischemia. Another positive effect of warm induction beside optimal oxygen delivery and energy metabolism is the effective arrest in diastole before start of cooling.

2.3
Summary and Closing Remarks

After an exciting period of experimentation and early clinical application cardioplegia has in the last 20–25 years undergone further developments, first of all based on thorough analyses of its practical adaptation both in general and as applied in different intraoperative situations. Especially, the necessity of providing homogenous distribution of both arrest and cooling has led to the rediscovery (Lillehei et al. 1956; Menasché et al. 1982) of retrograde coronary sinus perfusion, and combined antegrade and retrograde delivery has become a familiar technique for administration of both blood- and crystalloid-based solutions. More recently, the advent of warm heart surgery (Barner 1995; Salerno 2007) has reopened an old debate of optimal temperature of the myocardium as well as other tissues during CPB.

Blood cardioplegia with major advances in surgical application now seems to be the choice of a majority of surgical centres but crystalloid cardioplegia, as it was conceived 30 years ago, is still in broad clinical use. Whereas meta-analyses based on minor clinical studies indicate that blood cardioplegia is superior (Guru et al 2006; Jacob et al. 2008), this has been more difficult to prove in larger groups of patients (Ovrum et al. 2004). In closing this review on selected issues and concepts from the first period of cardioplegia research, we are still left with pro's and con's concerning techniques to be used, and it is apparent that an in-depth knowledge of both surgical procedures and the pathophysiology of myocardial ischemia is imperative. Of particular interest for the early future will be to see how surgical protection can be combined with pre- and postconditioning with regard to reperfusion and long term recovery. By invoking these endogenous and general responses cardioplegia can no longer be seen as a separate entity but as an integral part of perioperative myocardial protection.

References

Ambrosio G, Weisfeldt ML, Jacobus WE, Flaherty JT (1987) Evidence for a reversible oxygen radical-mediated component of reperfusion injury: reduction by recombinant human superoxide dismutase administered at the time of reflow. Circulation 75(1): 282–291.

Archie JP and Kirklin JW (1973) Effect of hypothermic perfusion on myocardial oxygen consumption and coronary resistance. Surg Forum 24: 186–188.

Barner HB, Laks H, Codd JE, Standeven J, Pennington DG, Hahn JAW, Willman VL (1979) Cold blood as the vehicle for potassium cardioplegia. Ann Thor Surg 28: 604–617.

Barner HB (1995). Historical aspects and current review of myocardial protection. In: Warm heart surgery. Ed. Salerno, TA. Arnold, London, pp 1–15.

Bigelow WG, Lindsey WK, Greenwood WF (1950). Hypothermia: Its possible role in cardiac surgery. Ann Surg 132: 849–856.

Bleese N, Døring V, Gercken G, Kalmar P, Lierse W, Pokar H, Polonius MJ, Steiner D, Rodewald G (1976) Langzeitherzstillstand durch cardioplegische Coronarperfusion. Thoraxchirurgie 24: 468–475.

Bleese N, Døring V, Kalmar P, Pokar H, Polonius MJ, Steiner D, Rodewald G. (1978) Intraoperative myocardial protection by cardioplegia in hypothermia. J Thorac Cardiovasc Surg 75: 405–413.

Brachfeld N (1974) Maintenance of myocardial cell viability. Circulation (Suppl.4) 39 and 40: 202–219.

Braimbridge MV, Chayen J, Bitensky L, Hearse DJ, Jynge P, Cankovic-Darracott S (1977) Cold cardioplegia or continuous coronary perfusion? J Thorac Cardiovasc Surg 74: 900–906.

Braunwald E (1969) The determinants of myocardial oxygen consumption. Physiologist 12: 65–93.

Brazier J, Hottenrott C, Buckberg GD (1975) Noncoronary collateral myocardial blood flow. Ann Thor Surg 19: 426–435.

Bretschneider HJ (1964) Überlebenszeit und Wiederbelebungszeit des Herzens bei Normo- und Hypothermie. Verh Deutsch Ges Kreislaufforschung 30: 11–34.

Bretschneider HJ, Hübner G, Knoll D, Lohr B, Spieckermann PG (1975) Myocardial resistance and tolerance to ischemia: physiological and biochemical basis. J Cardiovasc Surg 16: 241–260.

Bretschneider HJ (1980) Myocardial protection. Thorac Cardiovasc Surg 28: 295–302.

Buckberg GD (1977) Left ventricular subendocardial necrosis. Ann Thorac Surg 24: 278–393.

Buckberg GD, Brazier JR, Nelson RH, Goldstein SM, McConnell DH, Cooper N (1977). Studies on the effects of hypothermia on regional myocardial blood flow and metabolism during cardiopulmonary bypass. I. The adequately perfused beating, fibrillating, and arrested heart. J Thorac Cardiovasc Surg 73: 87–94.

Buckberg GD (1979). A solution to the cardioplegic controversy. J Thorac Cardiovasc Surg 77: 803–815.

Buckberg GD (1995) Update on current techniques of myocardial protection. Ann Thorac Surg 60: 805–814.

Challoner DR (1968) Respiration in myocardium. Nature 217: 78–79.

Chambers DJ, Braimbridge MV (1993) Cardioplegia with an extracellular formulation. In: Ischemia-Reperfusion in Cardiac Surgery, Eds HM Piper, CJ Preusse. Kluwer Academic Publishers, Dordrecht, The Netherland, p.135–179

Cooley DA, Beall AC, Grondin P (1962) Open-heart operations with disposable oxygenators, 5 per cent dextrose and normothermia. Surgery 52: 713–719.

Cooley DA, Reul GJ, Wukasch DC (1972) Ischemic contracture of the heart: "stone heart". Am J Cardiol 29: 575–577.

Coraboeuf D, Weidmann S (1954) Temperature effects on the electrical activity of Purkinje fibres. Helv Physiol Acta 12: 32–41.

Danforth WH, Naegle S, Bing RJ (1960) Effects of ischemia and reoxygenation on glycolytic reations and adenosinetriphosphate in heart muscle. Circ Res 8(5): 865–971.

Ebashi S, Lippman F (1962) Adenosine triphosphate-linked concentration of calcium ions in a particulate fraction of rabbit muscle. J Cell Biol 14: 389–400.

Endo M (1977) Calcium release from sarcoplasmic reticulum. Physiol Rev 57: 71–108.

Engelmann RM, Auvil J, O'Donghue MJ, Levitsky S (1978) The significance of multidose cardioplegia and hypothermia in myocardial preservation during ischemic arrest. J Thorac Cardiovasc Surg 75: 555–563.

Fabiani JN (1976) The no-reflow phenomenon following early reperfusion of myocardial infarction and its preventions by various drugs. Heart Bull 7: 134–142.

Fleckenstein A (1971) Specific inhibitors and promoters of calcium action in the excitation-contraction coupling of heart muscle and their role in the prevention or production of myocardial lesions. In: Calcium and the Heart. Eds P Harris, LP Opie. Academic Press, London, pp 135–188

Follette D, Steed DL, Foglia R, Fey K, Buckberg DG (1978) Advantages of intermittent blood cardioplegia over intermittent ischemia during prolonged hypothermic aortic clamping. Circulation 58(Suppl. 1): 200–209.

Follette DM, Fey K, Steed DL, Foglia RP, Buckberg GD (1978) Reducing reperfusion injury with hypocalcemic, hyperkalemic, alkalotic blood during reoxygenation. Surg Forum 29: 284–286.

Frank JS, Langer GA, Nudd LM, Seraydarian K (1977) The myocardial cell surface, its histochemistry and the effect of sialic acid and calcium removal on its structure and cellular ionic exchange. Circ Res 41: 702–714.

Fridovich A (1974) Hypoxia and oxygen toxicity. Adv Neurol 26: 255–259

Gallagher KP, Buda AJ, Pace D, Gerren RA, Shlafer M (1986) Failure of superoxide dismutase and catalase to alter size of infarction in conscious dogs after 3 hours of occlusion followed by reperfusion. Circulation 73: 1065–1076.

Gardner TJ, Stewart JR, Casale JM, Chambers DE (1983) Reduction of myocardial ischemic injury with oxygen-derived free radical scavengers. Surgery 94(3):23–427.

Gay WA, Ebert PA (1973) Functional, metabolic and morphological effects of potassium induced cardioplegia. Surgery 74: 287–290.

Gebhard MM, Bretschneider HJ, Gersing E, Preusse CJ, Schnabel A, Ulbricht LJ (1983) Calcium-free cardioplegia. Proc Eur Heart J 4(Suppl. H): 151–160.

Gibbon (1954) Application of mechanical heart and lung apparatus to cardiac surgery. Minn Med 37: 171–180.

Goldfarb D, Bahnson HT (1963) Early and late effects on the heart of small amounts of air in the coronary circulation. J Thorac Cardiovasc Surg 46: 368–372.

Gordon LM, Sauerheber RD, Esgate JA (1978) Spin label studies on rat liver and heart plasma membranes: Effects of temperature, calcium and lanthanum on membrane fluidity. J Supramol Structure 9: 299–326.

Guru V, Omura J, Alghandi AA, Fremes SE (2006) Is blood superior to crystalloid cardioplegia? A meta-analysis of randomized clinical trials. Circulation 114 (Suppl 1): 1331–1338.

Hausenloy DJ, Yellon DM (2008) Time to take myocardial reperfusion injury seriously. N Engl J Med 359(5): 518–520.

Hearse DJ, Stewart DA, Chain EB (1974) Recovery from bypass and elective cardiac arrest. Circ Res 35: 448–457.

Hearse DJ, Stewart DA, Braimbridge MV (1975) Hypothermic arrest and potassium arrest, metabolic and myocardial protection during elective cardiac arrest. Circ Res 36: 481–489

Hearse DJ, Stewart DA, Braimbridge MV (1976) Cellular protection during myocardial ischemia. The development and characterization of a procedure for the induction of reversible cardiac arrest. Circulation 54: 193–202.

Hearse DJ, Stewart DA, Braimbridge MV (1976) Myocardial protection during bypass and arrest, a possible hazard with lactate containing infusates. J Thorac Cardiovasc Surg 72: 880–884.

Hearse DJ, Garlick PB, Humphrey SM (1977) Ischemic contracture of the myocardium: mechanisms and prevention. Am J Cardiol 39: 986–993.

Hearse DJ, Stewart DA, Braimbridge MV (1978) Myocardial protection during ischemic cardiac arrest. The importance of magnesium in coronary infusates. J Thorac Cardiovasc Surg 75: 877–885.

Hearse DJ, Stewart DA, Braimbridge MV (1978) Myocardial protection during ischemic cardiac arrest. Possible deleterious effects of glucose and mannitol in coronary infusates. J Thorac Cardiovasc Surg 76: 16–23.

Hearse DJ, Humphrey SM and Bullock GR (1979) Reoxygenation, reperfusion and the calcium paradox: studies of cellular damage and enzyme release. In: Enzymes in Cardiology. Diagnosis and Research. Eds DJ Hearse and J de Leiris. John Wiley & Sons (New York): p 417–444

Hearse DJ, Braimbridge MV, Jynge P (1981) Basic concepts. In: Protection of the Ischemic Myocardium: Cardioplegia. Eds: Hearse DJ, Braimbridge MV, Jynge P. Raven, New York, pp 151–166.

Hearse DJ, Braimbridge MV, Jynge P (1981) Hypothermia. In: Protection of the Ischemic Myocardium: Cardioplegia. Eds: Hearse DJ, Braimbridge MV, Jynge P. Raven, New York, pp 167–208

Hearse DJ, Braimbridge MV, Jynge P (1981) Formulation and administration. In: Protection of the Ischemic Myocardium: Cardioplegia. Eds: Hearse DJ, Braimbridge MV, Jynge P. Raven, New York, pp 300-326

Hearse DJ (1982) Myocardial protection during open heart surgery: Pre-ischemic, ischemic and post-ischemic considerations. In: Advances in Studies on Heart Metabolism. Eds: Caldarera CM and Harris P. Editrice CLUEB, Bologna, pp 329–344

Helmsworth JA, Kaplan S, Clark LC, McAdams AJ, Matthews EC, Edwards FK (1959) Myocardial injury associated with asystole induced with potassium citrate. Ann Surg 149: 200–206.

Hölscher B (1960). Über lichtmikroskopische Frühveränderungen des Kaninchen- und des Hundeherzens bei verschiedenen Formen des induzierten Herzstillstandes. Langenbecks Arch Klin Chir 295: 745–748.

Hölscher B (1967) Studies by electron microscopy on the effects of magnesium chloride, procaine amide and potassium citrate on the myocardium in induced cardiac arrest. J Cardiovasc Surg 8: 163–166.

Ibrahim MF, Venn GE, Young CP, Chambers DJ (1999) A clinical comparative study between crystalloid and blood-based St. Thomas' Hospital cardioplegic solution. Eur J Cardiothorac Surg 15: 75–83.

Illes RW, Silverman NA, Krukenkamp IB, Levitsky S (1989) Upgrading acellular to sanguineous cardioplegic efficacy. J Surg Res 46(6): 543–548.

Illes RW, Silverman NA, Krukenkamp IB, Yusen RD, Chausow DD, Levitsky S (1989) The efficacy of blood cardioplegia is not due to oxygen delivery. J Thorac Cardiovasc Surg 98(6): 1051–1056.

Inesi G, Millman M, Eletr S (1973) Temperature induced transitions of function and structure in sarcoplasmic reticulum membranes. J Mol Biol 81: 483–504

Jacob S, Kallikourdis A, Sellke F, Dunning J (2008) Is blood cardioplegia superior to crystalloid cardioplegia? Interact Cardiovasc Thorac Surg 7: 491–498.

Jennings RB, Sommers HM, Smyth GA, Flack HA, Linn H (1960). Myocardial necrosis induced by temporary occlusion of a coronary artery in the dog. AMA Arch Pathol 70: 68–78.

Jennings RB and Reimer KA (1979) Biology of experimental, acute myocardial ischemia and infarction. In: DJ Hearse and J de Leiris (eds) Enzymes in cardiology. Diagnosis and research. John Wiley & Sons, New York, pp 21–58.

Jynge P, Hearse DJ, Braimbridge MV (1977) Myocardial protection during ischermic cardiac arrest. A possible hazard with calcium-free cardioplegic infusates. J Thorac Cardiovasc Surg 73: 846–855.

Jynge P, Hearse DJ, Braimbridge MV (1978) Protection of the ischemic myocardium: volume-duration relationships and the efficacy of myocardial infusates. J Thorac Cardiovasc Surg 76: 698–705.

Jynge P (1980) Protection of the ischemic myocardium. Cold chemical cardioplegia, coronary infusates and the importance of cellular calcium control. J Thorac Cardiovasc Surg 28: 310–321.

Jynge P, Hearse DJ, Feuvray D, Muhale W, Cankovic-Darracott S, O-Brien K, Braimbridge MV (1981) The St. Thomas' Hospital cardioplegic solution: a characterization in two species. Scand J Cardiovasc Surg Suppl. 30: 1–28.

Jynge P (1982) Cardioplegic solutions and sodium-calcium relationships.In: Advances in Studies on Heart Metabolism. Eds: Caldarera CM and Harris P. Editrice CLUEB, Bologna, pp 369–374.

Jynge P (1983) Calcium-free cardioplegia contra. Eur Heart J 4(Suppl): 161–168.

Karlsson JOG, Brurok H, Eriksen M, Towart R, Toft KG, Moen O, Engebretsen B, Jynge P, Refsum H (2001) Cardioprotective effects of the MR contrast agent MnDPDP and its metabolite MnPLED upon reperfusion of the ischemic procine myocardium. Acta Radiologica 42: 540–547.

Katz AM, Repke DI (1967) Quantitative aspects of dog cardiac microsomal calcium binding and calcium uptake. Circ Res 21: 153–162.

Katz AM, Tada (1972) The stone heart a challenge to the biochemist. Am J Cardiol 29: 578–580.

Kay EB, Head LR, Nogueira C (1958) Direct coronary artery perfusion for aortic valve surgery: Report of technique. JAMA 168: 159–164.

Kirklin JW (1979) Nature of the problem. In: Proceedings Cardioplegia Workshop: An International Exchange of Ideas, New York 1979: pp 1–5.

Kirklin JW (1990) The science of cardiac surgery. Eur J Cardiothorac Surg 4: 63–71.

Kirsch U, Rodewald G, Kalmar P (1972) Induced ischemic arrest and clinical experience with cardioplegia in open heart surgery. J Thorac Cardiovasc Surg 63: 121–130.

Kukreja RC, Kearns AA, Zweier JL (1991) Singlet oxygen interaction with Ca^{2+}-ATPase of cardiac sarcoplasmic reticulum. Circ Res 69: 1003–1014.

Lam CR, Geoghagan T, Lepore A (1955) Induced cardiac arrest for intracardiac surgical procedures. J Thorac Surg 30: 620–625.

Langer GA (1977) Ionic basis of myocardial contractility. Ann Rev Med 28: 13–20.

Lazar HL, Buckberg GD, Manganaro AM, Becker H (1980) Reversal of ischemic damage with amino acid substrate enhancement during reperfusion. Surgery 88: 702–709.
Lazar HL, Buckberg GD, Manganaro AM, Becker H (1980) Myocardial energy replenishment and reversal of ischemic damage by substrate enhancement of secondary blood cardioplegia with amino acids during reperfusion. J Thorac Cardiovasc Surg 80: 350–359.
Leaf A (1973) Cell swelling. A factor in ischemic tissue injury. Am J Med 49: 291–295.
Levitsky S (1977). Intracoronary perfusates for myocardial protection. Ann Thorac Surg 24: 297–298.
Lillehei CW, deWall RA, Gott VL, Varco RL (1956) The direct vision correction of calcific aortic stenosis by means of a pump-oxygenator and retrograde sinus perfusion. Chest 30: 123–132.
Lindal S, Gunnes S, Lund I, Straume BK, Jørgensen L, Sørlie D (1995) Myocardial and microvascular injury following coronary surgery and its attenuation by mode of reperfusion. Eur J Cardiothorac Surg 9(2): 83–89.
McFarland DG, Dreyer B, Bentall HH, Baker JBE (1960) Myocardial necrosis following elective cardiac arrest induced with potassium citrate. J Thorac Cardiovasc Surg 40: 200–208.
Melrose DG, Dreyer B, Bentall HH, Baker JBE (1955) Elective cardiac arrest: preliminary communication. Lancet 2: 21–22.
Melrose DG (1980). The first 25 years of cardioplegia (1980). In: Proceedings Symposium Cardioplegia: The First Quarter Century, London June 1980. p 1–5.
Menasché P, Kural S, Fauchet M, Lavergne A, Commins P, Bercot N, Touchot B, Georgiopolous G, Piwnica A (1982) Retrograde coronary sinus perfusion: A safe alternative for insuring cardioplegic delivery in aortic valve surgery. Ann Thorac Surg 34: 647–658.
Mitchell P (1966) Chemiosmotic coupling in oxidative and photosynthetic phosphorylation. Biol Rev Cam Philos Soc 41: 445–502.
Murry CE, Jennings RB, Reimer KA (1986) Preconditioning with ischemia: a delay of lethal cell injury in ischemic myocardium. Circulation 74:1124–1136.
Najafi H, Henson D, Dye WS, Javid H, Hunte JA, Callaghan R, Einstein R, Julian OC (1969). Left ventricular hemorrhagic necrosis. Ann Thor Surg 71:550–561.
Nelson RL, Fey KH, Follette DM, Livesay JJ, De Land EC, Maloney JV, Buckberg GD (1976) Intermittent infusion of cardioplegic solution during aortic cross-clamping. Surg Forum 27: 241–243.
Nordbeck, Bretschneider HJ, Fuchs C, Knoll D, Kohl FV, Sakai K, Spieckermann PG, Stapenhorst K (1974) Methode und Ergebnisse einer neuen Form des Künstlichen Herzstillstandes im Tierexperiment und unter Klinischen Bedingungen. Thoraxchirurgie 22: 582–587.
Ovrum E, Tangen G, Tollofsrud S, Øystese R, Ringdal MAL, Istad R (2004) Cold blood cardioplegia: A prospective randomized study of 1440 pateints undergoing coronary artery bypass grafting. J Thorac Cardiovas Surg 128 (6): 860–865.
Preusse CJ, Gebhard MM, Breschneider HJ (1979) Recovery of myocardial metabolism after a 210 minute cardiac arrest induced by Bretschneider cardioplegia. J Mol Cell Cardiol 11(Suppl. 2): 46.
Preusse CJ, Bretschneider HJ, Gebhard MM (1980) Myocardial equilibration procedures during cardioplegic coronary perfusion. In: Proceedings Symposium Cardioplegia: The First Quarter Century, London, pp 97–106.
Preusse CJ (1993) Cardioplegia with an intracellular formulation. In: Ischemia-Reperfusion in Cardiac Surgery, Eds HM Piper, CJ Preusse. Kluwer Academic Publishers, pp 107–134.
Proctor E (1972) Early sinus rhythm in dog hearts preserved for 96 hours and assessed ex vivo. Transplantation 13: 437–438.
Rahn H, Reeves RB, Howell BJ (1975) Hydrogen ion regulation, temperature and evolution. Am Rev Resp Dis 112: 165–172.
Reidemeister KR, Heberer G, Bretschneider HJ (1967) Induced cardiac arrest by sodium and calcium depletion and application of procaine. Intern Surg 47: 535–540.
Ringer S (1883) A further contribution regarding the influence of the different constituents of the blood on the contraction of the heart. J Physiol (Lond.) 4: 29–42.

Roe BB, Hutchinson JC, Fishman NH, Ullyot DJ, Smith DL (1977) Myocardial protection with cold, ischemic, potassium-induced cardioplegia. J Thorac Cardiovasc Surg 73: 366–374.

Rosenfeldt FL, Hearse DJ, Cankovic-Darracott S, Braimbridge MV (1980) The additive protective effects of hypotehermia and chemical cardioplegia during ischemic cardiac arrest in the dog. J Thorac Cardiovasc Surg 79: 29–38.

Rosenkranz ER, Buckberg GD, Mulder DG, Laks H (1986) Warm induction of cardioplegia with glutamate-enriched blood in coronary patients with cardiogenic shock who are dependent on inotropic drugs and intraaortic balloon support: initial experience and operative strategy. J Thorac Cardiovasc Surg 86: 507–518.

Ruigrok TJC, de Moes D, Borst C (1983) Bretschneider's histidine-buffered cardioplegic solution and the calcium paradox. J Thorac Cardiovasc Surg 86(3): 412–417.

Rygg IH and Kyvsgaard E (1958) Further development of the heart-lung machine with the Rygg-Kyvsgaard plastic bag oxygenator. Minerva Chir 13(23): 1402–1404.

Salerno TA (2007) Warm heart surgery: Reflections on the history of its development. J Card Surg 22: 257–259.

Senning Å (1952) Ventricular fibrillation during extracorporeal circulation, used as a method to prevent air embolism and to facilitate intracardiac operations. Acta Chir Scand 171: 1–79.

Shlafer M, Kane PF, Kirsh MM (1982) Superoxide dismutase plus catalase enhances the efficacy of hypothermic cardioplegia to protect the globally ischemic, reperfused heart. J Thorac Cardiovasc Surg 83(6): 830–839.

Shumway NE, Lower RR, Stofer RC (1959) Selective hypothermia of the heart in anoxic cardiac arrest. Surg Gyn Obst 109: 750–754.

Swan H (1973) Clinical hypothermia: A lady with a past and some promise for the future. Surgery 73: 736–758.

Söndergaard T, Berg E, Staffeldt I, Szczepanski K (1975) Cardioplegic arrest in aortic surgery. J Cardiovasc Surg 16: 288–290.

Taber RE, Morales AR, Fine G (1967) Myocardial necrosis and the postoperative low-cardiac-output syndrome. Ann Thor Surg 4: 12–28.

Tanguy S, Boucher FR, Malfroy B, de Leiris JG (1996) Free radicals in reperfusion-induced arrhythmias: study with EUK 8, a novel nonprotein catalytic antioxidant. Free Radic Biol Med 21(7): 945–954.

Tyers GFO, Manley NJ, Williams GH, Schaffer CW, Williams DR, Kurusz M (1977) Preliminary clinical experience with isotonic hypothermic potassium induced arrest. J Thorac Cardiovasc Surg 74: 674–681.

Uraizee A, Reimer KA, Murry CE, Jennings RB (1987) Failure of superoxide dismutase to limit size of myocardial infaction after 40 min of ischemia and 4 days of reperfusion in dogs. Circulation 75: 1237–1248

Warnecke H, Hetzer R, Iversen S, Franz P, Borst HG (1981) Re-excitation of the cardioplegic heart: a possible hazard in clinical cardioplegic arrest. Thorac Cardiovasc Surg 29: 163–167.

Yamamoto F, Braimbridge MV, Hearse DJ (1984) Calcium and cardioplegia. J Thorac Cardiovasc Surg 87: 902–912.

Ytrehus K, Gunnes S, Myklebust R, Mjøs OD (1987) Protection by superoxide dismutase and catalase in the isolated rat heart reperfused after prolonged cardioplegia: a combined study of metabolic, functional and morphometric ultrastructural variables. Cardiovasc Res 21: 492–499.

Zhao ZQ, Coevera JS, Halkos ME, Kerendi F, Wang NP, Guyton RA, Vinten-Johansen J (2003) Inhibition of myocardial injury by ischemic postconditioning during reperfusion: comparison with ischemic preconditioning. Am J Physiol 285: H579–H588.

Zimmerman ANE, Daems W, Hülsmann S, Snijder J, Wisse E, Durrer D (1967) Morphological changes of heart muscle caused by successive perfusion with calcium-free and calcium-containing solutions (calcium paradox). Cardiovasc Res 1: 201–209.

Sites of Injury: Myocyte

3

David J. Chambers

3.1 Introduction

As a surgeon, it is important to understand the pathophysiology of the disease process that causes the requirement for surgery. The predominant pathophysiologies influencing adult patients to require surgery is ischaemic heart disease, and myocardial hypertrophy as a result of valvular problems such as stenosis and regurgitation. Inevitably, there will be a certain degree of overlap in the effect of these pathophysiologies on the heart as a whole, and also on different components of the heart: the myocyte, the endothelium and the conductance system. This chapter will briefly describe effects of the pathology on the myocyte, how these pathologies may be affected by the additional stresses imposed by the surgery and by the cardioprotective methods used during the surgery.

3.2 Ischaemic Heart Disease

Ischaemic heart disease develops, usually over a relatively prolonged period, by atherosclerosis of the coronary arteries, with the resultant atherosclerotic plaque gradually narrowing the arterial lumen. Depending on the oxygen demand of the myocardium, and the ability (or inability) of the diseased artery to supply sufficient blood flow, the myocardium will become ischaemic for varying periods and then be "re-oxygenated" or "reperfused" when demand decreases. This ischaemia-reperfusion causes myocyte injury; the injury can be mild, inducing a "reversible" injury when the ischaemic duration is relatively short, with no lasting damage but potential transient dysfunction caused by myocardial stunning (Bolli and Marban 1999). Alternatively, more severe narrowing of the artery will limit oxygen delivery even at rest, and will lead to an "irreversible" injury causing myocardial

D.J. Chambers
Cardiac Surgical Research/Cardiothoracic Surgery, The Rayne Institute (King's College London), Guy's & St. Thomas' NHS Foundation Trust, St. Thomas' Hospital, London, SE1 7EH, UK
e-mail: david.chambers@kcl.ac.uk, david.chambers@gstt.nhs.uk

infarction, cell death (necrosis) and significant reduction in myocardial function (Schaper and Schaper 1988; Jennings et al. 1995). The development of collateral vessels into infarcted tissue may alleviate some of the ischaemic injury; however, this occurs over a relatively prolonged period. If an acute narrowing/occlusion occurs as a result of plaque rupture and/or thrombotic event, severe ischaemia and an irreversible injury will occur (collateral recruitment will be too slow to provide any benefit). Rapid intervention by primary angioplasty or thrombolysis, to reperfuse the ischaemic myocardium can, however, avoid severe injury and result in minimal cell death. Thus, reperfusion is an absolute requirement to prevent cell death, but reperfusion can exacerbate myocyte injury; "reperfusion-induced" injury (Hearse and Bolli 1992; Piper et al. 2003; Heyndrickx 2006).

3.2.1
Metabolic Effects of Ischaemia Reperfusion

Myocytes are highly aerobic cells, with a constant requirement for delivery of sufficient oxygen to maintain oxidative phosphorylation for energy production. This energy, in the form of adenosine triphosphate (ATP), is derived from a variety of substrates (predominantly from fatty acids and carbohydrates, but also from lactate, amino acids and ketone bodies depending on availability) that are ultimately metabolised via oxidative phosphorylation in the abundant mitochondria (around 25–35% by volume) found in the myocyte (Solaini and Harris 2005; Powers et al. 2007; Doenst et al. 2008). The contractile apparatus of the myocyte utilises the majority (around 60–70%) of ATP produced, with a further 25–35% used to maintain ionic balance by active transport pumps in the membranes. Interruption or restriction of the blood supply (ischaemia) to the myocytes will prevent oxidative metabolism and lead to a series of cellular events that can be damaging to the myocyte. Oxidative phosphorylation rapidly stops, but ATP can be maintained for a short period by glycolysis. However, an increased cytosolic NADH (without NAD regeneration), together with increases in lactate and protons that induce a cellular acidosis, inhibit glycolytic flux, and lead to a gradual decrease in ATP levels (being buffered by the more rapid utilisation of creatine phosphate content).

3.2.2
Ionic Effects of Ischaemia-Reperfusion

3.2.2.1
Cytoplasmic Effects

The cardiac myocyte contains numerous ion channels, pumps and transporters in the membranes of the cell (sarcolemma), the sarcoplasmic reticulum (SR) and the mitochondria (Fig. 1), that serve to maintain ionic homeostasis throughout the phases of excitation-contraction coupling (Bers 2002). During ischaemia, multiple ionic changes occur that cause an ionic imbalance within the myocyte. The decline in cellular ATP levels causes the ATP-dependent pumps (sarcolemmal Na^+/K^+-ATPase and Ca^{2+}-ATPase and the SR Ca^{2+}-ATPase) to become ineffective, which leads to increases in intracellular Na^+ and Ca^{2+}

3 Sites of Injury: Myocyte   43

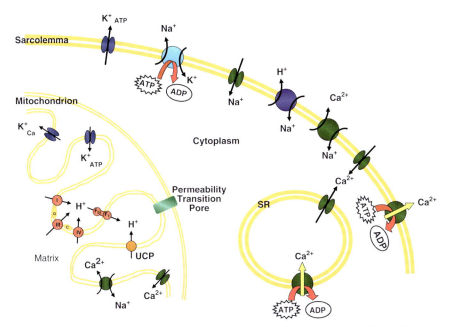

Fig. 1 Diagram of ion channels, exchangers and energy-dependent pumps involved in cardiac ionic fluxes occurring in the sarcolemma, sarcoplasmic reticulum (SR) and mitochondria. The mitochondrial inner membrane respiratory chain complexes are labelled I, III and IV, as is the FlF0-ATP synthase, Q is ubiquinone and c is cytochrome c complex, UCP denotes non-specific uncoupling proteins

concentrations. An increase in K^+ efflux leads to a depolarisation of the resting cell membrane, initiating non-inactivating Na^+ and Ca^{2+} "window" currents (Murphy and Steenbergen 2008; Murphy and Eisner 2009) that further increases intracellular Na^+ and Ca^{2+}. The rise in intracellular pH due to the metabolic acidosis activates the Na/H-exchanger, attempting to alleviate the accumulation of protons, will also cause an increase in Na^+ ion concentrations.

In an attempt to alleviate the rise in intracellular Na^+ concentrations, the Na^+/Ca^{2+} exchanger (which usually acts to remove Ca^{2+} from the cell in exchange for Na^+ during the normal action potential) will reverse and remove Na^+ in exchange for Ca^{2+}, thus again exacerbating the intracellular Ca^{2+} concentrations (Murphy and Steenbergen 2008; Murphy and Eisner 2009). The sarcolemmal L-type Ca^{2+}-channel participates in the action potential by voltage-activation after membrane depolarisation (by rapid Na^+ influx); the resultant Ca^{2+} influx initiates Ca^{2+} release from the SR (Ca^{2+}-induced Ca^{2+} release) to increase cytoplasmic Ca^{2+} levels to 0.6–2.0 µmol/L (generating the Ca^{2+} transient), which binds to troponin C and initiates contraction (Bers 2002). However, during ischaemia it may directly contribute to increased Ca^{2+} influx (Hool 2007; Hool and Corry 2007) via a conformational change of the channel protein that is caused by reactive oxygen species (ROS) generated during ischaemia-reperfusion. ROS, as well as the decreased ATP levels, will also inhibit the transport of Ca^{2+} out of the cell by the sarcolemmal Ca^{2+}-ATPase.

In contrast to the above, activation of the ATP-dependent K^+-channel (which occurs when ATP levels are decreased) will tend to reduce Ca^{2+} influx by shortening the action potential (Gross and Peart 2003), favouring a repolarisation of the membrane potential (by increasing the permeability of the membrane to K^+). Pharmacological activation of these channels improves cardioprotection by reducing Ca^{2+} entry and, thus, Ca^{2+} overload.

3.2.2.2 Mitochondria Effects

Mitochondria are critical for both life and death of the myocyte. During normal function, they provide ATP, the high-energy phosphate compound generated during oxidative phosphorylation, which is constantly in demand by the beating myocardium (Solaini and Harris 2005). Strategic location of mitochondria throughout the myocyte ensures efficient provision of this ATP where it is required. Since there is very little ATP storage in the myocyte, constant production is essential. Hence, it is not surprising that increasing evidence supports the importance of mitochondria in determining the fate of the myocyte, with various stimuli (such as ischaemia-reperfusion, cardiomyopathy and heart failure) triggering responses such as apoptosis and necrosis (Gustafsson and Gottlieb 2008).

Mitochondrial membranes have similar ion channels, pumps and transporters to those seen in the myocyte sarcolemma (Fig. 1) (O'Rourke et al. 2005; Solaini and Harris 2005), controlling tight regulation of ionic homeostasis within the mitochondria. This is necessary to maintain the pH gradient set up by proton translocation across the inner membrane via the electron transport chain complexes, together with the mitochondrial membrane potential ($\Delta\Psi_m$), establishing a proton driving force used by mitochondrial ATP synthase that generates ATP within the mitochondria (O'Rourke et al. 2005; Solaini and Harris 2005). Any change in the mitochondrial membrane permeability will influence this energy production (O'Rourke et al. 2005; Solaini and Harris 2005). Interestingly, the mitochondria can accumulate considerable quantities of Ca^{2+}, thus allowing the mitochondria to assist in preventing cytosolic Ca^{2+} overload. This increase in mitochondrial matrix Ca^{2+} is also thought to have a role in increasing ATP production through a direct effect on the mitochondrial ATP synthase (Solaini and Harris 2005; Gustafsson and Gottlieb 2008). The interplay between Ca^{2+} entry via the Ca^{2+} uniporter and Ca^{2+} efflux via the Na^+/Ca^{2+} exchanger in regulating mitochondrial Ca^{2+} levels eventually reaches a threshold whereby mitochondrial Ca^{2+} overload occurs; this causes activation (opening) of the mitochondrial permeability transition pore (mPTP).

The mPTP has been shown to be crucial in determining the fate of the myocyte during ischaemia and reperfusion (Solaini and Harris 2005; Di Lisa and Bernardi 2006; Halestrap 2006). Ischaemia primes the mPTP to open; utilisation of ATP briefly maintains $\Delta\Psi_m$ and mitochondrial pH but when ATP levels decline the $\Delta\Psi_m$ collapses (depolarises). This allows the membrane to become more permeable and the increased cytosolic Ca^{2+} accumulation during ischaemia-reperfusion (as described above) can enter the mitochondria and lead to mitochondrial Ca^{2+} overload; in addition, there is an increase in ROS (see later) that also have a large impact on myocyte injury. The mPTP is inhibited by acidotic conditions and so remains closed during ischaemia whilst the intracellular mileu remains acidotic (Halestrap 2006).

Reperfusion leads to mitochondrial membrane repolarisation, at which time there is a major increase in mitochondrial Ca^{2+} influx and this can lead to Ca^{2+} overload and mitochondrial dysfunction. A return to normal cytosolic pH occurs within a few minutes of reperfusion; at this time the mPTP can open and cause mitochondrial damage, constituting significant reperfusion injury if the open state of mPTP is maintained (Halestrap 2006). Studies using 2-deoxyglucose (DOG) have demonstrated that mPTP that open during reperfusion can subsequently close, with extent of closure correlating to recovery of the heart (Halestrap 2006). Opening of mPTP during reperfusion can lead to membrane depolarisation and ATP utilisation in an attempt to maintain $\Delta\Psi_m$ (Powers et al. 2007). This appears to be the important factor in myocyte death or survival. Prolonged opening of the mPTP allows entry of water into the mitochondrial matrix, leading to swelling and potential membrane rupture. Different degrees of injury (correlating to duration of mPTP opening) will determine the fate of the myocyte. Thus, if the pore opens briefly but then closes again, there will be no significant damage and the cell will recover (Fig. 2). However, moderate or localised mPTP opening could lead to release of apoptotic factors (such as cytochrome c and apoptosis-inducing factor) (Honda et al. 2005), resulting in programmed cell death (apoptosis) despite adequate energy metabolism (Valen 2003), whereas more prolonged pore opening will cause significant damage, with cessation of ATP production, cell swelling and cell death by necrosis (Honda et al. 2005; Halestrap 2006; Javadov and Karmazyn 2007; Powers et al. 2007).

3.2.3
Oxidative Injury During Ischaemia-Reperfusion

In aerobic organisms, molecular O_2 is utilised as the final electron acceptor in the metabolism of organic carbon for energy provision. This respiratory process involves consumption of substrates and O_2 to generate the high-energy compound ATP, water and carbon dioxide. During normal respiratory chain oxidative phosphorylation in the mitochondria, the use of O_2 to oxidise redox carriers can occur by 2 pathways; ~95% of O_2 is reduced tetravalently directly to water without production of ROS. The other approximately 5% of electron flow is reduced univalently, generating superoxide radicals as a byproduct of the process, making mitochondria a major site of ROS production (Becker 2004; O'Rourke et al. 2005; Solaini and Harris 2005; Gustafsson and Gottlieb 2008). ROS (superoxide anion ($O_2^{-\bullet}$), hydrogen peroxide (H_2O_2) and hydroxyl radical (OH^-)) can be extremely damaging molecules to their local environment, but are normally rapidly removed (detoxified) by the endogenous antioxidants (such as superoxide dismutase, which converts $O_2^{-\bullet}$ to H_2O_2, and catalase and glutathione peroxidase, which converts H_2O_2 to water) present in mitochondria, cytoplasm and blood plasma. Thus, oxidative tissues, such as the myocardium, have developed a considerable tolerance to ROS under normal conditions. However, under conditions of ischaemia and reperfusion, this homeostasis becomes altered; the antioxidant defence mechanisms become depleted and the

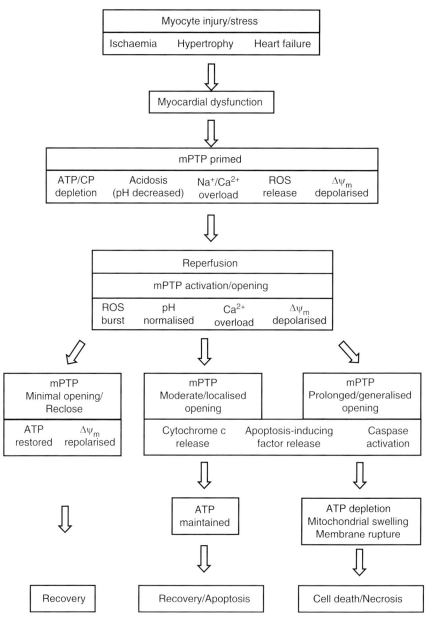

Fig. 2 Schematic flow diagram indicating the potential involvement of the mitochondria, and in particular the mitochondrial permeability transition pore (mPTP), in determining the outcome of the myocyte after injury or stress. ROS (reactive oxygen species)

increasing levels of H_2O_2 (together with ischaemia-induced free metal ions) can lead to the induction of the highly reactive and damaging hydroxyl radical. These radicals can lead to direct damage of the cell membrane, proteins, sulfhydryl bonds and lipid peroxidation. Additional free radicals, such as peroxynitrite can also be produced from nitric oxide (Becker 2004).

ROS generation occurs predominantly during reperfusion, when O_2 is reintroduced to the ischaemic tissue. Direct measurement of this oxidative burst has been measured using electron spin resonance techniques, demonstrating a peak release of ROS within seconds (Zweier et al. 1987) or minutes (Garlick et al. 1987) of reperfusion. However, the majority of evidence has been demonstrated by indirect measurement of improvements in recovery of hearts (or survival of myocytes) when antioxidants were incorporated into the reperfusion procedure (Becker 2004), suggesting the presence of a "reperfusion-induced" injury that occurs over and above that of the ischaemic process. It is important to realise that antioxidant therapy is only efficacious when applied at the time of reperfusion, emphasising the rapidity of the oxidative burst at this time.

Recently, the production of ROS during ischaemia has been demonstrated (Becker 2004). Clinical ischaemia is highly unlikely to cause complete anoxia, with sufficient molecular O_2 remaining in the cell such that the univalent pathway is increased, generating considerable superoxide radical. The evidence suggests that radical generation during ischaemia is predominantly derived from mitochondria. Inhibitors of specific electron transport sites in the electron transport chain suggest that complexes I–III are involved in this radical production, whereas complex IV does not seem to be involved (Becker 2004). Interestingly, the oxidative burst seen at reperfusion does not respond to these specific mitochondrial inhibitors, suggesting that this oxidant radical burst occurs from some other (currently unknown) source; this is an ongoing focus of research. Recently, it has been reported (Becker 2004; Gustafsson and Gottlieb 2008) that there is a positive feedback process of ROS-induced ROS release (RIRR) in which a low level of ROS production induces a secondary burst of ROS from the electron transport chain. There appear to be two RIRR pathways that involve either the mPTP or the inner membrane anion channel (IMAC). Both mechanisms induce a collapse of the $\Delta\Psi_m$, with a destabilisation influence on the myocyte action potential that combine to form an important mediator of ischaemia-reperfusion injury.

It has been known for some years that ROS can have a dual effect on cell function. Although excess ROS production that exceeds the detoxification mechanisms can lead to cellular injury, ROS have also been shown to have a physiological role in signal transduction mechanisms when produced at low levels. These small quantities of ROS can trigger protective mechanisms, and studies into the signal transduction pathways of ischaemic preconditioning protection provided much of the insight for this role of ROS (Downey et al. 2008). It was known that antioxidants could block ischaemic preconditioning protection (Becker 2004), and that opening the mitochondrial ATP-sensitive potassium channel (mK_{ATP}-channel) is involved in inducing protection whereas inhibition prevented protection (Garlid et al. 2003). It is now thought that opening mK_{ATP}-channel initiates a release of ROS from the mitochondria (occurring during the reperfusion phase of the preconditioning protocol when O_2 is returned to the myocyte) that activates protein kinase C (PKC) and constitutes the trigger phase of preconditioning. This activated PKC participates in the mediator phase of preconditioning comprised of multiple downstream kinases that result in the blockade of mPTP activation, and hence protection (Downey et al. 2008).

The influence of ROS on opening of mPTP remains an important factor in myocyte injury. Many studies have demonstrated that inhibition of mPTP opening is a protective event, whereas ischaemia and reperfusion that causes mPTP opening can proceed to a number of consequences (Fig. 2). If the ischaemia and reperfusion is mild, the mPTP opens only briefly before closing again, and this will result in a recovery of the myocyte. More prolonged injury from ischaemia-reperfusion can cause opening in a greater number of mitochondria which can initiate swelling of the mitochondrial matrix causing release of cytochromes, as well as apoptotic signalling proteins from the mitochondria; maintained ATP levels in those mitochondria less injured will provide the energy required for the apoptotic process to occur (Valen 2003). In contrast, severe ischaemia-reperfusion injury causes irreversible mPTP opening in a majority of mitochondria leading to massive swelling with membrane rupture, severe ATP utilisation and necrosis (Honda et al. 2005; Javadov and Karmazyn 2007).

3.3
Ventricular Pressure Overload and Hypertrophy

Clinically, pressure overload-induced ventricular hypertrophy (such as aortic valve stenosis) leads to progressive ventricular dilatation, contractile dysfunction, heart failure and increased vulnerability to ischemia-reperfusion injury (Friehs and del Nido 2003); hence, the mechanisms described above relating to metabolic and ionic effects associated with ischaemia-reperfusion will also apply to hypertrophic myocardium. Hypertrophy is a well-recognised risk factor, and has been identified as an important contributor to cardiovascular morbidity and mortality. This is particularly relevant for cardiac surgery, as LV hypertrophy often leads to post-operative contractile dysfunction (Mehta et al. 2001) as a result of the decreased ischaemic tolerance.

3.3.1
Myocyte Signalling Pathway Changes

The processes by which cardiac hypertrophy progress to heart failure are multifactorial, but the mechanism(s) involved remain unclear. Hypertrophy should, theoretically, provide improved function; the increase in the number of contractile elements (sarcomeres) within the myocyte should reduce wall stress by increasing wall thickness in concentric hypertrophy (additional sarcomeres in parallel, giving thicker myocytes) and increase stroke volume in eccentric hypertrophy (additional sarcomeres in series, giving longer myocytes) (Kempf and Wollert 2004). Signalling pathways that control the hypertrophic response of the myocyte have been investigated; pathological conditions increase levels of growth factors that stimulate G-protein-coupled receptors (GPCR) and/or mechanoreceptors. These signals progress downstream to the nucleus via networks of protein kinases, phospholipid kinases and protein phosphatases. These stimulate gene expression that affect contractile proteins, ion pumps and channels, cardiac energetics, matrix components and cell survival regulators (such as apoptosis) (Kempf and Wollert 2004). These effects perpetuate the activation, contributing to the vicious circle of hypertrophic maladaption. There is evidence, however, that certain signalling pathways are associated with either adaptive (protective) hypertrophic effects or maladaptive (detrimental) influences.

It would appear that excess activation of the GPCR, $G\alpha_q$, by growth factors such as angiotensin II or norepinephrine, promotes a hypertrophic effect that rapidly progresses to heart failure associated with aortic stenosis; angiotensin-converting enzyme (ACE) inhibitors or adrenoreceptor blockers can attenuate the adverse effects of heart failure (Kempf and Wollert 2004). Calcineurin, a Ca^{2+}-sensitive protein phosphatase, is another important hypertrophic signalling molecule that is activated by pressure overload. This is influenced by increased Ca^{2+} influx through the L-type Ca^{2+}-channels, and results in nuclear translocation of cytoplasmic NFAT (nuclear factor of activated T cells) transcription factors; $G\alpha_q$ can also link in with this mechanism to activate calcineurin (Kempf and Wollert 2004). Other factors, such as melusin or muscle LIM protein (MLP) appear to be involved in a more adaptive type of hypertrophy (such as that seen with cardiac growth during childhood, pregnancy or as a result of regular exercise). Hence, there may be a balance between adaptive and maladaptive signals leading to hypertrophy that can be exploited for therapeutic considerations (Kempf and Wollert 2004).

3.3.2
Myocyte Metabolic Changes

Energy metabolism in hypertrophic myocardium shifts towards increased glycolysis, with impaired fatty acid oxidation, representing a reversion to a more foetal metabolism. Unexpectedly, this results in a reduced tolerance to ischaemia-reperfusion, a finding that can be explained by the complexity of glucose regulation. Glucose transport into the myocyte is dependent on concentration gradient and is facilitated by specific transport proteins, GLUT-1 (responsible for basal transport) and GLUT-4 (insulin-regulated) (Friehs and del Nido 2003). GLUT-4 is the predominant transporter in cardiac myocytes, and is usually stored in intracellular vesicles, but stimulation (insulin, ischaemia, cardiac work) translocates the GLUT-4 to the plasma membrane, promoting glucose transport. However, hypertrophied myocardium was shown to have a reduced glucose uptake but no difference in transporter protein expression. This suggests either a reduction in translocation of the GLUT-4 to the membrane or an impaired delivery of substrate to the myocyte, possibly as a result of relative decrease in capillary density between myocytes (and thus increased diffusion distances); both of these options have been demonstrated in experimental studies (Friehs and del Nido 2003).

Other metabolic changes in hypertrophic myocytes have also been reported (Braunwald and Bristow 2000). Heart failure resulting from ischaemic heart disease and cardiomyopathy demonstrates a number of biochemical abnormalities; the efficiency of the myocytes acting as a "pump" is decreased as a result of relative ischaemia arising from hypertrophy. Levels of intracellular creatine phosphate are depressed; this can influence the transfer of ATP from the mitochondria to the myofibrils and is associated with reduced activity of creatine kinase. A deficiency in high-energy phosphate (ATP) provision will influence the involvement of Ca^{2+} in excitation-contraction coupling (Fig. 1), particularly the energy dependent uptake of Ca^{2+} into the SR, which will impair myocardial relaxation and hence increase diastolic stiffness (Braunwald and Bristow 2000).

3.4
Cardioprotection During Surgery

Conducting surgery on myocardium that has been injured by the variety of processes described above will necessarily impose additional stresses on this tissue. Predominantly, this stress will occur as an elective ischaemia that is imposed by the surgeon for various durations to allow the lesion to be corrected. Consequently, it is essential that any additional injury to this tissue be minimised. The current gold standard for myocardial protection during cardiac surgery is to use a hyperkalaemic cardioplegic solution that induces rapid cardiac arrest and thereby delays any additional irreversible ischaemia-induced injury to the already compromised myocytes. Cardioplegic solutions have now been used for over 3 decades with considerable success. However, there has been little change in the basic clinical formulation, despite innumerable experimental studies into methods to improve the protection achieved with these solutions. The advance in knowledge of the events that precipitate myocyte injury, some of which are described above, should be translated into an examination of the basic concept of myocardial protective techniques. Only fairly recently has it been fully appreciated just what a major role the mitochondria plays in determining the fate of the myocyte during the pathophysiology of the heart that constitutes ischaemic heart disease, hypertrophy and heart failure. The surgeon has to operate on these hearts knowing that they are compromised, and yet the techniques for cardiac protection during cardiac surgery have not progressed in line with these advances. It should be a matter of urgency for researchers and surgeons to collaborate in producing a cardioprotective regime that targets the events described above, and improve therapeutic myocardial protection during cardiac surgery. This has increasing urgency with the changing epidemiology of the patients coming for surgery in the era of increasing percutaneous coronary intervention (PCI) conducted by the cardiologist. Patients are older, sicker and have more severe and diffuse disease, and this requires improved myocardial protection during the surgery that minimises any exacerbation of the myocardial injury already present.

3.4.1
Endogenous Protection: Preconditioning and Postconditioning

Cardiac surgery, because of its elective nature, lends itself to the possibility of employing the endogenous protective mechanisms inherent in "preconditioning" (see earlier) and in the more recently described "postconditioning". The mechanisms of these techniques have been intensively studied and are the subject of a number of excellent recent reviews (Vaage and Valen 2003; Yellon and Downey 2003; Downey et al. 2007, 2008; Ferdinandy et al.

2007; Hausenloy and Yellon 2007; Vinten-Johansen 2007; Vinten-Johansen et al. 2007; Venugopal et al. 2009). Ischaemic preconditioning (IPC) refers to the phenomenon, first described by Murry and colleagues (Murry et al. 1986) in 1986, whereby brief episodes of ischaemia and reperfusion prior to a more prolonged ischaemic period paradoxically protects the myocardium against this potentially lethal ischaemic duration. Similarly, preconditioning can be initiated by pharmacological agents that stimulate components of the complex signalling pathways when used in the same way as that of the brief ischaemia (Downey et al. 2007). Cardiac surgery is potentially suitable for the application of preconditioning protection because the timing of the prolonged ischaemic duration is known in advance. However, the benefit of preconditioning in the context of cardiac surgery (particularly in association with cardioplegic protection) is controversial.

Experimental studies in isolated rat hearts were unable to demonstrate enhanced protection with both ischaemic preconditioning and cardioplegic protection (Kolocassides et al. 1994). In contrast, pharmacological preconditioning with a potassium channel opener, nicorandil, improved protection in hearts protected with potassium cardioplegic arrest (Menasche et al. 1995). Subsequently, many other experimental and clinical studies have confirmed these controversial and conflicting results (Venugopal et al. 2009). In the clinical setting, an explanation for these differences involves the concept that cardiopulmonary bypass per se can induce a preconditioning protection (Burns et al. 1995; Ghosh and Galinanes 2003). Additionally, the volatile inhalation anaesthetics often used during cardiac surgery (such as propofol, sevoflurane, and desflurane) have been shown to induce cardiac protection, although this also remains controversial (Venugopal et al. 2009).

An interesting recent development relates to the potential for remote ischaemic preconditioning of a different organ to promote protection in the heart. Remote preconditioning was first noted when protection was obtained in the occluded left anterior descending (LAD) territory of the heart by brief preconditioning episodes of ischaemia and reperfusion in the circumflex territory (Przyklenk et al. 1993). This has potential significant implications for cardiac surgery; the possibility of inducing remote limb ischaemic preconditioning was shown to occur in humans, and to reduce infarction in experimental studies (Kharbanda et al. 2002). Subsequently, remote limb ischaemic preconditioning was shown to be effective during cardiac surgery in both children (Cheung et al. 2006) and adults (Hausenloy et al. 2007). The mechanism whereby remote ischaemic preconditioning occurs is currently unknown; the pathways involved are likely to be similar to conventional ischaemic preconditioning, with initiation attributed to hormonal and/or neural stimulation (Hausenloy and Yellon 2008; Venugopal et al. 2009). Planned large-scale multicentre randomised clinical trials in the cardiac surgery arena should demonstrate whether this procedure has any real beneficial potential.

The phenomenon of ischaemic postconditioning, whereby improved protection is observed after a number of very brief episodes (seconds) of reperfusion followed by ischaemia initiated at the onset of reperfusion, was first described by Vinten-Johansen's group (Zhao et al. 2003). Postconditioning protection in humans has been demonstrated to reduce infarct size and improve myocardial function up to 6 months post-PCI (Thibault et al. 2008). Studies (from a single unit) on cardiac surgery patients undergoing bypass and cardioplegic arrest, showed that ischaemic postconditioning (by repeated cross clamping and removal) reduced myocardial injury (as measured by enzyme release and lower inotropic requirement) in both children and adults (Luo et al. 2007; Luo et al. 2008a, b). However, recent experimental studies from our group (Maruyama and Chambers 2008) failed to demonstrate enhanced cardioprotection with postconditioning when cardioplegia was used.

Thus, the potential for ischaemic postconditioning protection during cardiac surgery remains controversial; there is a need for more experimental and clinical studies, but the invasive technique of multiple rapid cross clamping is likely to pose a limitation to its acceptance during cardiac surgery. Nevertheless, postconditioning does represent an interesting possibility for reducing myocardial ischaemia-reperfusion injury in all patients, as a prior knowledge of the onset of the ischaemic event is not required. Although the mechanism by which postconditioning protection occurs is currently unclear, there is evidence suggesting the involvement of the mPTP (Boengler et al. 2009; Granfeldt et al. 2009). Other factors relevant to the clinical situation also require consideration, such as the apparent loss of endogenous preconditioning and postconditioning cardioprotection with ageing (Boengler et al. 2009; Downey and Cohen 2009) and with patient comorbidities such as diabetes (Downey and Cohen 2009). In addition, outcomes from experimental studies have to be reconciled with the fact that most use healthy hearts, and these may respond very differently to the hearts of aged and diseased patients (Downey and Cohen 2009). Despite these concerns, it is encouraging that the possibilities for endogenous protection mechanisms are increasingly being examined in the patients to which they are relevant.

3.5
Conclusions

Injury to the myocyte is a multifactorial process, involving all components of the myocyte. However, it would appear that mitochondria play a controlling role in determining the outcome of the myocyte. There are three potential scenarios; (1) the injury may be sufficiently mild that the injury is reversible and the myocyte recovers, (2) the injury is sufficiently severe that a cascade of enzymes are initiated that results in the energy-dependent process of apoptosis, causing a number of myocytes to enter into programmed cell death, or (3) the injury is so severe that cellular energy molecules are completely depleted, the myocyte swells causing membrane disruption and initiation of an inflammatory process that can affect adjacent cells and lead to cell necrosis. All these processes have common characteristics, and it is merely the severity of these processes that determines the fate of the myocyte.

References

Becker LB (2004). New concepts in reactive oxygen species and cardiovascular reperfusion physiology. Cardiovasc Res 61(3): 461–470.
Bers DM (2002). Cardiac excitation-contraction coupling. Nature 415(6868): 198–205.

Boengler K, Schulz R, Heusch G (2009). Loss of cardioprotection with ageing. Cardiovasc Res 83 (2): 247–261.

Bolli R, Marban E (1999). Molecular and cellular mechanisms of myocardial stunning. Physiol Rev 79(2): 609–634.

Braunwald E, Bristow MR (2000). Congestive heart failure: fifty years of progress. Circulation 102 (20 Suppl 4): IV14–IV23.

Burns PG, Krukenkamp IB, Caldarone CA, Gaudette GR, Bukhari EA, Levitsky S (1995). Does cardiopulmonary bypass alone elicit myoprotective preconditioning? Circulation 92(9 Suppl): II447–II451.

Cheung MM, Kharbanda RK, Konstantinov IE, Shimizu M, Frndova H, Li J, Holtby HM, Cox PN, Smallhorn JF, Van Arsdell GS, Redington AN (2006). Randomized controlled trial of the effects of remote ischemic preconditioning on children undergoing cardiac surgery: first clinical application in humans. J Am Coll Cardiol 47(11): 2277–2282.

Di Lisa F, Bernardi P (2006). Mitochondria and ischemia-reperfusion injury of the heart: fixing a hole. Cardiovasc Res 70(2): 191–199.

Doenst T, Bugger H, Schwarzer M, Faerber G, Borger MA, Mohr FW (2008). Three good reasons for heart surgeons to understand cardiac metabolism. Eur J Cardiothorac Surg 33(5): 862–871.

Downey JM, Cohen MV (2009). Why do we still not have cardioprotective drugs? Circ J 73(7): 1171–1177.

Downey JM, Davis AM, Cohen MV (2007). Signaling pathways in ischemic preconditioning. Heart Fail Rev 12(3–4): 181–188.

Downey JM, Krieg T, Cohen MV (2008). Mapping preconditioning's signaling pathways: an engineering approach. Ann N Y Acad Sci 1123: 187–196.

Ferdinandy P, Schulz R, Baxter GF (2007). Interaction of cardiovascular risk factors with myocardial ischemia/reperfusion injury, preconditioning, and postconditioning. Pharmacol Rev 59(4): 418–458.

Friehs I, del Nido PJ (2003). Increased susceptibility of hypertrophied hearts to ischemic injury. Ann Thorac Surg 75(2): S678–S684.

Garlick PB, Davies MJ, Hearse DJ, Slater TF (1987). Direct detection of free radicals in the reperfused rat heart using electron spin resonance spectroscopy. Circ Res 61(5): 757–760.

Garlid KD, Dos Santos P, Xie ZJ, Costa AD, Paucek P (2003). Mitochondrial potassium transport: the role of the mitochondrial ATP-sensitive K(+) channel in cardiac function and cardioprotection. Biochim Biophys Acta 1606(1–3): 1–21.

Ghosh S, Galinanes M (2003). Protection of the human heart with ischemic preconditioning during cardiac surgery: role of cardiopulmonary bypass. J Thorac Cardiovasc Surg 126(1): 133–142.

Granfeldt A, Lefer DJ, Vinten-Johansen J (2009). Protective ischaemia in patients: preconditioning and postconditioning. Cardiovasc Res 83(2): 234–246.

Gross GJ, Peart JN (2003). KATP channels and myocardial preconditioning: an update. Am J Physiol Heart Circ Physiol 285(3): H921–H930.

Gustafsson AB, Gottlieb RA (2008). Heart mitochondria: gates of life and death. Cardiovasc Res 77(2): 334–343.

Halestrap AP (2006). Calcium, mitochondria and reperfusion injury: a pore way to die. Biochem Soc Trans 34(Pt 2): 232–237.

Hausenloy DJ, Yellon DM (2007). Preconditioning and postconditioning: united at reperfusion. Pharmacol Ther 116(2): 173–191.

Hausenloy DJ, Yellon DM (2008). Remote ischaemic preconditioning: underlying mechanisms and clinical application. Cardiovasc Res 79(3): 377–386.

Hausenloy DJ, Mwamure PK, Venugopal V, Harris J, Barnard M, Grundy E, Ashley E, Vichare S, Di Salvo C, Kolvekar S, Hayward M, Keogh B, MacAllister RJ, Yellon DM (2007). Effect of remote ischaemic preconditioning on myocardial injury in patients undergoing coronary artery bypass graft surgery: a randomised controlled trial. Lancet 370(9587): 575–579.

Hearse DJ, Bolli R (1992). Reperfusion induced injury: manifestations, mechanisms, and clinical relevance. Cardiovasc Res 26(2): 101–108.

Heyndrickx GR (2006). Early reperfusion phenomena. Semin Cardiothorac Vasc Anesth 10(3): 236–241.

Honda HM, Korge P, Weiss JN (2005). Mitochondria and ischemia/reperfusion injury. Ann NY Acad Sci 1047: 248–258.

Hool LC (2007). What cardiologists should know about calcium ion channels and their regulation by reactive oxygen species. Heart Lung Circ 16(5): 361–372.

Hool LC, Corry B (2007). Redox control of calcium channels: from mechanisms to therapeutic opportunities. Antioxid Redox Signal 9(4): 409–435.

Javadov S, Karmazyn M (2007). Mitochondrial permeability transition pore opening as an endpoint to initiate cell death and as a putative target for cardioprotection. Cell Physiol Biochem 20(1–4): 1–22.

Jennings RB, Steenbergen C, Jr., Reimer KA (1995). Myocardial ischemia and reperfusion. Monogr Pathol 37: 47–80.

Kempf T, Wollert KC (2004). Nitric oxide and the enigma of cardiac hypertrophy. Bioessays 26(6): 608–615.

Kharbanda RK, Mortensen UM, White PA, Kristiansen SB, Schmidt MR, Hoschtitzky JA, Vogel M, Sorensen K, Redington AN, MacAllister R (2002). Transient limb ischemia induces remote ischemic preconditioning in vivo. Circulation 106(23): 2881–2883.

Kolocassides KG, Galinanes M, Hearse DJ (1994). Ischemic preconditioning, cardioplegia or both? J Mol Cell Cardiol 26(11): 1411–1414.

Luo W, Li B, Lin G, Huang R (2007). Postconditioning in cardiac surgery for tetralogy of Fallot. J Thorac Cardiovasc Surg 133(5): 1373–1374.

Luo W, Li B, Chen R, Huang R, Lin G (2008). Effect of ischemic postconditioning in adult valve replacement. Eur J Cardiothorac Surg 33(2): 203–208.

Luo W, Li B, Lin G, Chen R, Huang R (2008). Does cardioplegia leave room for postconditioning in paediatric cardiac surgery? Cardiol Young 18(3): 282–287.

Maruyama Y, Chambers DJ (2008). Does ischemic postconditioning improve myocardial protection after conventional cardioplegia? J Mol Cell Cardiol 44: 761.

Mehta RH, Bruckman D, Das S, Tsai T, Russman P, Karavite D, Monaghan H, Sonnad S, Shea MJ, Eagle KA, Deeb GM (2001). Implications of increased left ventricular mass index on in-hospital outcomes in patients undergoing aortic valve surgery. J Thorac Cardiovasc Surg 122(5): 919–928.

Menasche P, Kevelaitis E, Mouas C, Grousset C, Piwnica A, Bloch G (1995). Preconditioning with potassium channel openers. A new concept for enhancing cardioplegic protection? J Thorac Cardiovasc Surg 110(6): 1606–1613; discussion 1613–1604.

Murphy E, Eisner DA (2009). Regulation of intracellular and mitochondrial sodium in health and disease. Circ Res 104(3): 292–303.

Murphy E, Steenbergen C (2008). Ion transport and energetics during cell death and protection. Physiology (Bethesda) 23: 115–123.

Murry CE, Jennings RB, Reimer KA (1986). Preconditioning with ischemia: a delay of lethal cell injury in ischemic myocardium. Circulation 74(5): 1124–1136.

O'Rourke B, Cortassa S, Aon MA (2005). Mitochondrial ion channels: gatekeepers of life and death. Physiology (Bethesda) 20: 303–315.

Piper HM, Meuter K, Schafer C (2003). Cellular mechanisms of ischemia-reperfusion injury. Ann Thorac Surg 75(2): S644–648.

Powers SK, Murlasits Z, Wu M, Kavazis AN (2007). Ischemia-reperfusion-induced cardiac injury: a brief review. Med Sci Sports Exerc 39(9): 1529–1536.

Przyklenk K, Bauer B, Ovize M, Kloner RA, Whittaker P (1993). Regional ischemic 'preconditioning' protects remote virgin myocardium from subsequent sustained coronary occlusion. Circulation 87(3): 893–899.

Schaper J, Schaper W (1988). Time course of myocardial necrosis. Cardiovasc Drugs Ther 2(1): 17–25.

Solaini G, Harris DA (2005). Biochemical dysfunction in heart mitochondria exposed to ischaemia and reperfusion. Biochem J 390(Pt 2): 377–394.

Thibault H, Piot C, Staat P, Bontemps L, Sportouch C, Rioufol G, Cung TT, Bonnefoy E, Angoulvant D, Aupetit JF, Finet G, Andre-Fouet X, Macia JC, Raczka F, Rossi R, Itti R, Kirkorian G, Derumeaux G, Ovize M (2008). Long-term benefit of postconditioning. Circulation 117(8): 1037–1044.

Vaage J, Valen G (2003). Preconditioning and cardiac surgery. Ann Thorac Surg 75(2): S709–714.

Valen G (2003). The basic biology of apoptosis and its implications for cardiac function and viability. Ann Thorac Surg 75(2): S656–S660.

Venugopal V, Ludman A, Yellon DM, Hausenloy DJ (2009). 'Conditioning' the heart during surgery. Eur J Cardiothorac Surg 35(6): 977–987.

Vinten-Johansen J (2007). Postconditioning: a mechanical maneuver that triggers biological and molecular cardioprotective responses to reperfusion. Heart Fail Rev 12(3–4): 235–244.

Vinten-Johansen J, Zhao ZQ, Jiang R, Zatta AJ, Dobson GP (2007). Preconditioning and postconditioning: innate cardioprotection from ischemia-reperfusion injury. J Appl Physiol 103(4): 1441–1448.

Yellon DM, Downey JM (2003). Preconditioning the myocardium: from cellular physiology to clinical cardiology. Physiol Rev 83(4): 1113–1151.

Zhao ZQ, Corvera JS, Halkos ME, Kerendi F, Wang NP, Guyton RA, Vinten-Johansen J (2003). Inhibition of myocardial injury by ischemic postconditioning during reperfusion: comparison with ischemic preconditioning. Am J Physiol Heart Circ Physiol 285(2): H579–H588.

Zweier JL, Flaherty JT, Weisfeldt ML (1987). Direct measurement of free radical generation following reperfusion of ischemic myocardium. Proc Natl Acad Sci USA 84(5): 1404–1407.

Sites of Injury: The Endothelium

4

Johann Wojta

4.1
Introduction

An estimated 6×10^{13} endothelial cells form the inner surface of blood vessels in man. As such, in an adult human being they cover a total area of approximately 3,000 m^2 and have a total volume comparable to that of the liver (Huttner and Gabbiani 1982; Münzel et al. 2008). Traditionally, the endothelium has been assumed to be a passive barrier between the blood and the surrounding tissue; however, over the past 2–3 decades numerous additional roles for the endothelium have been described. These findings challenge the concept of the endothelium as a passive interface and leads to the notion of the endothelium being a highly active organ involved in the regulation and modulation of a vast number of physiological and pathophysiological processes. Endothelial cells are essential in the regulation of vascular tone, control of transendothelial movement of fluid, solutes and macromolecules, modulation of inflammation and leukocyte adhesion, promotion and inhibition of growth of new blood vessels and regulation of blood fluidity and platelet aggregation, fibrinolysis and coagulation.

Endothelial cells can respond to certain stimuli with "endothelial activation" (Cotran and Pober 1989). Such activated endothelial cells acquire new functions; for example, when exposed to inflammatory cytokines endothelial cells express new surface molecules and cytokines that promote leukocyte accumulation, adhesion and transmigration through the endothelial layer (Cotran and Pober 1989). Activated endothelial cells also display a prothrombotic phenotype by expressing tissue factor (TF) (Nawroth and Stern 1986). In contrast to endothelial activation, which is mainly caused by inflammatory stimuli related to host defence, "endothelial dysfunction" is caused by endothelial injury. In such injured endothelial cells NO-production is impaired resulting in increased vascular tone and high blood pressure (Panza et al. 1990). Dysfunctional endothelial cells also loose their ability to block intravascular coagulation and their barrier function to retain plasma proteins (Aird 2003; Joris et al. 1990). It is self-evident that severe forms of injury can result in endothelial cell death and dead endothelial cells are completely dysfunctional.

J. Wojta
Department of Internal Medicine, Allgemeines Krankenhaus der Stadt Wien, Medical University of Vienna, Währinger Güertel 18–20, 1090 Vienna, Austria

It is important to note that endothelial activation and endothelial dysfunction are key processes in many disease states in general, and in the development and progression of cardiovascular pathologies in particular.

The following sections will focus on mechanisms of endothelial activation, different forms of endothelial injury resulting in endothelial dysfunction and various forms of endothelial cell death. The last chapter will describe how ischemia reperfusion during heart surgery could lead to endothelial injury and dysfunction.

4.2
Endothelial Cell Activation

4.2.1
Quiescent Endothelium

Non-activated endothelium displays antithrombotic and antiadhesive properties. Quiescent, non-activated, endothelial cells express prostacyclin (PGI2) and NO, which inhibit platelet activation, adhesion and aggregation (Sessa 2004). In addition, non-activated endothelial cells display thrombomodulin on their surface, which converts procoagulant thrombin to an anticoagulant activator of protein C, which in turn inactivates several components of the coagulation cascade (Busse and Fleming 2006). Furthermore, such endothelial cells express proteoglycans on their surfaces that increase the inhibitory activity of antithrombin-III towards thrombin (Busse and Fleming 2006). More recently, it was discovered that quiescent endothelial cells also express tissue factor pathway inhibitors (TFPI), which inhibit the coagulation cascade (Pober and Sessa 2007).

Non-activated endothelium does not interact with leukocytes. Such endothelial cells do not express adhesion molecules such as E-selectin and vascular cell adhesion molecule-1 (VCAM-1) and, at least to a large extent, also intercellular adhesion molecule-1 (ICAM-1) on their surface (Ley and Reutershan 2006). Furthermore, they sequester chemokines, known to attract leukocytes to the endothelium, in their Weibel-Palade bodies (Middleton et al. 1997). Also basal NO production by non-activated endothelium seems to play a role in the regulation of leukocyte-endothelium interaction by inhibiting leukocyte activation and by counteracting the expression of proinflammatory genes in endothelial cells (De Caterina et al. 1995).

4.2.2
Acutely Inflamed Endothelium

In acute inflammation two different responses of the endothelium are evident. A fast activation, which is independent of new gene expression and a more delayed effect, which requires changes in gene expression and protein synthesis. Acute inflammation is a rapid response initiated by infection with pathogens or by tissue damage, which, if successful, will result in the eradication and elimination of the eliciting stimulus and the restoration of normal tissue architecture or the formation of scar tissue. The process of acute inflammation is characterized by an increase in local blood flow (resulting in red colour and warmth of the inflamed area), a localized leakage of fluid into the affected tissue (resulting in swelling) and recruitment of leukocytes to the site of inflammation (which by releasing various mediators cause pain).

The rapid response of endothelial cells in acute inflammation is generally triggered by mediators such as histamine, which bind to receptors coupled to Gq-proteins. Activation of such Gq proteins in turn leads to activation of phospholipase C-γ (PLC-γ) that results in the formation of inositol-1,4,5-triphosphate (IP3). IP3 subsequently leads to elevation of cytosolic Ca^{2+} by releasing Ca^{2+} from the endoplasmic reticulum. This Ca^{2+} influx into the cytosol of endothelial cells results in their contraction, in the appearance of gaps between adjacent endothelial cells and thus in the leakage of plasma and plasma proteins from the blood vessels into the surrounding tissue (De Caterina et al. 1995; Pober and Cotran 1990). The rise in intracellular Ca^{2+} also results in the expression of P-selectin and platelet activating factor (PAF), which subsequently cause tethering and extravasation of leukocytes (Birch et al. 1992; Lorant et al. 1991; Prescott et al. 1984).

The classical mediators of the more delayed reaction of endothelial cells in the setting of acute inflammation are the inflammatory cytokines tumour necrosis factor-α (TNF-α) and interleukin-1 (IL-1), which are both produced by activated leukocytes (Pober and Cotran 1990). After binding to their respective receptors, both cytokines initiate a cascade of intracellular signaling events finally resulting in the activation of particular genes responsible for the expression of a pro-adhesive and prothrombotic endothelial cell phenotype. TNF-α binds to its membrane receptor, TNF receptor-1 (TNFR-1). This binding recruits TNFR-associated via death domain protein (TRADD) to the cytoplasmic death domain of the receptor, which in turn recruits receptor interacting protein-1 (RIP-1) and TNFR-associated factor-2 (TRAF-2) to the complex. This entire complex then leads to activation of the transcription factor activator protein-1 (AP-1) and the dissociation of inhibitor of κB (IκB) from the transcription factor nuclear factor-κB (NF-κB); these changes lead to translocation of AP-1 and NF-κB into the nucleus of the activated cell where both bind to respective binding sequences on AP-1 and NF-κB responsive genes. IL-1 binds to its surface receptor IL-1 receptor (IL-1R), which initiates signaling through myeloid differentiation response gene 88 (MyD88), Toll/IlL-1 receptor accessory protein (TRIAP), IL-1R associated kinase-1 (IRAK-1) and IRAK-4 and TRAF-6. TRAF-6, similar to TRAF-2, causes translocation of AP-1 and NF-κB to the nucleus, which then results in increased transcription of specific genes (Pober and Sessa 2007). These genes include the genes for chemokines such as IL-8 and adhesion molecules such as E-selectin, ICAM-1 and VCAM-1 (Ley and Reutershan 2006). Increased expression of these proteins results in enhanced leukocyte migration to the inflamed area, and subsequently to increased leukocyte adhesion to the endothelium and extravasation into the inflamed tissue. TNF-α and IL-1 also induce leakage of fluid and plasma proteins into the affected tissue in an NF-κB-dependent manner. The precise mechanism, however, remains to be elucidated (Clark et al. 2007; Petrache et al. 2003; Pober et al. 1987). In addition, the genes for TF also responsive to NF-κB and thus to TNF-α and IL-1. TNF-α and IL-1 also increase the levels of plasminogen activator inhibitor-1 (PAI-1) produced by endothelial cells (Dellas and Loskutoff 2005). Thus inflammatory activation of endothelial cells through these mediators results in a prothrombotic and antifibrinolytic phenotype of the affected endothelial cells (Nawroth and Stern 1986).

4.2.3
Chronically Inflamed Endothelium

Chronic inflammation develops if the acute inflammatory response fails to eliminate the original stimulus. The chronic inflammatory response is characterized by the activation of special effector cells of the immune system. The discovery that endothelial cells express, on their surface, not only MHC class I molecules but also MHC class II molecules provided indirect evidence that endothelial cells might present antigen to T-cells (Hancock et al. 1982; Hart et al. 1981). In addition, it has been shown that, in a positive feedback loop, endothelial cells respond to interferon-γ (IFN-γ) which is produced by T helper-1 (T_H1) cells with the sustained expression of E-selectin which favours the recruitment of such T_H1 cells (Austrup et al. 1997; Doukas and Pober 1990). On the other hand, endothelial cells respond to IL-4 and IL-13, which are secreted by T_H2 cells, with the expression of eotaxin and VCAM-1 on their surface which in turn favour the local recruitment of T_H2 to these sites (Chaplin 2002).

Chronic inflammation is also associated with angiogenesis. The development of new blood vessels and thus increased blood flow is needed for the survival of inflammatory cells in such chronically inflamed tissues. This newly vascularized tissue is typical for chronic inflammatory pathologies such as the pannus in rheumatoid arthritis or the atheroma in atherosclerosis. The best characterized angiogenic factors involved in this process are vascular endothelial growth factor-A (VEGF-A), which binds to VEGF receptor-1 (VEGFR-1) and VEGFR-2, fibroblast growth factor-2 (FGF-2), which binds to FGF receptor-1 (FGFR-1) and angiopoietin-1 (Ang-1) and Ang-2, which signal through tyrosine kinase receptor-2 (TIE-2). All these receptor tyrosine kinases multimerize in response to ligand binding, and crossphosphorylate tyrosine residues in the other receptors of the complex formed by multimerization. In endothelial cells, the RAS-extracellular-signal regulated kinase-1 (ERK1)/ERK2 pathway, the phosphoinositide 3-kinase (PI3K) pathway and the Ca^{2+}-PLCγ pathway are activated by angiogenic growth factors (Shibuya and Claesson-Welsh 2006). The involvement of the latter pathway in VEGF-A signaling also explains vascular leakage caused by VEGF-A (Dvorak 2002). All three pathways initiate three key processes in angiogenesis, namely endothelial cell survival, proliferation and migration. VEGF-A binding to VEGFR-2 and FGF-2 binding to FGFR-1 activate all three pathways and thus stimulate survival, proliferation and migration of endothelial cells. In contrast, Ang-1 is thought to activate exclusively the PI3K pathway through binding to TIE-2 and to stabilize newly formed blood vessels, whereas Ang-2 destabilizes existing blood vessels (Pfaff et al. 2006). TNF-α, by binding to its receptor TNFR-2, also has pro-angiogenic properties (Zhang et al. 2003). In addition, chemokines are also involved in the regulation of angiogenesis. IL-8 induces angiogenesis whereas CXCL10 inhibits this process (Coughlin et al. 1998; Strieter 2005).

4.2.4
Overlap Between Acute and Chronic Inflammation

Overlap between events characteristic for either one of these inflammatory responses occur because particular mediators are differentially involved in the modulation of both processes. As mentioned above, TNF-α (by binding to TNFR-1) initiates events characteristic for acute inflammation; however, when TNF-α signals through TNFR-2 it stimulates angiogenesis, a process typical for chronic inflammation. VEGF-A is a potent angiogenic factor, but by causing vascular leakage it also supports extravasation of leukocytes and it enhances the effects of TNF-α in acute inflammation such as upregulation of adhesion molecules and TF (Clauss et al. 1990). A similar effect has been described for Ang-2 (Fiedler et al. 2006). In addition, Ang-2 promotes oxidant-induced injury and inflammation whereas Ang-1 counteracts the proinflammatory effects by inhibiting VEGF-A-induced vascular leakage and TF expression (Bhandari et al. 2006; Kim et al. 2002; Thurston et al. 2000). Thus, it becomes more and more evident that certain mediators play a key role in the regulation of acute as well as chronic inflammation thereby blurring the strict theoretical separation between the two events.

4.3
Endothelial Dysfunction

4.3.1
Endothelial Dysfunction: Definition

The term endothelial dysfunction was first used when it was discovered that the presence of uninjured endothelium is required for acetylcholine-induced smooth muscle cell relaxation. It had been observed that this endothelium dependent relaxation was impaired in hypertensive and hypercholesteremic animals as well as in coronary arteries in humans suffering from atherosclerosis (Furchgott and Zawadzki 1980; Ibengwe and Suzuki 1986; Ludmer et al. 1986; Verbeuren et al. 1986; Winquist et al. 1984). NO was then identified as the so-called endothelium derived relaxing factor (EDRF), responsible for endothelium dependent relaxation of the vessel wall (Palmer et al. 1987). NO also inhibits platelet aggregation, neutrophil adhesion to the endothelium and smooth muscle cell proliferation (Garg and Hassid 1989; Radomski et al. 1987). Since these discoveries, endothelial dysfunction has been suggested to be a key event in the initiation, progression and development of atherosclerosis (Suwaidi et al. 2000). In the following years evidence has accumulated supporting the notion that endothelial dysfunction is not only associated with atherosclerosis but also with physiological processes and pathologies such as aging, heart and renal failure, obesity, type I and type II diabetes, glucose intolerance, insulin resistance, inflammation, infections, sepsis, trauma, smoking etc. (Félétou and Vanhoutte 2006).

The underlying cause for endothelial dysfunction seems to be multifactorial. However evidence suggests that by decreasing bioavailability of NO in the vascular compartment increased production of reactive oxygen species (ROS) and oxidative stress are critically involved in the development of endothelial dysfunction.

4.3.2
L-Arginine, NO and Cyclic AMP as Modulators of Vascular Tone

The potent vasodilator NO is generated from L-arginine and O_2 by endothelial NO synthase (eNOS) when healthy endothelial cells are activated by mediators such as acetylcholine, bradykinin or adenosine triphosphate (ATP), or when these cells are exposed to shear stress or stretch or by inducible NOS (iNOS) by endothelial cells, macrophages or vascular smooth muscle cells under inflammatory conditions (Fleming and Busse 2003; Sodha et al. 2009). NO then diffuses into the vessel wall and in smooth muscle cells, activates soluble guanylate cyclase (sGC). This enzyme will then synthesize cyclic guanosine monophosphate (cGMP) which, by activating cGMP-dependent kinase I (cGK-I), will result in an increased open probability of K^+-channels, and thus in hyperpolarization of the affected smooth muscle cells. Moreover, cGK-I also phosphorylates the IP3-receptor-associated G-kinase substrate (IRAG) and thus inhibits Ca^{2+} release and contraction of the smooth muscle cells (Fleming and Busse 2003). In addition to its vasorelaxant properties, eNOS also inhibits platelet aggregation and leukocyte adhesion to the endothelium, whereas iNOS acts in a proinflammatory manner (Naseem 2005; Sodha et al. 2009).

4.3.3
Oxidative Stress as the Underlying Mechanism of Endothelial Dysfunction

As mentioned above, oxidative stress is generally seen as the underlying mechanism, which induces endothelial dysfunction (Griendling and Fitzgerald 2003a, b). Reactive oxygen species such as NO, $O_2^{-\bullet}$, $^\bullet OH$, H_2O_2 or $ONOO^{-\bullet}$ are produced by vascular cells in response to inflammation or injury. Enzymes such as cytochrome p450 monooxygenases, NADPH oxidase, NO synthases, and xanthine oxidase can generate $O_2^{-\bullet}$, which can then be reduced to H_2O_2 by superoxide dismutase (SOD), which subsequently can be converted to H_2O and O_2 by catalase or glutathione peroxidase. H_2O_2 through the Fenton- or the Haber-Weiss reactions, can generate $^\bullet OH$ which causes peroxidation of lipids and results in severe cell damage. $O_2^{-\bullet}$ can react with NO, thereby reducing the amount of this vasodilator, to form $ONOO^{-\bullet}$ another potent oxidant, which has been shown to cause oxidative damage to lipids, proteins and DNA (Zou et al. 2004).

ROS have been shown to impair endothelium-dependent vasorelaxation not only by reducing the level of available NO but also by inhibiting its target GC and the production of PGI2 (Griendling and Fitzgerald 2003a; Münzel et al. 2005; Price et al. 2000). Furthermore, ROS increases the expression of adhesion molecules and chemokines and activates matrixmetalloproteinases (MMPs) (Griendling and Fitzgerald 2003a). As these biomolecules are critically involved in the modulation of endothelial activation and injury, these findings demonstrate that the border between endothelial activation, described above, and endothelial injury may be heuristically useful but has to be considered to be somewhat artificial.

4.4
Endothelial Cell Death

Endothelial cells can undergo two forms of cell death, namely necrosis and apoptosis. Whereas necrosis is often accompanied by inflammation and is characterized by cellular and nuclear swelling, the latter process is associated with loss of membrane polarity, membrane vesiculation, nuclear condensation and fragmentation. Apoptotic cells are often taken up by phagocytic cells and usually, in contrast to necrotic cells, do not elicit an inflammatory response (Kerr 2002; Majno and Joris 1995; Saraste and Pulkki 2000).

When endothelial cells undergo apoptosis, they create a procoagulatory environment. Under apoptosis they shed membrane vesicles with prothrombotic properties into the circulation (Bombeli et al. 1997; Mallat et al. 2000). Furthermore, intracellular TF is also released into the blood stream (Greeno et al. 1996). Extensive cell death results in detachment of the endothelial layer from the vascular wall thereby exposing subendothelial basement membrane to the blood stream. Platelets will bind to this exposed surface and coagulation will be activated at such sites of extensive endothelial cell death (Walker et al. 1983). Endothelial cell necrosis will result in inflammatory activation of the surrounding endothelium as described above.

4.5
Endothelial Cell Injury in Cardiac Surgery

Despite considerable progress in medical research in recent years, cardiovascular disease is the leading cause of morbidity and mortality in the Western world. Besides pharmacotherapy and catheter-based interventions using new generations of stents, cardiac surgical techniques such as coronary artery bypass grafting remain an important therapeutic option in the treatment of cardiovascular disease. Most of cardiac surgical procedures, however, require a motionless operative field. Cardioplegic arrest, used to achieve these conditions, despite ongoing intensive research in this area, is associated with impairment of vasomotor function and vascular permeabilty in the coronary circulation. These events most likely result from endothelial injury caused by ischemia and subsequent reperfusion. The development of vascular dysfunction after cardioplegia is multifactorial. It involves inflammatory activation of the endothelium, impaired vasomotor response characteristic for endothelial dysfunction and finally endothelial cell death.

4.5.1
Inflammatory Activation of the Endothelium During Cardioplegia

During ischemia-reperfusion, the heart generates a host of inflammatory cytokines such as TNF-α, IL-1, IL-6, IL-8, and IL-18 (Chandrasekar et al. 1999; Deten et al. 2003; Matsumori et al. 1999; Pomerantz et al. 2001; Sawa et al. 1998; te Velthuis et al. 1995). As outlined above, these inflammatory cytokines activate endothelial cells. Such activation leads to increased expression of adhesion molecules such as E-selectin, ICAM-1 and VCAM-1 (Ley and Reutershan 2006). Increased expression of these proteins results in enhanced leukocyte migration and adhesion to the inflamed endothelium and to subsequent extravasation of leukocytes to the inflamed tissue. TNF-α and IL-1 also induce leakage of fluid and plasma proteins into the affected tissue and increase the levels of TF and PAI-1 produced by endothelial cells (Clark et al. 2007; Dellas and Loskutoff 2005; Nawroth and Stern 1986; Petrache et al. 2003; Pober et al. 1987). Thus, inflammatory activation of endothelial cells through ischemia-reperfusion results in a proadhesive, prothrombotic, and antifibrinolytic phenotype of the affected endothelial cells.

Increasing evidence suggests that VEGF is also involved in vascular changes and endothelial impairment in response to ischemia-reperfusion. Besides its angiogenic properties, VEGF is a potent vasodilator and induces vascular permeability. The expression of VEGF and its receptor VEGFR-1 are increased after reperfusion resulting in enhanced coronary vasorelaxation and vascular leakage (Tofukuji et al. 1998).

4.5.2
Endothelial Dysfunction and Cardiac Surgery

As described above the key feature of endothelial dysfunction is impaired endothelium dependent NO-induced vasorelaxation. After cardioplegic arrest, the expression of the antiinflammatory NOS, namely eNOS, in the affected tissue is reduced leading locally to a diminished production of NO and subsequently to impaired vasorelaxation (Engelman et al. 1995). The local vasorelaxation is further affected by the reduction of NO through its interaction with free radicals generated in response to ischemia-reperfusion (Becker et al. 2000; Guzik et al. 2003).

In contrast to eNOS, increased levels of iNOS are found in the heart after cardioplegic arrest. Whereas low concentrations of NO generated by eNOS, besides its vasorelaxant properties, inhibit leukocyte adhesion, the production of inflammatory cytokines and the agregation of platelets, large amounts of NO generated by iNOS are toxic and proinflammatory. This results from $O_2^{-\bullet}$ released under inflammatory conditions from various cells which in turn reacts with NO to form the potent oxidant $ONOO^{-\bullet}$. $ONOO^{-\bullet}$ has been shown to cause oxidative damage to lipids, proteins and DNA (Zou et al. 2004). It should be pointed out that a vicious inflammatory circle exists under these conditions: Inflammatory cytokines such as TNF-α, IL-1, IL-6, and IL-8 are upregulated by ischemia-reperfusion and subsequently induce proinflammatory iNOS which then in turn leads to increased production of these cytokines (Aktan 2004; Chandrasekar et al. 1999; Deten et al. 2003; Kleinert et al. 2004; Matsumori et al. 1999; Sawa et al. 1998; te Velthuis et al. 1995).

4.5.3
Endothelial Cell Apoptosis and Cardiac Surgery

Endothelial cell apoptosis in the coronary circulation as a consequence of cardiac surgery cannot reliably be measured in the patient. It is believed, however, that this ultimate form of endothelial injury occurs in the setting of cardiac surgery. This notion is supported by indirect evidence. It was shown that serum collected from patients after cornary artery bypass grafting induced apoptosis in cultured endothelial cells, whereas serum from patients undergoing surgical procedures other than cardiac surgery did not show this activity (Birdi et al. 1997).

4.6
Summary

Within the last 2–3 decades the notion that endothelium represents only a passive barrier between the blood and the surrounding tissue has been seriously challenged. Numerous additional roles for the endothelium have been described. Endothelial cells play a critical and essential role in the regulation of vascular tone, they control transendothelial movement of fluid, solutes and macromolecules, they modulate inflammation and leukocyte adhesion, promotion and inhibition of growth of new blood vessels and they regulate blood fluidity and platelet aggregation, fibrinolysis and coagulation. Through this multitude of physiological and pathophysiological functions it is evident that endothelial injury might have serious consequences for homeostasis and might impact on the pathogenesis of various diseases. Endothelial cells can respond to injury with "endothelial activation" and/or "endothelial dysfunction". Whereas the former is characterized by a switch of the endothelium from a antiadhesive, antithrombotic phenotype to a proadhesive, prothrombotic phenoytpe, the main characteristic of the latter is impaired NO-production.

Pharmacotherapy and catheter-based interventions provide increasingly successful treatment for patients suffering from cardiovascular disease. Besides these therapies, cardiac surgical techniques such as coronary artery bypass grafting remain an important therapeutic option in the treatment of these patients. In most of these surgical procedures cardioplegic arrest is used to create a motionless operative field. Despite ongoing intensive research in this area, cardioplegic arrest and ischemia reperfusion are associated with impairment of vasomotor function and vascular permeabilty of the affected vasculature. The development of these vascular defects after cardioplegia is a multifactorial process involving inflammatory activation of the endothelium, endothelial dysfunction and finally endothelial cell death.

References

Aird WC (2003) The role of the endothelium in severe sepsis and multiple organ dysfunction syndrome. Blood 101: 3765–3777

Aktan F (2004) iNOS-mediated nitric oxide production and its regulation. Life Sci 75: 639–653

Austrup F, Vestweber D, Borges E, Löhning M, Bräuer R, Herz U, Renz H, Hallmann R, Scheffold A, Radbruch A, Hamann A (1997) P- and E-selectin mediate recruitment of T-helper-1 but not T-helper-2 cells into inflamed tissues. Nature 385: 81–83

Becker BF, Kupatt C, Massoudy P, Zahler S (2000) Reactive oxygen species and nitric oxide in myocardial ischemia and reperfusion. Z Kardiol 89 Suppl 9: IX/88–91

Bhandari V, Choo-Wing R, Lee CG, Zhu Z, Nedrelow JH, Chupp GL, Zhang X, Matthay MA, Ware LB, Homer RJ, Lee PJ, Geick A, de Fougerolles AR, Elias JA (2006) Hyperoxia causes angiopoietin 2-mediated acute lung injury and necrotic cell death. Nat Med 12: 1286–1293

Birch KA, Pober JS, Zavoico GB, Means AR, Ewenstein BM (1992) Calcium/calmodulin transduces thrombin-stimulated secretion: studies in intact and minimally permeabilized human umbilical vein endothelial cells. J Cell Biol 118: 1501–1510

Birdi I, Angelini GD, Bryan AJ (1997) Biochemical markers of myocardial injury during cardiac operations. Ann Thorac Surg 63: 879–884

Bombeli T, Karsan A, Tait JF, Harlan JM (1997) Apoptotic vascular endothelial cells become procoagulant. Blood 89: 2429–2442

Busse R, Fleming I (2006) Vascular endothelium and blood flow. Handb Exp Pharmacol 176: 43–78

Chandrasekar B, Mitchell DH, Colston JT, Freeman GL (1999) Regulation of CCAAT/Enhancer binding protein, interleukin-6, interleukin-6 receptor, and gp130 expression during myocardial ischemia/reperfusion. Circulation 99: 427–433

Chaplin DD (2002) Cell cooperation in development of eosinophil-predominant inflammation in airways. Immunol Res 26: 55–62

Clark PR, Manes TD, Pober JS, Kluger MS. (2007) Increased ICAM-1 expression causes endothelial cell leakiness, cytoskeletal reorganization and junctional alterations. J Invest Dermatol 127: 762–774

Clauss M, Gerlach M, Gerlach H, Brett J, Wang F, Familletti PC, Pan YC, Olander JV, Connolly DT, Stern D (1990) Vascular permeability factor: a tumor-derived polypeptide that induces endothelial cell and monocyte procoagulant activity, and promotes monocyte migration. J Exp Med 172: 1535–1545

Cotran RS, Pober JS (1989) Effects of cytokines on vascular endothelium: their role in vascular and immune injury. Kidney Int 35: 969–975

Coughlin CM, Salhany KE, Gee MS, LaTemple DC, Kotenko S, Ma X, Gri G, Wysocka M, Kim JE, Liu L, Liao F, Farber JM, Pestka S, Trinchieri G, Lee WM (1998) Tumor cell responses to IFNgamma affect tumorigenicity and response to IL-12 therapy and antiangiogenesis. Immunity 9: 25–34

De Caterina R, Libby P, Peng HB, Thannickal VJ, Rajavashisth TB, Gimbrone MA Jr, Shin WS, Liao JK (1995) Nitric oxide decreases cytokine-induced endothelial activation. Nitric oxide selectively reduces endothelial expression of adhesion molecules and proinflammatory cytokines. J Clin Invest 96: 60–68

Dellas C, Loskutoff DJ (2005) Historical analysis of PAI-1 from its discovery to its potential role in cell motility and disease. Thromb Haemost 93: 631–640

Deten A, Volz HC, Holzl A, Briest W, Zimmer HG (2003) Effect of propranolol on cardiac cytokine expression after myocardial infarction in rats. Mol Cell Biochem 251: 127–137

Doukas J, Pober JS (1990) IFN-gamma enhances endothelial activation induced by tumor necrosis factor but not IL-1. J Immunol 145: 1727–1733

Dvorak HF (2002) Vascular permeability factor/vascular endothelial growth factor: a critical cytokine in tumor angiogenesis and a potential target for diagnosis and therapy. J Clin Oncol 20: 4368–4380

Engelman DT, Watanabe M, Engelman RM, Rousou JA, Flack JE 3rd, Deaton DW, Das DK (1995) Constitutive nitric oxide release is impaired after ischemia and reperfusion. J Thorac Cardiovasc Surg 110:1047–1053

Félétou M, Vanhoutte PM (2006) Endothelial dysfunction: a multifaceted disorder (The Wiggers Award Lecture). Am J Physiol Heart Circ Physiol 291: H985–H1002

Fiedler U, Reiss Y, Scharpfenecker M, Grunow V, Koidl S, Thurston G, Gale NW, Witzenrath M, Rosseau S, Suttorp N, Sobke A, Herrmann M, Preissner KT, Vajkoczy P, Augustin HG (2006) Angiopoietin-2 sensitizes endothelial cells to TNF-alpha and has a crucial role in the induction of inflammation. Nat Med 12: 235–239

Fleming I, Busse R (2003) Molecular mechanisms involved in the regulation of the endothelial nitric oxide synthase. Am J Physiol Regul Integr Comp Physiol 284: R1–R12

Furchgott RF, Zawadzki JV. The obligatory role of endothelial cells in the relaxation of arterial smooth muscle by acetylcholine (1980) Nature 288: 373–376

Garg UC, Hassid A (1989) Nitric oxide-generating vasodilators and 8-bromo-cyclic guanosine monophosphate inhibit mitogenesis and proliferation of cultured rat vascular smooth muscle cells. J Clin Invest 83: 1774–1777

Greeno EW, Bach RR, Moldow CF (1996) Apoptosis is associated with increased cell surface tissue factor procoagulant activity. Lab Invest 75: 281–289

Griendling KK, FitzGerald GA (2003a) Oxidative stress and cardiovascular injury: Part I: basic mechanisms and in vivo monitoring of ROS. Circulation 108: 1912–1916

Griendling KK, FitzGerald GA (2003b) Oxidative stress and cardiovascular injury: Part II: animal and human studies. Circulation 108: 2034–2040

Guzik TJ, Korbut R, Adamek-Guzik T (2003) Nitric oxide and superoxide in inflammation and immune regulation. J Physiol Pharmacol 54: 469–487

Hancock WW, Kraft N, Atkins RC (1982) The immunohistochemical demonstration of major histocompatibility antigens in the human kidney using monoclonal antibodies. Pathology 14: 409–414

Hart DN, Fuggle SV, Williams KA, Fabre JW, Ting A, Morris PJ (1981) Localization of HLA-ABC and DR antigens in human kidney. Transplantation 31: 428–433

Huttner I, Gabbiani G (1982) Vascular endothelium: recent advances and unanswered questions. Lab Invest 47: 409–411

Ibengwe JK, Suzuki H (1986) Changes in mechanical responses of vascular smooth muscles to acetylcholine, noradrenaline and high-potassium solution in hypercholesterolemic rabbits. Br J Pharmacol 87: 395–402

Joris I, Cuénoud HF, Doern GV, Underwood JM, Majno G (1990) Capillary leakage in inflammation. A study by vascular labeling. Am J Pathol 137: 1353–1363

Kerr JF (2002) History of the events leading to the formulation of the apoptosis concept. Toxicology 181–182: 471–474

Kim I, Oh JL, Ryu YS, So JN, Sessa WC, Walsh K, Koh GY (2002) Angiopoietin-1 negatively regulates expression and activity of tissue factor in endothelial cells. FASEB J 16: 126–128

Kleinert H, Pautz A, Linker K, Schwarz PM (2004) Regulation of the expression of inducible nitric oxide synthase. Eur J Pharmacol 500: 255–266

Ley K, Reutershan J (2006) Leucocyte-endothelial interactions in health and disease. Handb Exp Pharmacol 176: 97–133

Lorant DE, Patel KD, McIntyre TM, McEver RP, Prescott SM, Zimmerman GA (1991) Coexpression of GMP-140 and PAF by endothelium stimulated by histamine or thrombin: a juxtacrine system for adhesion and activation of neutrophils. J Cell Biol 115: 223–234

Ludmer PL, Selwyn AP, Shook TL, Wayne RR, Mudge GH, Alexander RW, Ganz P (1986) Paradoxical vasoconstriction induced by acetylcholine in atherosclerotic coronary arteries. N Engl J Med 315: 1046–1051

Majno G, Joris I (1995) Apoptosis, oncosis, and necrosis. An overview of cell death. Am J Pathol 146: 3–15

Mallat Z, Benamer H, Hugel B, Benessiano J, Steg PG, Freyssinet JM, Tedgui A (2000) Elevated levels of shed membrane microparticles with procoagulant potential in the peripheral circulating blood of patients with acute coronary syndromes. Circulation 101: 841–843

Matsumori A, Igata H, Ono K, Iwasaki A, Miyamoto T, Nishio R, Sasayama S (1999) High doses of digitalis increase the myocardial production of proinflammatory cytokines and worsen myocardial injury in viral myocarditis: a possible mechanism of digitalis toxicity. Jpn Circ J 63: 934–940

Middleton J, Neil S, Wintle J, Clark-Lewis I, Moore H, Lam C, Auer M, Hub E, Rot A (1997) Transcytosis and surface presentation of IL-8 by venular endothelial cells. Cell 91: 385–395

Münzel T, Daiber A, Ullrich V, Mülsch A (2005) Vascular consequences of endothelial nitric oxide synthase uncoupling for the activity and expression of the soluble guanylyl cyclase and the cGMP-dependent protein kinase. Arterioscler Thromb Vasc Biol 25: 1551–1557

Münzel T, Sinning C, Post F, Warnholtz A, Schulz E (2008) Pathophysiology, diagnosis and prognostic implications of endothelial dysfunction. Ann Med 40: 180–196

Naseem KM (2005) The role of nitric oxide in cardiovascular diseases. Mol Aspects Med 26: 33–65

Nawroth PP, Stern DM (1986) Modulation of endothelial cell hemostatic properties by tumor necrosis factor. J Exp Med 163: 740–745

Palmer RM, Ferrige AG, Moncada S (1987) Nitric oxide release accounts for the biological activity of endothelium-derived relaxing factor. Nature 327: 524–526

Panza JA, Quyyumi AA, Brush JE Jr, Epstein SE (1990) Abnormal endothelium-dependent vascular relaxation in patients with essential hypertension. N Engl J Med 323: 22–27

Petrache I, Birukova A, Ramirez SI, Garcia JG, Verin AD (2003) The role of the microtubules in tumor necrosis factor-alpha-induced endothelial cell permeability. Am J Respir Cell Mol Biol 28: 574–581

Pfaff D, Fiedler U, Augustin HG (2006) Emerging roles of the Angiopoietin-Tie and the ephrin-Eph systems as regulators of cell trafficking. J Leukoc Biol 80: 719–726

Pober JS, Lapierre LA, Stolpen AH, Brock TA, Springer TA, Fiers W, Bevilacqua MP, Mendrick DL, Gimbrone MA Jr (1987) Activation of cultured human endothelial cells by recombinant lymphotoxin: comparison with tumor necrosis factor and interleukin 1 species. J Immunol 138: 3319–3324

Pober JS, Cotran RS (1990) The role of endothelial cells in inflammation. Transplantation 50: 537–544

Pober JS, Sessa WC (2007) Evolving functions of endothelial cells in inflammation. Nat Rev Immunol 7: 803–815

Pomerantz BJ, Reznikov LL, Harken AH, Dinarello CA (2001) Inhibition of caspase 1 reduces human myocardial ischemic dysfunction via inhibition of IL-18 and IL-1beta. Proc Natl Acad Sci U S A 98: 2871–2876

Prescott SM, Zimmerman GA, McIntyre TM (1984) Human endothelial cells in culture produce platelet-activating factor (1-alkyl-2-acetyl-sn-glycero-3-phosphocholine) when stimulated with thrombin. Proc Natl Acad Sci USA 81: 3534–3538

Price DT, Vita JA, Keaney JF Jr (2000) Redox control of vascular nitric oxide bioavailability. Antioxid Redox Signal 2: 919–935

Radomski MW, Palmer RM, Moncada S (1987) The anti-aggregating properties of vascular endothelium: interactions between prostacyclin and nitric oxide. Br J Pharmacol 92: 639–646

Saraste A, Pulkki K (2000) Morphologic and biochemical hallmarks of apoptosis. Cardiovasc Res 45: 528–537

Sawa Y, Ichikawa H, Kagisaki K, Ohata T, Matsuda H (1998) Interleukin-6 derived from hypoxic myocytes promotes neutrophil-mediated reperfusion injury in myocardium. J Thorac Cardiovasc Surg 116: 511–517

Sessa WC (2004) eNOS at a glance. J Cell Sci 117: 2427–2429

Shibuya M, Claesson-Welsh L (2006) Signal transduction by VEGF receptors in regulation of angiogenesis and lymphangiogenesis. Exp Cell Res 312: 549–560

Sodha NR, Clements RT, Sellke FW (2009) Vascular changes after cardiac surgery: role of NOS, COX, kinases, and growth factors. Front Biosci 14: 689–698

Strieter RM (2005) Masters of angiogenesis. Nat Med 11: 925–927

Suwaidi JA, Hamasaki S, Higano ST, Nishimura RA, Holmes DR Jr, Lerman A (2000) Long-term follow-up of patients with mild coronary artery disease and endothelial dysfunction. Circulation 101: 948–954

te Velthuis H, Jansen PG, Oudemans-van Straaten HM, Sturk A, Eijsman L, Wildevuur CR (1995) Myocardial performance in elderly patients after cardiopulmonary bypass is suppressed by tumor necrosis factor. J Thorac Cardiovasc Surg 110: 1663–1669

Thurston G, Rudge JS, Ioffe E, Zhou H, Ross L, Croll SD, Glazer N, Holash J, McDonald DM, Yancopoulos GD (2000) Angiopoietin-1 protects the adult vasculature against plasma leakage. Nat Med 6: 460–463

Tofukuji M, Metais C, Li J, Franklin A, Simons M, Sellke FW (1998) Myocardial VEGF expression after cardiopulmonary bypass and cardioplegia. Circulation 98(19 Suppl): II242–II246

Verbeuren TJ, Jordaens FH, Zonnekeyn LL, Van Hove CE, Coene MC, Herman AG (1986) Effect of hypercholesterolemia on vascular reactivity in the rabbit. I. Endothelium-dependent and endothelium-independent contractions and relaxations in isolated arteries of control and hypercholesterolemic rabbits. Circ Res 58: 552–564

Walker LN, Ramsay MM, Bowyer DE (1983) Endothelial healing following defined injury to rabbit aorta. Depth of injury and mode of repair. Atherosclerosis 47: 123–130

Winquist RJ, Bunting PB, Baskin EP, Wallace AA (1984) Decreased endothelium-dependent relaxation in New Zealand genetic hypertensive rats. J Hypertens 2: 541–545

Zhang R, Xu Y, Ekman N, Wu Z, Wu J, Alitalo K, Min W (2003) Etk/Bmx transactivates vascular endothelial growth factor 2 and recruits phosphatidylinositol 3-kinase to mediate the tumor necrosis factor-induced angiogenic pathway. J Biol Chem 278: 51267–51276

Zou MH, Cohen R, Ullrich V (2004) Peroxynitrite and vascular endothelial dysfunction in diabetes mellitus. Endothelium 11: 89–97

Part III
Special Focus

Intraoperative Protection of the Myocardium: Effects of Age and Gender

5

James D. McCully and Sidney Levitsky

5.1
Background

5.1.1
Myocardial Protection in the Aged

Myocardial infarction is the leading cause of death worldwide and affects both men and women. Each year more than 5.3 million patients in the United States present to emergency departments with chest pain and related symptoms and ultimately, more than 1.4 million individuals are hospitalized and require either interventional cardiologic procedures and/or coronary artery bypass surgery (CABG) (Nashef et al. 1999; Ferguson et al. 2002; Society of Thoracic Surgeons National Database to 2004).

In the U.S.A. there has been a dramatic shift in aging. In 1960, 9.2% of the population was over 65 years of age and it is projected that the percentage of those over 65 years of age will increase by 21.6% to 86.7 million by 2050 (Guralnik and Fitzsimmons 1986; U.S. Census Bureau, 2007, http://www.census.gov/). The percentage of those over 85 years of age, the "oldest old"; is also projected to increases form 2.7 million in 1987 to 16 million by 2030 and to 20 million by 2050 (Wenger et al. 1987; U.S. Census Bureau, 2007, http://www.census.gov/). This group is now the fastest growing segment in the U.S.A. As a consequence of these demographic changes, there has been an increase in cardiac surgical procedures performed on the elderly, where age over 70 years is an incremental risk factor (Edmunds et al. 1988; Fremes et al. 1989; Gersh et al. 1993).

Studies investigating the efficacy of coronary artery bypass surgery in the elderly have shown that elderly patients have more co-morbidities and more acute presentations

---

J.D. McCully (✉)
Division of Cardiothoracic Surgery, Beth Israel Deaconess Medical Center, Harvard Medical School, 33 Brookline Avenue, DA-0734, Boston, MA 02115, USA
e-mail: james_mccully@hms.harvard.edu

S. Levitsky
Division of Cardiothoracic Surgery, Beth Israel Deaconess Medical Center, Harvard Medical School, 110 Francis Street, Suite 2A, Boston, MA 02115, USA
e-mail: slevitsk@bidmc.harvard.edu

and higher in hospital mortality than younger patients (Christenson et al. 1994; Likosky et al. 2008). It has also been shown that operative mortality is increased with age and operative complexity. Bridges et al. (2003) have reported that in patients undergoing CABG, operative mortality was 11.8% for patients aged greater than 90 years as compared to 2.8% for those aged 50–79 years. In those patients undergoing CABG and valve replacement/repair operative mortality was increased to 12.0% for those aged greater than 90 years compared to 7.6% for those aged 50–79 years. Median survival following CABG in patients aged ≥85 years was greater than 5 years in all these studies and quality of life outcome studies have shown no observable statistical differences as compared to normative data for individuals aged 75 years or older (Ullery et al. 2008). In total, these studies show that CABG in the elderly (>85 years of age) is justified and has an acceptable early mortality and long-term survival.

5.1.2
Myocardial Ischemia/Reperfusion Injury

The initiation of myocardial infarction involves an ischemic episode which, by itself, may induce reversible and (but not necessarily) irreversible (necrosis) cellular injury. To limit myocardial injury following ischemia, reperfusion must be re-instated as soon as is feasible. The individual or collaborate contributions of ischemia and/or reperfusion to the mechanisms leading to myocardial cell injury and/or post-ischemic functional recovery remain controversial and current hypothetical mechanisms suggest that both ischemia and reperfusion contribute to myocardial cell injury (Lesnefsky et al. 2004; Vinten-Johansen et al. 2005; Gross and Auchampach 2007).

At least two morphologically distinct pathways, namely necrosis and apoptosis, have been shown to contribute significantly to myocardial ischemia/reperfusion injury. Necrosis is generally considered to be initiated by non-cellular mechanisms, such as ischemia, trauma and/or coronary artery thrombosis that ultimately lead to irreversible cell death with cell swelling, depletion of high energy stores, disruption of the cellular membrane involving fluid and electrolyte alterations and the loss of potassium and magnesium ions and accumulation of intracellular water, sodium, chloride, hydrogen and calcium (Saraste and Pulkki 2000).

In contrast, apoptosis is a highly regulated, evolutionarily conserved mode of cell death characterized by a discrete set of biochemical and morphological events resulting in the ordered disassembly of the cell, distinct from cell death provoked by external injury (Susin et al. 2000). Apoptosis is characterized by the activation of a family of aspartate-specific proteases identified as caspases (cysteinyl aspartate-specific proteinase), normally expressed as latent zymogens, containing heterologous pro-domains of ~5 kDa (caspase -3,-6,-7) or ~20 kDa (caspase -1,-2,-4,-5,-8,-9) which are cleaved and reassociated to generate catalytically active heterodimers. Apoptosis is marked by the fragmentation of nuclear DNA and the generation of inter-nucleosomal fragments (mono- and/or oligomers of 200 base pairs; DNA ladders), whereas DNA degradation in necrosis is random and nonspecific (McConkey 1998).

5.1.3
Apoptosis in Myocardial Ischemia/Reperfusion Injury

Apoptosis is induced by two main pathways, the extrinsic (death receptor) and the intrinsic (stress) pathways exhibiting differential sensitivity to the anti-apoptotic protein bcl2. The cellular induction pathways regulating these two modes of apoptosis are distinct. In the intrinsic apoptotic pathway, kinase-mediated signaling pathways control the post-translational modification and/or subcellular redistribution of bcl2 proteins to the mitochondria, with the indirect and subsequent activation of caspases, whereas in the extrinsic pathway, multi-protein complexes are assembled at the plasma membrane to orchestrate caspase activation directly (Susin et al. 2000; Nuess et al. 2001). Subtle variations on these modes of activation exist because cross-talk can occur between the mitochondrial and death receptor pathways (Aggarwal 2003). We have recently demonstrated that activation of the intrinsic apoptosis but not the extrinsic pathway occurs following ischemia and reperfusion in the myocardium (McCully et al. 2004; Hsieh et al. 2007).

Myocardial ischemia/reperfusion injury occurs as a continuum rather than an all or none phenomena, prior to the development of unequivocal irreversible ischemia/reperfusion injury (McCully et al. 2004; Stadler et al. 2001; Tansey et al. 2006; Toyoda et al. 2000). Dependent upon the severity and duration of the ischemic event, the myocardium may have decreased function without cellular injury. These states have been defined as myocardial stunning or hibernation. Stunning is a reversible mechanical dysfunction that persists immediately after reperfusion despite the absence of myocellular damage and despite the return of normal or near-normal perfusion (Bolli 1998). A second form of reversible ischemia/reperfusion injury is hibernation which is a syndrome of reversible, chronically reduced contractile function as a result of one or more recurrent episodes of acute or persistent ischemia, referred to as "chronic stunning" (Rahimtoola 1999). As in stunning, hibernating myocardium is viable but not functional and is reversible with coronary revascularization (Schinkel et al. 2007).

Our studies have shown that following 15 min of normothermic regional ischemia there is no detectable necrosis or apoptosis; however, as ischemia time is increased to 20 min and beyond, irreversible ischemia/reperfusion injury occurs (Stadler et al. 2001; Toyoda et al. 2000). Our data demonstrate that as ischemic time is increased from 15–30 to 45 or 60 min, infarct size and apoptosis are significantly increased and regional myocardial function is significantly decreased (Stadler et al. 2001; Toyoda et al. 2000).

The induction of pro-apototic protein cleavage occurs in a sequential manner and is evident prior to biochemical detection by TUNEL. The pro-apoptotic protein, bax, is significantly increased and the proteolytic cleavage of caspase-9 is evident following only 5 min of ischemia, caspase-3 cleavage is evident following 10 min of ischemia and poly ADP-ribose polymerase (PARP) cleavage is evident following 15 min of ischemia. These events precede increased caspase activity and detectable DNA cleavage and the generation of inter-nucleosomal fragments and the significant decrease in left ventricular peak developed pressure and systolic shortening (McCully et al. 2004).

The induction of apoptosis, and the resultant activation of caspases, is not only involved in apoptosis but also in the induction of inflammation. Initial conceptual mechanisms had suggested that apoptosis and inflammation are exclusive; however, evidence suggests that these processes are linked at various levels (Valentijn et al. 2003). Evidence exists to show that caspase-1 processes maturates the cytokine precursors, pro-IL-1β and pro-IL-18. The proinflammatory cytokine IL-18 requires cleavage of its precursor form by caspase 1 (also known as the IL-1β-converting enzyme). Previous studies have shown that IL-18 induces gene expression and synthesis of tumour necrosis factor (TNF), IL-1, Fas ligand (Fas-L) resulting in the induction of apoptosis. Recently, simulated ischemia/reperfusion studies using superfused human atrial myocardial trabeculae have shown that mRNA levels for IL-18 are elevated after ischemia/reperfusion and the concentration of IL-18 in myocardial homogenates is increased and is associated with depression in contractile force (Pomerantz et al. 2001).

5.1.4
Necrosis in Myocardial Ischemia/Reperfusion Injury

Both necrosis and apoptosis are initiated by events occurring during ischemia and executed during reperfusion and represent a continuum of overlapping rather than discriminant events contributing to myocellular injury following surgically-induced ischemia/reperfusion (Freude et al. 2000; McCully et al. 2004). The resultant effect of apoptosis or necrosis in the myocardium is similar, namely, the loss of cell viability and cellular contractile function. At present the modulation of apoptosis using caspase inhibitors is possible, however, the cost of these inhibitors makes their clinical use unfeasible.

In our studies we have found that the contribution of necrosis to infarct size is significantly greater than that of apoptosis. Our data have shown that necrosis represents approximately 90% of all cell death in ischemia/reperfusion injury and accounts for all decreased post-ischemic-functional recovery (McCully et al. 2004). These studies have shown that the inhibition of apoptosis using specific and non-specific irreversible tetrapeptide caspase inhibitors, either separately or in combination, significantly decreased TUNEL positive cell number and caspase activity below detectable limits and reduced infarct size by approximately 8.3%, however, this reduction in apoptosis and overall cell death failed to enhance post-ischemic-functional recovery (McCully et al. 2004). The mechanism(s) by which apoptosis and necrosis alter post-ischemic-functional recovery have yet to be fully elucidated and the effects of stunning and the relative proportion of cell death must be evaluated more fully prior to consensus. However, this area of investigation may provide insight for alternative modes of cardioprotection.

5.1.5
Morphological Alterations in Ischemia/Reperfusion Injury

The modulation of post-ischemic functional recovery may occur at many levels; however, it has been suggested that changes occurring at the intercalated disc may play an important role (Beardslee et al. 2000). The intercalated disc functions as the site of electromechanical coupling within the myocardium. Principal components of the intercalated disc include the gap junctions that allow for direct communication between adjacent cells, and the adherens junctions which provide cell-cell adhesion (Kostetskii et al. 2005; Zuppinger et al. 2000). N-cadherin is the primary cell adhesion molecule found in the adherens junction and appears critical in maintaining the integrity of the intercalated disc structure, while connexin 43 alpha 1 (C× 43[α1]) is the principal connexin expressed in the ventricle. C× 43[α1] exists primarily in the phosphorylated active state; however, it has been shown in animal models that, following ischemic injury, C× 43[α1] becomes dephosphorylated and non-functional (Huang et al. 1999).

The appropriate organization of each of these junctional complexes within the intercalated disc is essential for myocardial tissue development as well as the coordinated contractile function of the heart. Disruption of the intercalated disc and subsequent alterations in cell-cell interactions have been implicated in several human cardiovascular disease states, including ischemic and hypertrophic cardiomyopathy, atrial fibrillation and congestive heart failure (Dupont et al. 2001; Kostin et al. 2002; Peters et al. 1993). Apart from intercellular junctions, the interaction of cardiomyocytes with the extracellular matrix also serves an important role in both the structural and functional integrity of the myocardium and in the stabilization of force transmission during contraction (Katsumi et al. 2004).

Our studies have shown that coincident with the activation of apoptosis there are quantitative changes in myocardial structure (McCully et al. 2002, 2004; Wakiyama et al. 2002). These morphologic alterations are evident as changes in myocardial interfibrillar space that increase as post-ischemic functional recovery decreases (Tansey et al. 2006). These data have shown that changes in myocardial interfibrillar structure involve the cellular redistribution and the significant decrease in the active phosphorylated form of C× 43[α1], and a significant decrease in N-cadherin, the principal adherens junction protein. The use of specific or non-specific caspase inhibitors did not alter the occurrence or extent of these quantitative changes in myocardial structure suggesting that these alterations occur independent of apoptosis activation (Tansey et al. 2006).

Since connexins are fundamentally involved in the propagation of electrical activity from cell to cell, we sought to quantify whether the changes in C× 43[α1] phosphorylation and cellular redistribution following ischemia/reperfusion resulted in altered electrical conduction on a macroscopic scale. However; measurement of conduction velocity using extracellular epicardial electrograms did not demonstrate statistically different conduction velocity anisotropy in hearts subjected to ischemia as compared to non-ischemic controls. These findings may be attributed to the relatively large physiologic reserve of gap junctions that exists in the myocardium and an increase in discontinuous, or zig-zag, conduction between myofibrils imposed by the concomitant increase in interfibrillar spaces which was also observed (Tansey et al. 2006). It is important to note that our studies showed no alteration of integrin β1, an extracellular matrix attachment protein following ischemia and reperfusion. The maintenance of cell-matrix interactions during ischemia is clinically relevant as it affords the potential for full functional recovery after cardiac surgery. If extracellular matrix attachment was compromised, an irreversible end-point of cell death would occur, with no possibility of restoration of normal cell structure and function (Meredith et al. 1993).

5.1.6
Mitochondrial Alterations in Ischemia/Reperfusion Injury

Myocardial infarction does not evolve in a uniform manner. Based upon subjective macroscopic examination of infarction, we have observed that greater infarct is observed in the sub-endocardium rather than in the sub-epicardium (McCully et al. 2002, 2004; Wakiyama et al. 2002). Jennings et al. (1995) described these regional differences as a consequence of metabolism and energy requirements that render the endocardium more vulnerable to ischemic injury and that myocardial injury and necrosis migrate as a "wave front of cell death" towards to the epicardial surface.

The heart is an obligate aerobic organ and is dependent upon a continuous supply of oxygen to maintain normal function. Myocardial oxygen reserve is exhausted within 8 s following the onset of normothermic global ischemia (Kubler and Spieckermann 1970).

Previous studies have shown that myocardial oxygen consumption (MVO_2) is compartmentalized into the oxygen needed for external work of contraction (80–90%) and the unloaded contraction such as basal metabolism, excitation-contraction coupling and heat production (Krukenkamp et al. 1987). A unique aspect of myocardial energetics is that 75% of the coronary arterial oxygen presented to the myocardium is extracted during a single passage through the heart and, thus, depressed coronary venous oxygen content persists despite a wide range of cardiac workloads. Consequently, the heart is extremely susceptible to the limitations of oxygen delivery, whereby an increase in MVO_2 can only be met by augmentation of coronary blood flow. This is diametrically opposite to skeletal muscle, where increased oxygen demand can initially be met by an increase in oxygen extraction.

Under aerobic conditions, the heart derives its energy requirements primarily from the mitochondria that constitute 30% of the total myocardial cell volume. Mitochondria utilize a variety of substrates and provide for oxidative phosphorylation, aerobic metabolism of glucose and fat, modulation of intracellular calcium, calcium signaling and modulation of cellular viability/death signaling (Sternbergh et al. 1989).

In a series of studies, we have shown that mitochondria play a key role in the modulation of the effects of ischemia. Our studies, and those of others, have demonstrated that alterations in mitochondrial structure and function occur during ischemia and extend into reperfusion to severely compromise post-ischemic functional recovery and cellular viability (Faulk et al. 1995a; Lesnefsky et al. 2004; McCully et al. 2002; Rousou et al. 2004).

These studies have shown that ischemia detrimentally alters mitochondrial structure, volume and function (Rousou et al. 2004). In ischemic hearts, there is extensive sarcomere disruption with significantly increased longitudinal and transverse interfibrillar separation and the mitochondria are severely swollen and electron transparent, with numerous mitochondrial calcium granules (Fig. 1). In contrast, in control hearts sarcomere structure is preserved and mitochondria exhibit intact, electron dense intra-cristae matrix (Rousou et al. 2004).

We have quantified these changes in mitochondrial volume using both transmission electron microscopy and light scattering techniques. These studies have demonstrated that mitochondrial matrix and cristae area are significantly increased following ischemia as compared to non-ischemic controls, in agreement with previous studies demonstrating that 88% of cardiac mitochondria are swollen with increased intermembrane space and swollen

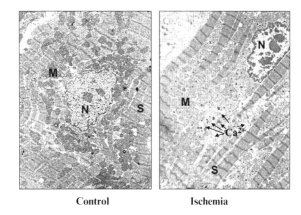

Fig. 1 Sarcomere and mitochondrial alterations following ischemia and reperfusion. Representative transmission electron microscopy (TEM) images ($\times$10,500) of left ventricular tissue samples for Control and Ischemic zones. (*Arrows*) calcium granules, (M) mitochondrion, (S) sarcomere, (N) nucleus

cristae and disrupted matrix following 20 min of anoxia-reoxygenation (Ozcan et al. 2001; Rousou et al. 2004).

These changes in mitochondrial structure and volume are associated with significantly increased mitochondrial calcium ($[Ca^{2+}]_{mito}$) accumulation during ischemia ($p < 0.05$ vs. control) (McCully et al. 2007; Rousou et al. 2004; Tsukube et al. 1996). The effects of increased $[Ca^{2+}]_{mito}$ on the electron transport chain and mitochondrial function are well documented (Suleiman et al. 2001). Under homeostatic conditions, the mitochondrial inner membrane (cristae), containing the electron transport chain, expels protons to the cytosol, creating a charge gradient that provides passive energy for Ca^{2+} influx by the Ca^{2+} uniporter. As calcium enters the mitochondria, water follows leading to mitochondrial matrix swelling (McCully et al. 1994). The increase in $[Ca^{2+}]_{mito}$ destabilizes the inner mitochondrial membrane, causing the inner membrane pore to open and permit further cation movement ("futile calcium cycling"), an energy dependent process requiring ATP to transport calcium against the electrochemical gradient out of the mitochondrion (McCully et al. 1994). These events result in collapse of the mitochondrial inner transmembrane potential and uncouple the respiratory chain.

Additional studies have shown that increased $[Ca^{2+}]_{mito}$ accumulation also significantly decreases the maximal velocity of cytochrome oxidase, the terminal enzyme complex of the inner mitochondrial electron transport chain which has been shown to be vital in the production of high energy phosphate (Faulk et al. 1995b; McCully et al. 2007; Rousou et al. 2004). This reduction in cytochrome oxidase is associated with a significant decrease in mitochondrial complex I and complex II oxygen consumption.

Recently, we have shown that both malate/glutamate (complex I) and succinate (complex II) dependent state 3 oxygen consumption is significantly decreased by ischemia and that these effects extend into reperfusion (McCully et al. 2007; Rousou et al. 2004). The reduction in complex I and complex II state 3 oxygen consumption would be expected to decrease high energy phosphate synthesis required for cell maintenance and mechanical function.

These observations have been confirmed by both serial ^{31}P nuclear magnetic resonance (NMR) and endpoint biochemical spectro-photochemical analysis (McCully et al. 2007;

Tsukube et al. 1997). Our studies using these techniques have shown that high energy phosphates are rapidly and significantly decreased during ischemia and that resynthesis during reperfusion is severely compromised. ^{31}P NMR studies have shown that βNTP area (ATP) is decreased to 66 ± 4% of control by 12 min ischemia and 36 ± 3% by 30 min ischemia and recovers to only 48 ± 3% of control following 60 min reperfusion (Tsukube et al. 1997). These findings agree with spectro-photochemical analysis showing that tissue ATP content (μM/gram tissue wet weight) recovers to only 39% of control following 15 min reperfusion and to only 47% of control by 120 min reperfusion (McCully et al. 2007). These changes in mitochondrial structure and function are associated with significantly decreased post-ischemic functional recovery and significantly increased infarct size and are exacerbated in the aged (McCully et al. 2006, 2007) (Fig. 2).

5.2
Cardioprotection

Cardioplegia is used as a cardioprotective solution for the attenuation of surgically induced ischemic injury incurred during cardiac operative procedures, to allow for the functional preservation of the myocardium. These solutions induce the rapid electromechanical arrest of the myocardium through alteration of cellular electrochemical gradients and provide a flaccid blood-free operating field.

Most cardioplegia solutions use high potassium to arrest the heart (Wright et al. 1978). The use of hypothermic potassium cardioplegia in adult open heart surgery increases the available intraoperative time, and has been correlated with improved postischemic myocardial functional recovery, and reduced postoperative mortality (Wright et al. 1978). Potassium-induced arrest maintains the heart in a depolarized state, significantly decreasing the energy demand of the myocardium (Sternbergh et al. 1989). Basal metabolic energy requirements are sustained under potassium-induced arrest and, thus, still constitutes a significant energy expenditure. In addition, depolarization leads to the alteration of the ion flux across the sarcolemmal membrane and is associated with both increased cytosolic calcium accumulation and the significant depletion of cellular ATP reserves (Tsukube et al. 1997).

In previous investigations we have shown that magnesium supplemented potassium cardioplegia (K/Mg, Deaconess Surgical Association) provides superior cardioprotection as compared to high potassium cardioplegia (Faulk et al. 1995a, b; Matsuda et al. 1997; Tsukube et al. 1994, 1997). In a series of reports, using the isolated perfused rabbit heart and the in situ blood perfused sheep and pig heart models, we have shown that K/Mg cardioplegia partially modifies the biochemical changes that lead to lethal myocardial ischemia/reperfusion injury. We have also shown that the mechanisms by which magnesium-supplemented potassium cardioplegia affords enhanced cardioprotection involve the amelioration of cytosolic, mitochondrial and nuclear calcium overload, enhanced preservation and resynthesis of high energy phosphates, and the modulation of nuclear and mitochondrial function (Faulk et al. 1995a; McCully et al. 1994; Tsukube et al. 1997). The end effector of these mechanisms remains to be elucidated; however, recent investigations have suggested that the mitochondrial ATP-sensitive potassium (mitoK$_{ATP}$) channels

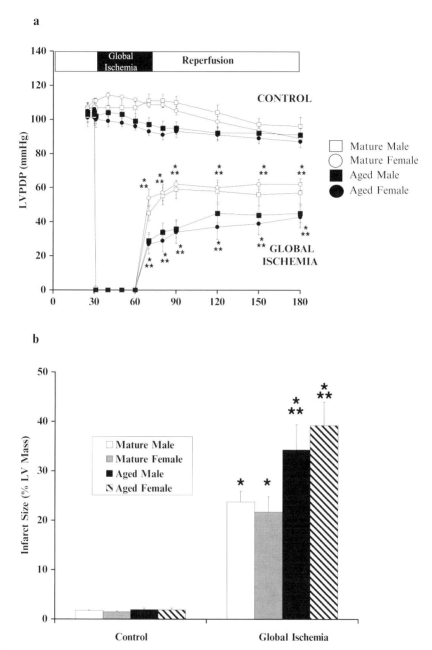

Fig. 2 Effects of ischemia and reperfusion on post-ischemic functional recovery and infarct size in the mature and aged heart Left ventricular peak developed pressure (LVPDP; mmHg) and (**b**) infarct size (%LV Mass) in Control (following 180 min of perfusion without ischemia) and in Global Ischemia (GI) hearts following 30 min equilibrium, 30 min global ischemia, and 120 min reperfusion. All results are shown as the mean ± standard error of the mean for n = 6–10 for each group. Significant differences at $p < 0.05$ versus control are indicated by *asterisk*. Significant difference mature versus aged are shown as *double asterisk*

play an important role in the cardioprotection afforded by K/Mg cardioplegia (Toyoda et al. 2001; Wakiyama et al. 2002).

Our studies have demonstrated that the addition of diazoxide, a specific mitoK$_{ATP}$ channel opener, to allow for the early or enhanced opening of mitoK$_{ATP}$ channels significantly enhances the cardioprotection afforded by K/Mg cardioplegia in both the isolated perfused and the in situ blood perfused heart models (Toyoda et al. 2001; Wakiyama et al. 2002). In these experiments we have used 50 μmol/L diazoxide, a concentration we and others have shown to significantly decrease infarct size independent of vasodilatation (Garlid et al. 1997). Our investigations (Toyoda et al. 2001; Wakiyama et al. 2002) have shown that the addition of 50 μmol/L diazoxide to K/Mg cardioplegia (K/Mg + DZX) has no significant effect on proximal, distal or proximal/distal coronary flow or on mean arterial pressure, but significantly decreased infarct size to $1.5 \pm 0.4\%$ ($p < 0.05$ vs. K/Mg) following 30 min of normothermic global ischemia and 120 min of reperfusion. This infarct size in K/Mg + DZX was not significantly different from that seen in non-ischemic control hearts.

It is important to note that, in our studies, diazoxide (50 μmol/L) was included with cold blood cardioplegia only during initial administration but was not included when cold blood cardioplegia was re-administered following 15 min global ischemia. This was based on preliminary results which showed that re-administration of diazoxide resulted in a significant decrease in mean arterial pressure upon reperfusion (Toyoda et al. 2001). Diazoxide is highly bound to albumin (predominately hydrophobic and to a lesser extent hydrogen bonding) and has a plasma half-life of 22 h (Sellers and Koch-Weser 1974). Diazoxide is used as an anti-hypertensive drug and has vasodilatory properties; however, at a concentration of 50 μmol/L we and others have shown that the infarct limiting effects of diazoxide are independent of vasodilatation (Garlid et al. 1997). Using only a single dose in the initial administration of cardioplegia and then cardioplegia without diazoxide in all subsequent administrations, no difference in heart rate, mean arterial pressure or coronary flow was observed between hearts receiving cold blood cardioplegia and hearts receiving cold blood cardioplegia + diazoxide.

No definitive study has been performed to indicate the exact diazoxide concentration to allow for clinical use; however, our studies suggest that, based on a total blood volume of 3–4 L in the pig, a circulating diazoxide concentration of approximately 7.5–10 μmol/L is adequate, in agreement with the investigations of Garlid et al. (1997) who have shown that diazoxide decreases cell injury in a dose-dependent manner at concentrations between 1 and 30 μmol/L.

Our studies have also demonstrated that the early or enhanced opening of the mitoK$_{ATP}$ channels significantly enhances cardioprotection by decreasing apoptosis and by modulating mitochondrial structure and function (McCully et al. 2002; Rousou et al. 2004). Mitochondrial modulation of apoptosis has been described earlier and our data substantiate these mechanisms in cardioprotection. Further studies show that diazoxide, when added to cardioplegia, preserves mitochondrial structure and significantly increases mitochondrial matrix and cristae area and matrix volume as compared to non-ischemic controls (Rousou et al. 2004). These results are in agreement with others (Dos Santos et al. 2002) who have suggested increased mitochondrial matrix volume allows for the maintenance of efficient energy transfer during reperfusion.

These results indicate that the addition of diazoxide to cardioplegia significantly decreases state 3 mitochondrial oxygen consumption (complex I and complex II) as compared to non-ischemic controls and preserves tissue ATP content. These effects in combination with depolarized arrest significantly decrease infarct size and significantly enhance cardioprotection.

5.3
Effects of Age and Gender in Ischemia/Reperfusion Injury

Presently, in the United States, the mean age of patients requiring coronary artery bypass surgery (CABG) is 68 years with approximately 44% of these patients being female (Capdeville et al. 2001; Koch et al. 2003; Vaccarino et al. 2003). Census-based projections indicate that both mean age and the proportion of females requiring cardiac surgery will increase in the coming years.

Recent studies have shown that patients aged 80 years or older are more likely to be female, more likely to be emergency priority and more likely to have associated comorbidities (Bridges et al. 2003). Women have been shown to have a significantly greater operative risk as compared to men, and to have worse outcomes after cardiac surgery (Abramov et al. 2000; Davis et al. 1995; Edwards et al. 1998; Koch et al. 2003; Vaccarino et al. 2003).

The etiologies for these differences are speculative and include surgical technical issues associated with anatomic size differences, differences in body mass and associated fat deposition (Blankstein et al. 2005; Kim et al. 2007) hormonal differences (Humphrey et al. 2002; Nelson et al. 2002) and specific molecular differences between male and female myocardial cells and their susceptibility to myocardial ischemia/reperfusion injury (Simkhovich et al. 2003; Vina et al. 2005).

Both the Society for Thoracic Surgeons (STS) National Cardiac Surgery Database (the largest clinical cardiac surgery database in the world) and the EuroSCORE algorithm (one of the best-established and validated models for contemporary practice in cardiac surgery) indicate female sex is an operative risk factor (Nashef et al. 1999; Ferguson et al. 2002; Society of Thoracic Surgeons National Database to 2004). The STS Database provides evidence that, in the United States, women undergoing CABG have a significantly higher operative mortality (4.5%) compared with that of men (2.6%; $P < 0.0001$). The Toronto Hospital study (Abramov et al. 2000), the Reykjavik Study (Jónsdóttir et al. 1998) the University of Michigan Study (Kim et al. 2007) and the Israeli Coronary Artery Study (Zitser-Gurevich et al. 2002) have all demonstrated that myocardial infarction in women is age-dependent with both incidence and prevalence increasing continuously and steeply with age.

In the analysis of co-morbidities and anatomy relating to early mortality, it has been noted that preoperative risk factors are more prevalent among women than men. These factors include age above 70, angina class 3 or 4, urgent operation, preoperative intraaortic balloon pump usage, congestive heart failure, previous percutaneous transluminal coronary angioplasty, diabetes, hypertension, peripheral vascular disease and smaller coronary artery size and smaller mean body surface area as compared to men (Abramov et al. 2000; Kim et al. 2007). However, in a contemporary data set analysis from 31 Midwestern hospitals it has been shown that after adjusting for all co-morbidities including body surface area, female gender is an independent predictor of increased mortality following coronary artery bypass surgery, with a risk adjusted operative mortality of 3.81% for women as compared to 2.43% for men (Blankstein et al. 2005).

It has also been shown that significant differences in in-hospital mortality for women persist (Tsukube et al. 1997) despite the fact that women have better cardiac function pre-operatively and fewer bypass grafts constructed as compared to men (Abramov et al. 2000; Kim et al. 2007). In a prospective study following 1,113 patients (804 men and 309 women) who underwent first CABG consecutively between February 1999 and February 2001, it was shown that women have a more difficult recovery compared with men, which cannot be explained by illness severity, pre-surgery health status, or other patient characteristics (Vaccarino et al. 2003). Multivariate analysis has also shown that women have higher mortality rates than equally matched men in low-risk and medium-risk groups. It is only among very high-risk patients that sex is not found to be an independent predictor of adverse outcomes.

5.4
Decreased Efficacy of Cardioprotection in the Aged Female

Our experimental studies indicated that current cardioprotective protocols are significantly less effective in the aged female as compared to the aged male (McCully et al. 2006, 2007). Analysis of age and gender, and age by gender, effects on the cardioprotection afforded by cardioplegia on post-ischemic myocardial functional recovery indicated that left ventricular peak developed pressure (LVPDP) was significantly decreased and left ventricular end diastolic pressure (LVEDP) and infarct size were significantly increased in the aged female as compared to the aged male heart (McCully et al. 2006, 2007).

Our results are consistent with clinical data showing that, following CABG, there is a significant depression in each parameter of cardiac function related to the heterogeneous myocardial stunning with a significant increase in LVEDP and a significant increase in myocardial infarction in females as compared to men (Abramov et al. 2000; Bolooki et al. 2004).

The mechanisms responsible for decreased cardioprotection in the aged, and in particular the aged female, remain to be fully elucidated but in a recent report we have shown that cardioplegia ± diazoxide modulates mitochondrial oxygen consumption and mitochondrial calcium accumulation. These effects are significantly decreased in the aged as compared to the mature heart and significantly decreased in the female as compared to the male heart (McCully et al. 2007). These data suggest that temporal changes specific to the female may modulate cardioprotection. One such mechanism is modulation through hormonal receptors.

5.5
Female Age and the Role of Estrogen

Young women have been shown to have a greater resistance to myocardial ischemic injury and that this resistance is lost following menopause (Bridgman et al. 2005; Mendelsohn et al. 2005; Willems et al. 2005). Aged women have also been shown to have a significant increase in the incidence of perioperative myocardial infarction as compared to men (4.5 vs.

3.1%; p < 0.05) suggesting that women have a greater incidence of ischemia/necrosis with aortic cross-clamping and surgically induced myocardial ischemia (Abramov et al. 2000). It has also been demonstrated that the incidence of cardiovascular disease increases in both aged women and in pre-menopausal women who have undergone previous oophorectomy (Barrett-Connor 1997; Crabbe et al. 2003). The mechanisms responsible for enhanced cardioprotection in the young as compared to the aged female have been hypothesized to include estrogen receptor activation and regulation of cardioprotective genes and modulation of mitochondrial function (Jovanovic et al. 2000; Mendelsohn et al. 2005; Murphy and Steenbergen 2007; Stirone et al. 2005).

The effect of estrogen on gene transcription has been well established (Edwards 2005; Vina et al. 2005) and it has been shown by several investigators that 17β-estradiol, the active form of estradiol, enhances cardioprotection through up-regulation of genes associated with cardioprotection (Beato and Klug 2000; Lee et al. 2000). However, it should be noted that these studies were not performed in the aged female heart- but rather in the young or mature heart using New Zealand white rabbits 50–250 days (Gilsanz et al. 1988), ~12 week (Booth et al. 2003, 2005) and 4–6 month (Hale et al. 1996); mouse 11 week (Otsuki et al. 2003); rat 6 day post-delivery (Too et al. 1999), 3 months (Stirone et al. 2005), 6 months (Bolego et al. 2005); dog, 10–15 kg (Tsai et al. 2002) or cell culture (Jovanovic et al. 2000).

While there is sufficient data to indicate that estrogen modulates genes associated with cardioprotection (Murphy and Steenbergen 2007; Mendelsohn and Karas 2005) a recent large clinical trial failed to show cardioprotection for post-menopausal females on hormone replacement therapy (HRT: estrogen–progestin) (Hayward et al. 2000; Rossouw et al. 2002). In fact, HRT was shown to increase cardiovascular risk in females (Hayward et al. 2000; Rossouw et al. 2002). These studies suggest that that chronic HRT therapy may not be an option and that alternate approaches must be initiated in order to delineate mechanisms to enhance cardioprotection in the aged female.

These data indicate that aged women may be more susceptible to ischemia/reperfusion injury and further suggest that current clinical myoprotective procedures may be inadequate to prevent this discrepancy. Further investigation is required to identify basic biologic mechanisms to reduce morbidity and mortality in the aged female cardiac surgical patient.

5.6
Future Directions for the Amelioration of Ischemia/Reperfusion Injury

We, and others, have shown that RNA transcription and translation are significantly decreased in the aged as compared to the mature heart (Faulk et al. 1995a; McCully et al. 1991; Simkhovich et al. 2003) and that the cardioprotection afforded by cardioplegia is modulated by de novo RNA synthesis (Matsuda et al. 1997). We have also shown that, with aging, mitochondrial DNA is susceptible to excision mechanisms following ischemia and reperfusion that delete 7.3 kb of mitochondrial DNA coding for the mitochondrial genes of oxidative phosphorylation (Levitsky et al. 2003). The incidence and prevalence of this deletion was increased in patients with clinical indications of poor recovery suggesting that this deletion may provide an important indicator to surgical outcome in the cardiac surgical patient (Levitsky et al. 2003).

These data suggest that the temporal differences in the cardioprotection afforded by cardioplegia in males and females may be associated with alterations in transcription and translation and in particular changes in fidelity of mitochondrial associated genes and gene products that directly affect high energy synthesis and regulation of mitochondrial function. The previous finding that mRNA levels in the female are significantly decreased as compared to males under normal and pathological conditions would support the hypothesis that decreased cardioprotection in the aged female as compared to the aged male is modulated by gene transcription mechanisms (Bridgman et al. 2005).

5.7
Conclusion

The mechanisms modulating cardioprotection are complex and cannot be investigated as a single entity but rather must be investigated as a system. Previously, we and others have used a variety of methods to identify the RNA's and proteins associated with global ischemia and with cardioprotection (Faulk et al. 1995a; Xu et al. 2001). These studies, while providing valuable information, utilized a targeted approach involving one or a few genes. The mostly static data garnered by these studies, while providing valuable information, did not allow for the interactive analysis of collateral, cognate gene and protein expression.

The advent of current technologies such as microarray and proteomic analysis has allowed for the co-identification of collateral and cognate gene expression and related protein biomarkers. Recent studies incorporating these methodologies have shown that the mechanisms of cardioprotection involve specific transcript/protein related alterations affecting metabolic and regenerative pathways (Ruel et al. 2003; Schomisch et al. 2005; White et al. 2005; McCully et al. 2009).

While still at initial stages it is expected that the elucidation and identification of specific transcript/protein modification associated with cardioprotection will allow for the development of designer cardioplegia solutions. These solutions could be developed to provide cardioprotection over a variety of conditions. In particular it would be possible to enhance cardioprotection and reduce morbidity and mortality in the aged female through directed pharmacological or methodological up-regulation of RNA and protein biomarkers.

Acknowledgement Support: This study was supported by the National Institutes of Health (HL29077).

References

Abramov D, Tamariz MG, Sever JY, Christakis GT, Bhatnagar G, Heenan AL, Goldman BS, Fremes SE (2000) The influence of gender on the outcome of coronary artery bypass surgery. Ann Thorac Surg 70: 800–805

Aggarwal, BB (2003) Signaling pathways of the superfamily: a double edged sword. Nat Rev Immunol 3: 745–756

Barrett-Connor E (1997) Sex differences in coronary heart disease. Why are women so superior? The 1995 Ancel Keys Lecture. Circulation 95: 252–264

Beardslee MA, Lerner DL, Tadros PN, Laing JG, Beyer EC, Yamada KA, Kléber AG, Schuessler RB, Saffitz JE (2000) Dephosphorylation and intracellular redistribution of ventricular connexin43 during electrical uncoupling induced by ischemia. Circ Res 87: 656–662

Beato M, Klug J (2000) Steroid hormone receptors: an update. Hum Reprod Update 6: 225–236

Blankstein R, Ward RP, Arnsdorf M, Jones B, Lou YB, Pine M (2005) Female gender is an independent predictor of operative mortality after coronary artery bypass graft surgery: contemporary analysis of 31 Midwestern hospitals. Circulation 112 (9 Suppl): I323–I327

Bolego C, Cignare A, Sanvito P, Pelosi V, Pellegatta F, Puglisi L, Pinna C (2005) The acute estrogenic dilation of rat aorta is mediated solely by selective estrogen receptor-α agonists and is abolished by estrogen deprivation. J Pharmacol Exp Ther 313: 1203–1208

Bolli R (1998) Why myocardial stunning is clinically important. Basic Res Cardiol 193: 169–172

Bolooki H, Green R, Vargas A, Kaiser GA, Ghahramani A (2004) Coronary artery surgery in women. Tex Heart Inst J 31: 410–417

Booth EA, Marchesi M, Kilbournee J, Lucchesi BR (2003) 17β-Estradiol as a receptor-mediated cardioprotective agent. J Pharmacol Exp Ther 307: 395–401

Booth EA, Obeid NR, Lucchesi BR (2005) Activation of estrogen receptor alpha protects the in vivo rabbit heart from ischemia-reperfusion injury. Am J Physiol Heart Circ Physiol 28: H2039–H2047

Bridgman P, Aronovitz MA, Kakkar R, Oliverio MI, Coffman TM, Rand WM, Konstam MA, Mendelsohn ME, Patten RD (2005) Gender-specific patterns of left ventricular and myocyte remodeling following myocardial infarction in mice deficient in the angiotensin II type 1a receptor. Am J Physiol Heart Circ Physiol 289: H586–H592

Bridges CR, Edwards FH, Peterson ED, Coombs LP, Ferguson TB (2003) Cardiac surgery in nonagenarians and centenarians. J Am Coll Surg 197: 347–356

Capdeville M, Chamogeogarkis T, Lee JH (2001) Effect of gender on outcomes of beating heart operations. Ann Thorac Surg 72: S1022–S1025

Christenson JT, Schmuziger M, Maurice J, Simonet F, Velebit V (1994) How safe is coronary bypass surgery in the elderly patient? Analysis of 111 patients aged 75 years or more and 2939 patients younger than 75 years undergoing coronary artery bypass grafting in a private hospital. Coron Artery Dis 5: 169–174

Crabbe DL, Dipla K, Ambati S, Zafeiridis A, Gaughan JP, Houser SR, Margulies KB (2003) Gender differences in post-infarction hypertrophy in end-stage failing hearts. J Am Coll Cardiol 41: 300–306

Davis KB, Chaitman B, Ryan T, Bittner V, Kennedy JW (1995) Comparison of 15 year survival for men and women after initial medical or surgical treatment for coronary artery disease: a CASS registry study. J Am Coll Cardiol 25: 1000–1009

Dos Santos P, Kowaltowski AJ, Laclau MN, Seetharaman S, Paucek P, Boudina S, Thambo JB, Tariosse L, Garlid KD (2002) Mechanisms by which opening of the mitochondrial ATP-sensitive K+ channel protects the ischemic heart. Am J Physiol Heart Circ Physiol 283: H284–H295

Dupont E, Matsushita T, Kaba RA, Vozzi C, Coppen SR, Khan N, Kaprielian R, Yacoub MH, Severs NJ (2001) Altered connexin expression in human congestive heart failure. J Mol Cell Cardiol 33: 359–371

Edmunds LH, Jr., Stephenson LW, Edie RN, Ratcliffe MB (1988) Open-heart surgery in octogenarians. N Engl J Med 319: 131–136

Edwards DP (2005) Regulation of signal transduction pathways by estrogen and progesterone. Annu Rev Physiol 67: 335–376

Edwards FH, Carey JS, Grover FL, Bero JW, Hartz RS (1998) Impact of gender on coronary bypass operative mortality. Ann Thorac Surg 66: 125–131

Faulk EA, McCully JD, Hadlow NC, Tsukube T, Krukenkamp IB, Federman M, Levitsky S (1995a) Magnesium cardioplegia enhances mRNA levels and the maximal velocity of cytochrome oxidase I in the senescent myocardium during global ischemia. Circulation 92: 405–412.

Faulk EA, McCully JD, Tsukube T, Hadlow NC, Krukenkamp IB, Levitsky S (1995b) Myocardial mitochondrial calcium accumulation modulates nuclear calcium accumulation and DNA fragmentation. Annal Thorac Surg 60: 338–344.

Ferguson TB Jr, Hammill BG, Peterson ED, DeLong ER, Grover FL (2002) A decade of change – risk profiles and outcomes for isolated coronary artery bypass grafting procedures, 1990–1999: a report from the STS National Database Committee and the Duke Clinical Research Institute. Society of Thoracic Surgeons. Ann Thorac Surg 73: 480–489

Fremes SE, Goldman BS, Ivanov J, Weisel RD, David TE, Salerno T (1989) Valvular surgery in the elderly. Circulation 80: 177–190

Freude B, Masters TN, Robicsek F, Fokin A, Kostin S, Zimmermann S, Ulmann, C, Lorenz-Meyer S, Schaper, U (2000) Apoptosis is initiated by myocardial ischemia and executed during reperfusion. J Mol Cell Cardiol 32: 197–208

Garlid KD, Paucek P, Yarov-Yarovoy V, Murray HN, Darbenzio RB, D'Alonzo AJ, Lodge NJ, Smith MA, Grover GJ (1997) Cardioprotective effect of diazoxide and its interaction with mitochondrial ATP-sensitive K+ channels: Possible mechanism of cardioprotection. Circ Res 81: 1072–1082

Gersh BJ, Kronmal RA, Schaff HV, Frye TJ, Myers WO, Atherarn MW, Gosselin AJ, Kaiser GC, Killip T, 3rd (1993) Long-term (5 year) results of coronary bypass surgery in patients 65 years old or older; a report from the Coronary Artery Surgery Study. Circulation 68(suppl II): II190–II199

Gilsanz V, Roe TF, Gibbens DT, Schulz EE, Carlson ME, Gonzalez O, Boechat MI (1988) Effect of sex steroids on peak bone density of growing rabbits. Am J Physiol 255: E416–E421

Gross GJ, Auchampach JA (2007) Reperfusion injury: does it exist? J Mol Cell Cardiol 4: 12–18

Guralnik JM, Fitzsimmons SC (1986) Aging in America: A demographic perspective. Cardiol Clin 4: 175–183

Hale SL, Birnbaum Y, Kloner RA (1996) beta-Estradiol, but not alpha-estradiol, reduced myocardial necrosis in rabbits after ischemia and reperfusion. Am Heart J 132: 258–262

Hayward CS, Kelly RP, Collins P (2000) The roles of gender, the menopause and hormone replacement on cardiovascular function. Cardiovasc Res 46: 28–49

Hsieh Y, Wakiyama H, Levitsky S, McCully JD (2007) Cardioplegia and diazoxide modulate STAT3 activation and DNA binding. Ann Thorac Surg 84: 1272–1278

Huang X-D, Sandusky GE, Zipes DP (1999) Heterogeneous loss of connexin43 protein in ischemic dog hearts. J Cardiovasc Electrophysiol 10: 79–91

Humphrey LL, Chan BK, Sox HC (2002) Postmenopausal hormone replacement therapy and the primary prevention of cardiovascular disease. Ann Intern Med 137: 273–284

Jennings RB, Steenbergen C Jr, Reimer KA (1995) Myocardial ischemia and reperfusion. Monogr Pathol 37: 47–80

Jovanovic S, Jovanovic A, Shen WK, Terzic A (2000) Low concentrations of 17beta-estradiol protect single cardiac cells against metabolic stress-induced Ca^{2+} loading. J Am Coll Cardiol 36: 948–952

Jónsdóttir LS, Sigfusson N, Sigvaldason H, Thorgeirsson G (1998) Incidence and prevalence of recognised and unrecognised myocardial infarction in women. The Reykjavik Study. Eur Heart J 19: 1011–1018

Katsumi A, Orr AW, Tzima E, Schwartz MA (2004) Integrins in mechanotransduction. J Biol Chem. 279: 12001–12004

Kim C, Redberg RF, Pavlic T, Eagle KA (2007) A systematic review of gender differences in mortality after coronary artery bypass graft surgery and percutaneous coronary interventions. Clin Cardiol 30: 491–495

Koch CG, Khandwala F, Nussmeier N, Blackstone EH (2003) Gender and outcomes after coronary artery bypass grafting: a propensity matched comparison. J Thorac Cardiovasc Surg 126: 2032–2043

Kostetskii I, Li J, Xiong Y, Zhou R, Ferrari VA, Patel VV, Molkentin JD, Radice GL (2005) Induced deletion of the N-cadherin gene in the heart leads to dissolution of the intercalated disc structure. Circ Res 96: 346–354

Kostin S, Klein G, Szalay Z, Hein S, Bauer EP, Schaper J (2002) Structural correlate of atrial fibrillation in human patients. Cardiovasc Res 54: 361–379

Krukenkamp IB, Silverman NA and Levitsky S (1987) The effect of cardioplegic oxygenation on the correlation between linearized Frank-Starling relationship and myocardial energetics in the ejecting postischemic heart. Circulation 76 (Suppl 5): 122–128

Kubler W, Spieckermann PG (1970) Regulation of glycolysis in the ischemic and anoxic myocardium. J Mol Cell Cardiol 1: 351–377

Lee TM, Su SF, Tsai CC, Lee YT, Tsai CH (2000) Cardioprotective effects of 17-beta-estradiol produced by activation of mitochondrial ATP-sensitive K(ATP) channels in canine hearts. J Mol Cell Cardiol 32: 1147–1158

Lesnefsky EJ, Chen Q, Slabe TJ, Stoll MS, Minkler PE, Hassan MO, Tander B, Hoppel CL (2004) Ischemia, rather than reperfusion inhibits respiration through cytochrome oxidase in the isolated perfused rabbit heart: role of cardiolipin. AM J Phys Heart Circ Phys 287: H258–H267

Levitsky S, Laurikka J, Stewart RD, Campos CT, Lahey SJ, McCully JD (2003) Mitochondrial DNA deletions in coronary artery bypass grafting patients. Eur J Cardiothorac Surg 24: 777–784

Likosky DS, Dacey LJ, Baribeau YR, Leavitt BJ, Clough R, Cochran RP, Quinn R, Sisto DA, Charlesworth DC, Malenka DJ, MacKenzie TA, Olmstead EM, Ross CS, O'Connor GT, Northern New England Cardiovascular Disease Study Group (2008) Long-term survival of the very elderly undergoing coronary artery bypass grafting. Ann Thorac Surg 85: 1233–1237

Matsuda H, McCully JD, Levitsky S (1997) Developmental differences in cytosolic calcium accumulation associated with global ischemia: Evidence for differential intracellular calcium channel receptor activity. Circulation 96(suppl II): II-233–II-239

McConkey DJ (1998) Biochemical determinants of apoptosis and necrosis. Toxicol Letts 99: 157–168

McCully JD, Wang RX, Kellam B, Sole MJ, Liew CC (1991) Isolation and characterization of a previously unrecognized myosin heavy chain gene present in the Syrian hamster myocardium. J Mol Biol 218: 657–665

McCully JD, Tsukube T, Ataka K, Krukenkamp IB, Feinberg H, Levitsky S (1994) Myocardial cytosolic calcium accumulation during ischemia/reperfusion: The effects of aging and cardioplegia. J Cardiothorac Surg 9: 449–452

McCully JD, Wakiyama H, Cowan DB, Federman M, Levitsky S (2002) Diazoxide amelioration of myocardial injury and mitochondrial damage during cardiac surgery. Ann Thorac Surg 74: 2138–2146

McCully JD, Wakiyama H, Hsieh Y-J, Jones M, Levitsky S (2004) Differential contribution of necrosis and apoptosis in myocardial ischemia/reperfusion injury. Am J Physiol Heart Circ Physiol 286: H1923–H1935

McCully JD, Toyoda Y, Wakiyama H, Rousou AJ, Parker RA, Levitsky S (2006) Age and gender related differences in ischemia/reperfusion injury and cardioprotection: Effects of diazoxide. Ann Thorac Surg 82: 117–123

McCully JD, Rousou AJ, Parker RA, Levitsky S (2007) Age and gender differences in mitochondrial oxygen consumption and free matrix calcium during ischemia/reperfusion and with cardioplegia and diazoxide. Ann Thorac Surg 83: 1102–1109

McCully JD, Bhasin MK, Wakiyama H, Daly C, Guerrero M, Dillon S, Libermann TA, Cowan DB, Mably JD, Parker RA, Ericsson M, McGowan FX, Levitsky S (2009) Transcriptomic and proteomic analysis of the Cardioprotection afforded by Cardioplegia. Physiol Genomics. 38: 125–137

Mendelsohn ME, Karas RH (2005) Molecular and cellular basis of cardiovascular gender differences Science 308: 1583–1587

Meredith JE, Fazeli B, Schwartz MA (1993) The extracellular matrix as a cell survival factor. Mol Biol Cell. 4: 953–961

Murphy E, Steenbergen C (2007) Gender-based differences in mechanisms of protection in myocardial ischemia-reperfusion injury. Cardiovasc Res 75: 478–486

Nashef SA, Roques F, Michel P, Gauducheau E, Lemeshow S, Salamon R (1999) European system for cardiac operative risk evaluation (EuroSCORE). Eur J Cardiothorac Surg 16: 9–13

Nelson HD, Humphrey LL, Nygren P, Teutsch SM, Allan JD (2002) Postmenopausal hormone replacement therapy: scientific review. J Am Med Assoc 288: 872–881

Nuess M, Crow MT, Chesley A, and Lakatta EG (2001)Apoptosis in cardiac disease-what is it-how does it occur. Cardiovasc Drugs Ther 15: 507–523

Otsuki M, Gao H, Dahlman-Wright K, Ohlsson C, Eguchi N, Urade Y, Gustafsson JA (2003) Specific regulation of lipocalin-type prostaglandin d synthase in mouse heart by estrogen receptor beta. Mol Endocrinol 17: 1844–1855

Ozcan C, Holmuhamedov EL, Jahangir A, Terzic A (2001) Diazoxide protects mitochondria from anoxic injury: implication for myopreservation. J Thorac Cardiovasc Surg 121: 298–306

Peters NS, Green CR, Poole-Wilson PA, Severs NJ (1993) Reduced content of connexin43 gap junctions in ventricular myocardium from hypertrophied and ischemic hearts. Circulation 88: 864-875

Pomerantz BJ, Reznikov LL, Harken AH, Dinarello CA (2001) Inhibition of caspase 1 reduces human myocardial ischemic dysfunction via inhibition of IL-18 and IL-1 beta. Proc Natl AcadlScil (USA) 98: 2871–2876.

Rahimtoola SH (1999) Concept and evaluation of hibernating myocardium. Annu Rev Med 50: 75–86

Rossouw JE, Anderson GL, Prentice RL, LaCroix AZ, Kooperberg C, Stefanick ML, Jackson RD, Beresford SA, Howard BV, Johnson KC, Kotchen JM, Ockene J, Writing Group for the Women's Health Initiative Investigators (2002) Risks and benefits of estrogen plus progestin in healthy postmenopausal women: principal results From the Women's Health Initiative randomized controlled trial. JAMA 288: 321–333

Rousou AJ, Ericsson M, Federman M, Levitsky S, McCully JD (2004) Diazoxide and cardioplegia ameliorate ischemia/reperfusion cell death through the modulation of mitochondrial volume and calcium accumulation and mitochondrial respiratory control index. Am J Physiol Heart Circ Physiol 287: H1967–H1976

Ruel M, Bianchi C, Khan TA, Xu S, Liddacott JR, Voisine P, Araujo E, Lyon H, Kohane IS, Libermann TA, Sellke FW (2003) Gene expression profile after cardiopulmonary bypass and cardioplegic arrest. J Thorac Cardiovasc Surg 126: 1521–1530

Saraste A, Pulkki K (2000) Morphologic and biochemical hallmarks of apoptosis. Cardiovasc Res 45: 528–537

Schinkel AF, Bax JJ, Poldermans D, Elhendy A, Ferrari R, Rahimtoola SH (2007) Hibernating myocardium: diagnosis and patient outcomes. Curr Probl Cardiol 32: 375–410

Schomisch SJ, Murdock DG, Hedayati N, Carino JL, Lesnefsky EJ, Cmolik BL (2005) Cardioplegia prevents ischemia-induced transcriptional alterations of cytoprotective genes in rat hearts: a DNA microarray study. J Thorac Cardiovasc Surg 130: 1151–1158

Sellers EM, Koch-Weser J (1974) Binding of diazoxide and other benzothiadiazines to human albumin. Biochem Pharmacol 23: 553–566

Simkhovich BZ, Marjoram P, Poizat C, Kedes L, Kloner RA (2003) Age-related changes of cardiac gene expression following myocardial ischemia/reperfusion. Arch Biochem Biophys 420: 268–278

Stadler B, Phillips J, Toyoda Y, Federman M, Levitsky, S, McCully JD (2001) Adenosine enhanced ischemic preconditioning modulates necrosis and apoptosis: Effects of stunning and ischemia/reperfusion. Ann Thorac Surg 72: 555–563

Sternbergh WC, Brunsting LA, Abd-Elfattah AS, Wechsler AS (1989) Basal metabolic energy requirements of polarized and depolarized arrest in rat heart. Am J Physiol 256: H846–H851

Stirone C, Duckles SP, Krause DN, Procaccio V (2005) Estrogen increases mitochondrial efficiency and reduces oxidative stress in cerebral blood vessels. Mol Pharmacol 68: 959–965

Suleiman MS, Halestrap AP, Griffiths EJ (2001) Mitochondria: a target for myocardial protection. Pharm Therap 89: 29–46

Susin SA, Daugas E, Ravagnan L, Samejima K, Zamzami N, Loeffler M, Costantini P, Ferri KF, Irinopoulou T, Prevost MC, Brothers G, Mak TW, Penninger J, Earnshaw WC, Kroemer G (2000) Two distinct pathways leading to nuclear apoptosis. J Exp Med 192: 571–579

Tansey EE, Kwaku KF, Hammer PE, Cowan DB, Federman M, Levitsky S, McCully JD (2006) Reduction and redistribution of gap and adherens junction proteins following ischemia/reperfusion. Ann Thorac Surg 82: 1472–1479

Too CK, Giles A, Wilkinson M (1999) Estrogen stimulates expression of adenine nucleotide translocator ANT1 messenger RNA in female rat hearts. Mol Cell Endocrinol 150: 161–167

Toyoda Y, Di Gregorio V, Parker RA, Levitsky S, McCully JD (2000) Anti-stunning and anti-infarct effects of adenosine enhanced ischemic preconditioning. Circulation 102: 326–331

Toyoda Y, Levitsky S, McCully JD (2001) Opening of mitochondrial ATP-sensitive potassium channels enhances cardioplegic protection. Ann Thorac Surg 71:1281–1289

Tsai CH, Su FS, Chou TF, Lee TM (2002) Differential effects of sarcolemmal and mitochondrial channels activated by 17β-estradiol on reperfusion arrhythmias and infarct size in canine hearts. J Pharmacol Exp Ther 301:234–240

Tsukube T, McCully JD, Faulk E, Federman M, LoCicero J, Krukenkamp IB, Levitsky S (1994) Magnesium cardioplegia reduces cytosolic and nuclear calcium and DNA fragmentation in the senescent myocardium. Annal Thorac Surg 58:1005–1011

Tsukube T, McCully JD, Federman M, Krukenkamp IB, Levitsky S (1996) Developmental differences in cytosolic calcium accumulation associated with surgically induced global ischemia: Optimization of cardioplegic protection and mechanism of action. J Thorac Cardiovasc Surg 112: 175–184

Tsukube T, McCully JD, Metz RM, Cook CU, Levitsky S (1997) Amelioration of ischemic calcium overload correlates with high energy phosphates in the senescent myocardium. Am J Physiol (Heart Circ Physiol) 42: H418–H427

Ullery BW, Peterson JC, Milla F, Wells MT, Briggs W, Girardi LN, Ko W, Tortolani AJ, Isom OW, Krieger KH (2008) Cardiac surgery in select nonagenarians: should we or shouldn't we? Ann Thorac Surg 85: 854–860

Vaccarino V, Lin ZQ, Casl SV, Mattera JA, Roumanis SA, Abramson JL (2003) Gender differences in recovery after coronary artery bypass surgery. J Am Coll Cardiol 41: 307–314

Valentijn AJ, Metcalfe AD, Kott J, Streuli CH, Gilmore AP (2003) Spatial and temporal changes in Bax subcellular localization during anoikis. J Cell Biol 162: 599–612

Vina J, Borras C, Gambini J, Sastre J, Pallardo FV (2005) Why females live longer than males? Importance of the upregulation of longevity-associated genes by oestrogenic compounds. FEBS Lett 579: 2541–2545

Vinten-Johansen J, Zhao ZQ, Jiang R, Zatta AJ (2005) Myocardial protection in reperfusion with postconditioning. Expert Rev Cardiovasc Ther 3: 1035–1045

Wakiyama H, Cowan DB, Toyoda Y, Federman M, Levitsky S, McCully JD (2002) Selective opening of mitochondrial ATP-sensitive potassium channels during cardiopulmonary bypass decreases apoptosis and necrosis in a model of acute myocardial infarction. Eur J Cardiothorac Surg 21: 424–433

Wenger NK, Marcus FI, O'Rourke RA (1987) Cardiovascular disease in the elderly. JACC 10: 80A–87A

White MY, Cordwell SJ, McCarron HC, Prasan AM, Craft G, Hambly BD, Jeremy RW (2005) Proteomics of ischemia/reperfusion injury in rabbit myocardium reveals alterations to proteins of essential functional systems. Proteomics 5: 1395–1410

Willems L, Zatta A, Holmgren K, Ashton KJ, Headrick JP (2005) Age-related changes in ischemic tolerance in male and female mouse hearts. J Mol Cell Cardiol 38: 245–256

Wright R, Levitsky S, Rao K, Holland C, Feinberg H (1978) Potassium cardioplegia. Arch Surg 113: 976–980

Xu X, Li J, Simons M, Li J, Laham RJ, Sellke FW (2001) Expression of vascular endothelial growth factor and its receptors is increased, but microvascular relaxation is impaired in patients after acute myocardial ischemia. J Thorac Cardiovasc Surg 121: 735–742

Zitser-Gurevich Y, Simchen E, Galai N, Mandel M, ISCAB Consortium (2002) Effect of perioperative complications on excess mortality among women after coronary artery bypass: the Israeli Coronary Artery Bypass Graft Study (ISCAB). J Thorac Cardiovasc Surg 123: 517–524

Zuppinger C, Eppenberger-Eberhardt M, Eppenberger HM (2000) N-cadherin: structure, function and importance in the formation of new intercalated disc-like cell contacts in cardiomyocytes. Heart Fail Rev 5: 251–257

Protection of the Right Heart

Gábor Szabó

6.1 Introduction

Until recently, right ventricular failure (RVF) was a relatively neglected medical condition. The right ventricle was considered as a moderately passive conduit between the systemic and pulmonary circulations. This belief was supported by studies showing that complete destruction of the right ventricular free wall in dogs had no detectable impairment on overall cardiac performance (Starr et al. 1943). However, precipitating factors for right ventricular failure are common in the clinical praxis of cardiothoracic surgery and intensive care medicine. These include increased pulmonary resistance, such as after cardiac transplantation, acute respiratory distress syndrome, the presence of left ventricular assist device, positive pressure mechanical ventilation and sepsis. Therefore it can be speculated that there is a higher incidence of right ventricular failure than generally recognized.

Right ventricular failure has a similar incidence as left sided heart failure, each affecting about 1 in 20 of the population (Health Central 2006). In particular, cardiocirculatory dysfunction associated with cardiopulmonary bypass and cardiac arrest is often caused by depressed right ventricular function (Boldt et al. 1989). This situation is aggravated by a transient pulmonary hypertension occurring frequently after cardiopulmonary bypass as a result of endothelial injury (Riedel 1999), decreased nitric oxide (Morita et al. 1996) or increased thromboxane (Cave et al. 1993) synthesis. The phenomenon of acute elevation of right ventricular afterload – as a main cause of early morbidity and mortality – in the setting of cardiac transplantation has been studied extensively (Szabó et al. 1998, 2005). These studies showed that the adaptation mechanisms of right ventricle to an increased afterload might be exhausted under certain pathophysiologic conditions.

The role of ischemia/reperfusion injury in perioperative right ventricular dysfunction has not been elucidated yet. A plethora of information is available on ischemia/reperfusion injury, nevertheless almost all functional studies focus on the left ventricle. Whether the protection of right ventricle requires different protection strategies during transient ischemia/reperfusion injury in the context of cardiac surgery remains to be clarified.

G. Szabó
Abteilung Herzchirurgie, Chirurgische Universitätsklinik, Im Neuenheimer Feld 110, 69120 Heidelberg, Germany

Right ventricular infarction, a more serious form of right heart ischemia is also a somewhat neglected area of cardiovascular research although the morbidity and mortality is considerably higher than left sided myocardial infarction. Typically, right ventricular infarction occurs when there is an occlusion of the right coronary artery proximal to the acute marginal branches, but it may also occur with an occlusion of the left circumflex artery in patients who have left-dominant coronary circulation. Although less common, occlusion of the left anterior descending artery may also result in infarction of the anterior right ventricle. The incidence of right ventricular infarction in association with left ventricular myocardial infarction ranges from 14 to 84%, depending on the population studied and the pathologic criteria (Ratliff and Hackel 1980). Isolated right ventricular infarction accounts for less than 3% of all cases of infarction but may result in considerable morbidity (Moreyra et al. 1986).

In the present chapter, the physiology and pathophysiology and protection strategies of the right heart will be discussed.

6.2
Physiology of the Right Ventricle

The primary function of the RV is to maintain a low right atrial pressure, optimising venous return and to provide sustained low-pressure perfusion through the lungs. To achieve this, the RV ejects blood quasi-continuously from the right atria to the lungs, continuously emptying the right atria. This "continuous" ejection is possible because of the favourable characteristics of the pulmonary vascular bed, which is a low pressure, low resistance and high compliance circuit with a pressure gradient of 5 mm Hg. Conversely, the left ventricle generates high-pressure pulsatile flow through arterial vessels with low compliance.

The RV is anatomically adapted for the generation of a sustained low-pressure perfusion. It comprises two anatomically and functionally different cavities, termed the sinus and the cone. The sinus generates pressure during systole and the cone regulates this pressure (Stephanazzi et al. 1997). Right ventricular contraction occurs in three phases; contraction of the papillary muscles, then movement of the right ventricular free wall towards the interventricular septum and, finally, contraction of the left ventricle causes a "wringing" which further empties the RV. The net effect is pressure generation in the sinus with a peristaltic motion starting at the apex moving towards the cone and, due to the compliance of the upper cone region of the thin-walled RV, the peak pressure is reduced and prolonged. Therefore, ejection into the pulmonary circulation is sustained until the RV has completed its emptying, end-diastolic pressure is minimal and venous return is optimal. Notably, right ventricular preload is determined by both the compliance of the RV and the venous return. The latter depends on the pressure gradient from the periphery to the right atria and the venous resistance. Despite the thin muscular walls of the RV, it adapts to small changes in venous return, such as those occurring during respiration, without altering cavity pressures or volumes. However, larger changes in venous return affect the right ventricular end-diastolic volume.

The pressure–volume characteristics for the RV differ markedly from those of the left ventricle (Fig. 1). The right ventricular pressure-volume loop has a more triangular shape

6 Protection of the Right Heart

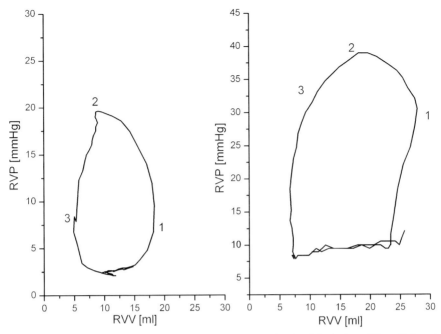

Fig. 1 Right ventricular pressure-volume loops are shown under physiological conditions (*left*) and after acute elevation of right ventricular afterload by pulmonary banding (*right*). The numbers indicate: (1) the opening of the pulmonary valve marking the start of the ejection phase; (2) the onset of relaxation; (3) the closing of the pulmonary valve marking the end of the ejection phase. Under physiological conditions, the pressure-volume loop is more triangular than that of the left ventricle. Ejection from the right ventricle starts early during the pressure increase and the isovolaemic contraction phase is consequently not well defined. It is interesting to note that ejection continued after the peak pressure during pressure decline (between points 2 and 3). After pulmonary banding, the pressure-volume loop resembles that of the left ventricle. There is a well defined end systolic shoulder and there is no ejection during the pressure decline

compared with that of the left ventricle, with only brief periods of isovolaemic contraction and relaxation. There is sustained ejection during pressure development that, more importantly, continues during pressure decline. This prolonged low-pressure emptying implies that right ventricular emptying is very sensitive to changes in afterload.

6.3
Pathophysiology of Right Heart Failure

6.3.1
Effects of an Elevation of Right Ventricular Afterload

In a patient with pulmonary hypertension, the right ventricular pressure-volume loop is not triangular and resembles that of the left ventricle (Fig. 1b). To compensate, the RV dilates to maintain the stroke volume, though the ejection fraction is reduced (Matthay et al. 1992), and the peristaltic contraction is lost, causing an accelerated increase in pulmonary artery pressure and flow.

The compensatory mechanisms maintaining RV performance during increased afterload are homeometric autoregulation with augmentation of contractility and the Frank-Starling mechanism (heterometric autoregulation) through increased myocardial stretch. The existence of the so-called homeometric autoregulation in the right heart was a matter of debate previously. For the first time, we described this autoregulatory mechanism in the right heart using pressure-length relationships (Szabó et al. 1998) and confirmed in a canine orthotopic heart transplantation model (Szabó et al. 2005) applying conductance catheter derived pressure-volume analysis. Meanwhile, the importance of right ventricular homeometric autoregulation was demonstrated in other settings of pulmonary constriction (Hon et al. 2001), respiratory distress syndrome (DeVroomen et al. 2001) and endotoxin shock (Lambermont et al. 2003). In a recent study (Wanthy et al. 2004) it was demonstrated that acute elevation of pulmonary resistance leads to an increase of right ventricular contractility regardless how pulmonary pressure has been increased (hypoxia vs. distal embolisation vs. pulmonary banding) and which species was used (goat vs. pig vs. dog).

Previously, we extensively studied, how pathophysiological states alters the adaptation of right ventricle to an increased afterload. In canine model of the brain dead organ donor (Szabó et al. 1998), the induction of brain death leads to myocardial injury and under certain circumstances hemodynamic instability. We observed that baseline right ventricular function remained unchanged but the adaptation potential of the right ventricle to an increased afterload became limited. There was no evidence of any deterioration in the RV pump performance in the brain dead animals: SW increased in the similar way as in the control group after a stepwise increase of afterload by pulmonary banding and cardiac output remained stable. However, the increase in SW, which was comparable to the control group, was associated with a greater rise in RVEDP. The greater rise in RVEDP with maintained pump performance compared to the control group indicates the utilization of the Frank-Starling mechanism as a primary form of adaptation to increased afterload (Fig. 2).

Similar phenomenon could be observed after cardioplegic arrest and reperfusion (Szabó et al. 2003), after orthotopic transplantation (Szabó et al. 2005) and in chronic heart failure (Szabó et al. 2006).

There are many possible mechanisms which may explain the missing homeometric regulation in different disease states. In the potential organ donor after brain death or after cardiac transplantation the sympathetic regulation of the heart is missing. The results of Rose et al. (Rose et al. 1983) using β-adrenergic blockade indicate that the β-adrenergic component of the sympathetic nervous system is important in the right ventricular response to afterload changes. Support for this could be found in the steeper rate of rise in the RVEDP with applied afterload during β-adrenergic blockade. The parallel increase of RVEDP with increased afterload after β-blockade was very similar to our observations in the brain death group. Abel and Waldhausen (1967) showed similar changes after surgical denervation of the heart.

Heart failure or acute dilation of the right ventricle lead to an enlargement of the right ventricle and thereby changes functional anatomy. In these ventricles the above described "peristaltic" contraction is lost causing an accelerated increase in pulmonary artery pressure and flow (Mebazaa et al. 2004). The altered ejection and contraction pattern may limit the inotropic adaptation potential of the right ventricle.

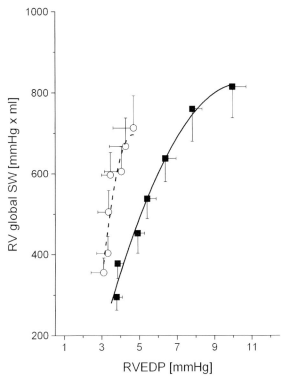

Fig. 2 Effects of increased right ventricular afterload on global cardiac function in healthy controls and in brain dead donors. Right ventricular stroke work (SW) is plotted against end-diastolic pressure (RVEDP) Significantly higher increase of right ventricular preload follows (i.e., RVEDP) elevations in RV afterload in the brain death fill (■, *solid line*) group in comparison to the controls (○, *dotted line*). Steeper increase of the SW-RVEDP relation in the control group indicates a higher contractile state than in the brain death group and in turn greater rise in RVEDP with maintained pump performance compared to the control group indicates the utilization of the Frank-Starling mechanism as a primary form of adaptation to increased afterload in brain dead donors

Alterations of cellular calcium handling and contractile proteins may also contribute to the changes of inotropic response (Alvarez et al. 1999). Several sarcolemmal proteins have been shown to be involved in the stretch-induced increase in the intracellular calcium transient, e.g., stretch activated calcium channels (Perez et al. 2001) and the Na^+/H^+ as well as the Na^+/Ca^{2+} exchanger. Stretching may also modulate the sarcoplasmatic reticulum calcium release via Pi(3) kinase-dependent phosphorylation of AKT-kinase stimulation of the endothelial NO-synthetase (Petroff et al. 2001). Thus, increasing muscle length may result in mechanisms increasing the sarcolemmal calcium influx, but may not support the sarcoplasmatic reticulum calcium uptake. In the chronically volume overloaded, the Anrep effect was almost absent. This finding is in concert with a novel study of Brixius et al. (2005), in which decreased homeometric autoregulation was associated with alterations of calcium homeostasis in muscle stripes isolated from terminally failing human hearts.

They proposed that both altered calcium sensitivity of the myofibrils and altered calcium supply to the myofibrils are responsible for these changes.

Beside direct changes of the right ventricular muscle mass (both anatomical and subcellular level) indirect factors may also contribute to altered response to afterload elevation. The changes of coronary perfusion may also play a role in the impairment of contractile response to increased afterload in the failing heart. In contrast to the left ventricle, in the right heart, coronary perfusion pressure is decoupled from afterload: an elevation of afterload is not associated with an automatic increase of coronary perfusion pressure. Even if coronary autoregulation is probably satisfactory to cover energy demand associated with increased contractility in the normal hearts, it may be exhausted earlier in the chronically volume overloaded animals after right ventricular afterload increase, especially at higher elevations. There are only very few data available even under physiological conditions which describe the effect of coronary perfusion pressure on right ventricular function and the results are controversial. Unfortunately we also do not have any evidence at this point.

If alterations in the phosphorylation status, mutations or alterations in the expressions of contractile proteins may influence contractile response remains also to be clarified.

6.3.2
Ventricular Interdependence

There is a high degree of ventricular interdependence due to the interaction of the inter-ventricular septum in the contraction of both ventricles, which is pronounced due to the existence of the pericardium (Visner et al. 1983). The load on a ventricle is dependent on the passive filling of the contralateral ventricle (Goto et al. 1985). Indeed, increases in the end-diastolic volume of the left ventricle are transmitted to the RV by movement of the inter-ventricular septum towards the right cavity, increasing the end-diastolic pressure of the RV. Similarly, when the right ventricular end-diastolic volume is increased, the inter-ventricular septum shifts towards the left cavity during diastole due to the restrictions imposed by the pericardium on the RV as the cavity volume increases. This leftward shift impairs the function of the left ventricle due to the reduction in left ventricular volume, decreasing both left ventricular filling and compliance, manifested as increased muscle stiffness. Thus, in a canine model, ischaemia and acute dilatation of the RV decreased the compliance of the left ventricle, resulting in decreased cardiac output due to a leftward shift in the inter-ventricular septum, which was attenuated by the opening of the pericardium.

Ventricular interdependence can also cause RVF during left ventricular assist device support. As the left ventricular assist device unloads the left ventricle, the inter-ventricular septum is shifted left. This alters the right ventricular compliance decreasing force and rate of contraction together with a decreased afterload and increased preload. In a healthy heart, cardiac output may be maintained but, with pre-existing pathology, the decrease in contractility may result in RVF (Santamore and Gray 1996). It is therefore crucial to support right ventricular function during the first days following insertion of a left ventricular assist device.

6.3.3
Vicious Cycle of Auto-Aggravation

Compared to the left ventricle, RVF progresses quickly from compensated to end-stage because of a vicious cycle of auto-aggravation. This is unique to the RV and is not a consequence of isolated left ventricular failure. The elevated right atrial and ventricular end-diastolic pressures eventually lead to an increased right ventricular end-diastolic volume, insufficiency of the tricuspid valve and regurgitation. The tricuspid insufficiency aggravates hepatic and kidney congestion and decreases cardiac output; the heart is, therefore, unable to maintain an adequate function. Thus, the auto-aggravation becomes an irreversible vicious cycle. In addition, decreased venous return to the left ventricle reduces left ventricular preload. This further exacerbates the situation as it causes decreased left ventricular output and systemic blood pressure and hence further impairment of organ perfusion, including the coronary arteries. This ischaemia further diminishes cardiac function and the cycle of worsening output, congestion and ischaemia continues. Therefore, any sign of RVF should result in immediate treatment to avoid the start of the vicious cycle of auto-aggravation.

6.3.4
Right Ventricular Infarction

The severity of the hemodynamic derangements associated with right ventricular infarction is related not only to the extent of right ventricular ischemia and consequent right ventricular dysfunction, but also to the restraining effect of the pericardium and the resulting interaction between the ventricles. Experimentally induced infarction of the right ventricle in dogs with an intact pericardium results in acute right ventricular dilatation and elevation of intrapericardial pressure caused by pericardial constraint (Calvin 1991). There is also a reduction in right ventricular systolic pressure, left ventricular end-diastolic size, cardiac output, and aortic pressure, as well as equalization of the right and left ventricular diastolic pressures. These hemodynamic abnormalities improve when the pericardium is incised.

It was initially postulated that, as right ventricular systolic function diminishes, the pressure gradient between the right atrium and the left becomes the driving force for pulmonary perfusion[5]. This mechanism seemed consistent with the clinical observations that the ischemic right ventricle is particularly sensitive to alterations in both preload and afterload (Fantidis et al. 1992). Augmented atrial contractility is necessary to overcome the increased myocardial stiffness associated with right ventricular infarction (Goldstein et al. 1990). Factors that impair filling of the noncompliant right ventricle, such as intravascular volume depletion due to the use of diuretics and nitrates or any diminution in atrial function caused by concomitant atrial infarction or the loss of atrioventricular synchrony, are likely to have profoundly adverse effects on hemodynamics in patients with large right ventricular infarctions. Interventricular forces, left ventricular function, and pericardial constraining factors are key determinants of the pathophysiology of right ventricular infarction.

6.4
Diagnosis of Right Heart Failure

Because the clinical presentation of right heart failure is very nonspecific, it is difficult to make a diagnosis of RVF by clinical examination alone. In the ICU scenario there are essentially two ways to assess right-sided function: pulmonary artery catheterization and echocardiography. The latter can be divided into transthoracic and transoesophageal methods. Magnetic resonance and radionuclide ventriculography are two other valid methods of assessment, but because their use at the bedside is difficult we do not consider them here. Electrocardiography and troponin assessment are also useful when MI is suspected.

6.4.1
Pulmonary Catheter

Pulmonary arterial catheterization is the most invasive and oldest method of assessing right-sided cardiac function. It is the only available continuous monitoring device that permits evaluation of the efficacy of treatment. In fact, it permits continuous monitoring of right atrial pressure, right ventricular pressure, pulmonary arterial pressure, pulmonary artery wedge pressure (PAWP), continuous cardiac output and mixed venous oxygen saturation. Modern PACs can also be used to measure RVEF and right ventricular end-diastolic volume. The diagnosis of RVF is made in situations of systemic hypotension, decreased cardiac output and low mixed venous saturation, and when there is a high right atrial pressure that is higher than a usually normal PAWP. Diagnosis of pulmonary artery hypertension (PAH) is easily made by assessing pulmonary pressure. Fluid loading in RVF can be dangerous.

New catheters permit continuous measurement of right ventricular end-diastolic volume index (RVEDVI) and RVEF. RVEDVI is a novel preload index. Interestingly, it seems that better understanding and use of RVEDVI result from its consideration together with RVEF, a parameter that can define the contractility status of the RV. Thus, it appears that correct interpretation of RVEDVI is strongly dependent on RVEF.

6.4.2
Echocardiography

The role of echocardiography has expanded in recent years. The most powerful characteristic of this technique is that it permits immediate qualitative diagnosis of heart disease, simultaneously allowing for estimation of flows and pressures. In order to explore the right side of the heart, transthoracic echocardiography can be used as long as the patient remains unventilated. When mechanical ventilation is being used, a transoesophageal approach should be used, resulting in better imaging. Transoesophageal echocardiography may confirm an initial suspicion of RVF (high central venous pressure) if absence of the respiratory variation in vena cava diameter is detected. Both transthoracic and transoesophageal echocardiography can be used to estimate pulmonary pressures. The qualitative aspect of echocardiography allows a diagnosis of RVF to be made along with recognition of its cause. It is possible to recognize RVF secondary to a PE, ARDS, or coronary obstruction simply by analyzing the different recorded images. Furthermore, echocardiography can assess both the right and left sides of the heart, and can allow measurements to be taken in systolic and diastolic phases that can be repeated, allowing intermittent monitoring of the efficacy of treatment.

6.5
Treatment Options: Protection Strategies

6.5.1
Treatment of Right Ventricular Infarction

Reperfusion of the occluded coronary is beneficial and should be a primary goal in proven right-sided infarction (Bowers et al. 1998). The goals suggested by Pfisterer (2003) for right ventricular infarction are as follows: early recognition, early reperfusion, maintenance of adequate preload, reduction in right ventricular afterload (inotropes, balloon counter-pulsation), preservation of right ventricular synchrony and avoidance of vasodilators, nitrates, morphine and β-blockers. It is very important that the left ventricular pressure be kept as close to normal as possible; this can help to restore the normal position of the interventricular septum and thereby improve contraction of the RV.

6.5.2
Fluid Management

Because of the interventricular dependence phenomenon, volume overload can dilate the RV so much that it may impair left ventricular function and the entire circulation. Conversely, adequate fluid loading is necessary to achieve optimal contraction. So what should happen at the bedside in a patient with RVF? In the ICU fluid therapy is often guided by fluid challenges. Mercat et al. (1999) discovered that, in acute pulmonary embolism, fluid challenges improve cardiac output, especially in patients with low baseline atrial pressure, who probably represent those in whom interventricular dependence is not yet playing a substantial role. Using mean pulmonary arterial pressure as a guide to fluid challenge, it seemed reasonable to stop filling beyond a mean pulmonary artery pressure of 30 mm Hg (Sibbald and Driedger 1983; Mebazaa et al. 2004).

Therefore, if a fluid challenge is followed by an increase in filling pressure without change in cardiac output, then fluid loading should be stopped. PAC is a valuable tool in this context because it allows the clinician to assess pulmonary pressure and CI on a continuous basis. The efficacy of fluid challenge can be monitored by watching changes in CI, SVI, RVEDVI, and RVEF. Fluid removal with diuretics or haemofiltration may then be beneficial (Mebazaa et al. 2004). However, fluid withdrawal is effected, it is important that cardiac output monitoring be used to assess the efficacy and safety of treatment.

6.5.3
Systemic Vasodilators

In the presence of elevated pulmonary vascular resistances, vasodilator therapy may reduce right ventricular afterload. This will improve right ventricular function by decreasing right ventricular myocardial oxygen consumption and improving left ventricular filling, which will eventually increase systemic blood pressure and right coronary artery perfusion pressure. This will, in turn, decrease right atrial pressure and organ congestion. Thus, intravenous vasodilators such as nitroglycerin, nitroprusside or prostaglandin E1 may be beneficial in patients with isolated RVF (Bundgaard et al. 1997; Vincent et al. 1992). However, systemic pulmonary vasodilators reverse hypoxic pulmonary vasoconstriction, worsening ventilation-perfusion matching within the lung and decreasing arterial oxygen saturation. Also, they decrease diastolic pressure, resulting in decreased right coronary artery perfusion, which worsens ischaemia (Packer 1985).

6.5.4
Inhaled Vasodilators

Inhalational vasodilatory agents, such as prostacyclin or its analogues and nitric oxide (NO), have a direct, selective effect on the pulmonary vasculature (Haraldsson et al. 1996; Galiè et al. 2003). NO diffuses into the pulmonary vascular smooth muscle cells, causing vasodilation, and its effects are localised as it rapidly binds to plasma proteins and haemoglobin. Following prolonged administration, rebound pulmonary hypertension has been frequently reported when NO inhalation is suddenly withdrawn. Despite its haemodynamic benefits, a survival advantage for patients with RVF who respond to NO therapy has not been proven (Borade et al. 1999).

An alternative to inhaled NO is inhaled prostacyclin (=prostaglandin I_2) (Langer et al. 2001). Besides its vasodilator properties, inhaled prostacyclin is the most potent platelet aggregation inhibitor known. Prostacyclin also stimulates endothelial release of NO, and vice versa. A potentially substantial advantage of inhaled, versus intravenous, prostacyclin is that rebound pulmonary hypertension after abrupt discontinuation has so far not been reported. This suggests that, in comparison with inhaled NO, inhaled prostacyclin may treat pulmonary hypertension more effectively.

6.5.5
Inotropes

Positive inotropic agents are also commonly used to improve right ventricular function. Left ventricular contraction assists the ejection from the RV; therefore, inotropic drugs that increase the contraction of the whole heart will improve right ventricular function both by directly enhancing right-sided contractility and by their effects on the entire myocardium. Positive inotropic agents – ß-adrenoceptor agonists and phosphodiesterase inhibitors – enhance myocardial contractility by increasing the intracellular calcium concentration in both ventricles due to their actions on cAMP. In the treatment of chronic heart failure patients, vasoactive ß-agonists produce a net increase in cardiac output providing a short-term benefit, but the increased contractility, working against a greater afterload, increases the workload of the heart, resulting in an increase in energy utilisation. Therefore, the oxygen consumption of the myocardium is increased without increasing oxygen supply, which may cause or worsen ischaemia and arrhythmias. Thus, the use of some of these agents has been associated with an increase in long-term mortality and, in the case of dobutamine, tolerance develops after a short time. The treatment of RVF is comparatively short and repeated dosing less common than for chronic heart failure, therefore tolerance may not be relevant in this setting. However, the effects of sympathomimetics on long-term outcome should perhaps be considered when selecting appropriate treatment for RVF.

A newer class of drugs, the calcium sensitisers, also improve cardiac function by increasing the contraction of the myocardium, but without significantly increasing intracellular calcium levels. Levosimendan, the first calcium sensitiser in clinical use, increases the sensitivity of the cardiac myofilaments to calcium during systole without affecting diastole. The increased calcium sensitivity increases the force and rate of contraction of the myocardium. Moreover, as it only increases systolic calcium sensitivity, it does not affect the relaxation kinetics, in contrast to the traditional inotropic drugs. Hence, levosimendan has no adverse effects on diastolic function and is not associated with a significant increase in myocardial oxygen consumption in patients with chronic heart failure (Ukkonen et al. 2000), though this result remains to be confirmed.

Levosimendan also induces dilatation of the pulmonary, systemic and coronary vasculature by activation of ATP-sensitive potassium channels resulting in a decreased systemic and pulmonary vascular resistance (Slawsky et al. 2000). This may cause under-perfusion of the myocardium, but the dilation of the coronary arteries results in improved myocardial blood flow (Ukkonen et al. 2000). Levosimendan improved haemodynamic performance and decreased the risk of worsening heart failure and mortality in different heart failure populations, compared with dobutamine or placebo (Follath et al. 2002). Indeed, all the evidence described comes from studies in patients with chronic heart failure, and the direct effects of levosimendan on RVF are currently unproven. However, from its known effects, including a demonstrated improvement in right ventricular contractile efficiency (Ukkonen et al. 2000), beneficial effects in RVF may also be expected. The haemodynamic effects of levosimendan may be sustained for days, or even weeks, due to an active metabolite with a half-life of over 3 days (Kivikko et al. 2002).

6.5.6
Vasopressors

Vasopressors directly increase arterial blood pressure and improve coronary artery perfusion, though also increasing afterload. They may be critical in the treatment of RVF, preventing the vicious cycle by improving right coronary artery perfusion and right ventricular contraction (Ghignone 1984). Norepinephrine, a potent α-adrenergic-agonist is recommended to improve right coronary artery perfusion pressure and right ventricular function, and it is more effective than phenylephrine, another selective α-adrenergic agonist. In patients with septic shock, norepinephrine increased mean arterial pressure, with a moderate increase in mean pulmonary artery pressure, improving right coronary artery perfusion pressure and right ventricular contraction (Ghignone 1984).

6.5.7
Novel Protective Strategies: Do They Already Exist?

The aforementioned therapeutic options aim to treat right ventricular dysfunction at the time as right heart failure is already exists. To our best knowledge, no established therapy exists which specifically protects the right heart from injury. Especially in cardiac surgery a preventive approach would be favourable to reduce mortality and morbidity associated with right ventricular failure.

A major cause of right ventricular failure is ischemia/reperfusion injury especially in the context of cardiac transplantation where extended times of ischemia occur. In general, any therapeutic option which reduce ischemia/reperfusion injury would improve right ventricular functions well.

We do believe however that some class of drugs may have a high potential to become agents which are used specifically to right heart protection. As mentioned above the stimulation of the NO/cGMP pathway is a central therapeutic option in the treatment of right heart failure caused by pulmonary hypertension. Phosphodiesterase-5 inhibitors such as Sildenafil or Vardenafil were initially used in the management of erectile dysfunction. Its effect is greater on pulmonary than on the systemic circulation because it inhibits phosphodiesterase-5 more than its analogous isoforms. This particular enzyme is expressed mainly in pulmonary vessels and in the corpora cavernosa. Oral administration has proven to reduce hypoxia-induced PAH. In cardiac surgery sildenafil has been used to wean patients from inhaled iNO (Mychaskiw et al. 2001). Its synergistic effects both with iNO and iloprost have been demonstrated.

Currently, we could show in a canine model of cardiopulmonary bypass, that pharmacologic preconditioning with vardenafil prevents the impairment of right ventricular contractility after ischemia/reperfusion (Szabó et al. 2010). As a preconditioning mimicking and pulmonary dilator agent phosphodiesterase-5 inhibitors may have an important role in the prevention of right ventricular dysfunction especially in the field of cardiac surgery.

6.6
Conclusions

It is now evident that the RV plays a pivotal role in haemodynamic homeostasis, and changes in right ventricular function can have profound effects on the pulmonary and systemic circulation. Therefore, it is important that RVF is diagnosed quickly and accurately before it degenerates into the vicious cycle of auto-aggravation with tricuspid deficiency, worsening cardiac ischaemia and multiple organ congestion. Diagnosis should include an assessment of the patient and the use of diagnostic tools that also enable the clinician to follow the progress of treatment.

The management of RVF should focus on restoring right ventricular function with the treatment dictated by the underlying aetiology. The primary cause of RVF should be corrected wherever possible. The right ventricular afterload should be reduced, if necessary, by decreasing the pulmonary artery pressure (e.g., by administering pulmonary vasodilators such as inhaled NO or prostacyclin) and limiting plateau pressure in mechanically ventilated patients, the preload should be increased cautiously with volume loading and an adequate right coronary artery perfusion maintained. Positive inotropic agents have an important role in the treatment of RVF by improving cardiac output and coronary perfusion. However, traditional inotropic drugs increase myocardial contractility by their sympathomimetic action at the expense of increasing myocardial intracellular calcium concentration and oxygen consumption. Calcium sensitisers, specifically levosimendan, enhance contractility without increasing myocardial oxygen consumption. If the beneficial effects that have been observed in chronic heart failure patients are validated in RVF in clinical studies, this class of agents may represent a valuable addition to the clinician's armamentarium for the management of this condition.

References

Abel FL, Waldhausen JA (1967) Effects of alterations in pulmonary vascular resistance on right ventricular function. J Thor Cardiovas Surg 54:886–894

Alvarez BV, Perez NG, Ennis IL et al. (1999) Mechanisms underlying the increase in force and Ca^{2+} exchange that follow stretch of cardiac muscle: a possible explanation of the Anrep effect. Circ Res 85:716–722

Boldt J, Kling D, Moosdorf R, Hempelmann G (1989) Influence of acute volume loading on right ventricular function after cardiopulmonary bypass. Crit Care Med 17:518–522

Borade S, Christenson J, O'Connor M, Lavoie A, Pohlman A, Hall JB (1999) Response to inhaled nitric oxide in patients with acute right heart syndrome. Am J Respir Crit Care Med 159:571–579

Bowers TR, O'Neill WW, Grines C, Pica MC, Safian RD, Goldstein JA (1998) Effect of reperfusion on biventricular function and survival after right ventricular infarction. N Engl J Med 338:933–940

Brixius K, Reuter H, Bloch W, Schwinger RHG (2005) Altered hetero- and homeometric autoregulation in the terminally failing human heart. Eur J Heart Fail 2:29–35

Bundgaard H, Boesgaard S, Mortensen SA, Arendrup H, Aldershvile J (1997) Effect of nitroglycerin in patients with increased pulmonary vascular resistance undergoing cardiac transplantation. Scand Cardiovasc J 31:339–342

Calvin JE (1991) Optimal right ventricular filling pressures and the role of pericardial constraint in right ventricular infarction in dogs. Circulation 84:852–861

Cave AC, Manche A, Derias NW, Hearse DJ (1993) Thromboxane A2 mediates pulmonary hypertension after cardiopulmonary bypass in the rabbit. J Thorac Cardiovasc Surg. 106:959–967

DeVroomen H, Steendijk P, Lopes Cardoso RH, Brouwers HH, Van Bel F, Baan J (2001) Enhanced systolic function of the right ventricle during respiratory distress syndrome in neonatal lambs. Am J Physiol 280:392–400

Fantidis P, Castejon R, Fernandez Ruiz A, Madero-Jarabo R, Cordovilla G, Sanz Galeote E (1992) Does a critical hemodynamic situation develop from right ventriculotomy and free wall infarct or from small changes in dysfunctional right ventricle afterload? J Cardiovasc Surg (Torino) 33:229–234

Follath F, Cleland JG, Just H, Papp JG, Scholz H, Peuhkurinen K, Harjola VP, Mitrovic V, Abdalla M, Sandell EP, Lehtonen L (2002) Efficacy and safety of intravenous levosimendan compared with dobutamine in severe low-output heart failure (the LIDO study): a randomised double-blind trial. Lancet 20:196–202

Galiè N, Manes A, Branzi A (2003) Prostanoids for pulmonary arterial hypertension. Am J Respir Med 2:123–137

Ghigone M, Girling L, Prewitt RM (1984) Effect of increased pulmonary vascular resistance on right ventricular systolic performance in dogs. Am J Physiol 246:H339–43.

Goldstein JA, Barzilai B, Rosamond TL, Eisenberg PR, Jaffe AS (1990) Determinants of hemodynamic compromise with severe right ventricular infarction. Circulation 82:359–368

Goto Y, Yamamoto J, Saito M, Haze K, Sumiyoshi T, Fukami K, Hiramori K (1985) Effects of right ventricular ischemia on left ventricular geometry and the end-diastolic pressure-volume relationship in the dog. Circulation 72:1104–1114

Haraldsson A, Kieler-Jensen N, Ricksten SE (1996) Inhaled prostacyclin for treatment of pulmonary hypertension after cardiac surgery or heart transplantation: a pharmacodynamic study. J Cardiothorac Vasc Anesth 10:864–868

Health Central (2006) General encyclopedia – right-sided heart failure http://www.healthcentral.com/mhc/top/000154.cfm. Accessed January 2006

Hon JK, Steendijk P, Khan H, Wong K, Yacoub M (2001) Acute effects of pulmonary artery banding in sheep on right ventricle pressure-volume relations: relevance to arterial switch operation. Acte Physiol Scand 172:97–106

Kivikko M, Antila S, Eha J, Lehtonen L, Pentikainen PJ (2002) Pharmacokinetics of levosimendan and its metabolites during and after a 24-hour continuous infusion in patients with sever heart failure. Int J Clin Pharmacol Ther 40:465–471

Lambermont B, Ghuysen A, Kohl P, et al. (2003) Effects of endototxin shick on right ventricular systolic function and mechanical efficiency. Cardiovasc Res. 59:412–418

Langer F, Wendler O, Wilhelm W, Tscholl D, Schafers HJ (2001) Treatment of a case of acute right heart failure by inhalation of iloprost, a long-acting prostacylclin analogue. Eur J Anaestheiol 18:770–773

Matthay RA, Arroliga AC, Wiedemann HP, Schulman DS, Mahler DA (1992) Right ventricular function at rest and during exercise in chronic obstructive pulmonary disease. Chest 101: 255S–262S

Mebazaa A, Karpati P, Renaud E, Algotsson L (2004) Acute right ventricular failure – from pathophysiology to new treatments. Int Care Med 30:185–196

Mercat A, Diehl JL, Meyer G, Teboul JL, Sors H (1999) Hemodynamic effects of fluid loading in acute massive pulmonary embolism. Crit Care Med 27:540–544

Moreyra AE, Wajnberg A, Byra W, Kostis JB (1986) Nondominant right coronary artery occlusion presenting with isolated right ventricular infarction and ventricular fibrillation. Am J Med 81:146–148

Morita K, Ihnken K, Buckberg GD, Sherman MP, Ignarro LJ (1996) Pulmonary vasoconstriction due to impaired nitric oxide production after cardiopulmonary bypass. Ann Thorac Surg. 61:1775–1780

Mychaskiw G, Sachdev V, Heath BJ (2001) Sildenafil (Viagra) facilitates weaning of inhaled nitric oxide following placement of a biventricular-assist device. J Clin Anesth 13:218–220

Packer M (1985) Vasodilator therapy for primary pulmonary hypertension. Limitations and hazards. Ann Intern Med 103:258–270

Perez NG, de Hurtado MC, Cingolani HE (2001) Reverse mode of Na^+–Ca^{2+} exchange after myocardial stretch: underlying mechanism of the slow force response. Circ Res 88:376–382

Petroff MG, Kim SH, Pepe S et al. (2001) Endogenous nitric oxide mechanisms mediate the stretch dependence of Ca^{2+} release in cardyomyocytes. Nat Cell Biol 3:867–373

Pfisterer M (2003) Right ventricular involvement in myocardial infarction and cardiogenic shock. Lancet 362:392–394

Ratliff NB, Hackel DB (1980) Combined right and left ventricular infarction: pathogenesis and clinicopathologic correlations. Am J Cardiol 45:217–221

Riedel B (1999) The pathophysiology and management of perioperative pulmonary hypertension with specific emphasis on the period following cardiac surgery. Int Anesthesiol Clin 37:55–79

Rose CE, Van Benthuysen K, Jackson JT, Tucker CE, Kaiser DL, Grover RF, Weil JV (1983) Right ventricular performance during increased afterload impaired by hypercapnic acidosis in coscious dogs. Circ Res 52:76–84

Santamore WP, Gray LA (1996) Left ventricular contributions to right ventricular systolic function during LVAD support. Ann Thorac Surg 61:350–356

Sibbald WJ, Driedger AA (1983) Right ventricular function in acute disease states: pathophysiologic considerations. Crit Care Med 11:339–345

Slawsky MT, Colucci WS, Gottlieb SS (2000) Acute hemodynamic and clinical effects of levosimendan in patients with severe heart failure. Circulation 102:2222–2227

Starr I, Jeffers WA, Meade RH (1943) The absence of conspicuous increments of venous pressure after sever damage to the RV of the dog, with discussion of the relation between clinical congestive heart failure and heart disease. Am Heart J 26:291–301

Stephanazzi J, Guidon-Attali C, Escarment J (1997) Right ventricular function: physiological and pathophysiological features. Ann Fr Anesth Reanim 16:165–186

Szabó G, Buhmann V, Andrsi TB, Stumpf N, Bährle S, Kékesi V, Hagl S, Szabó C, Juhsz-Nagy A (2003) Poly-ADP-Ribose polymerase (PARP)-inhibition protects against myocardial and endothelial reperfusion injury after hypothermic cardiac arrest. J Thorac Cardiovasc Surg 126:651–658

Szabó G, Radovits T, Veres G, Krieger N, Loganathan S, Sandner P, Karck M, Lichtenberg A (2010) Vardenafil protects against myocardial and endothelial injury after cardiopulmonary bypass. Eur J Cardiothorac Surg

Szabó G, Sebening C, Hagl C, Tochtermann U, Vahl CF, Hagl S (1998) Right ventricular function after brain death: response to an increased afterload. Eur J Cardiothorac Surg 13:449–459

Szabó G, Soos P, Bährle S, Radovits T, Weigang E, Kékesi V, Merkely B, Hagl S (2006). Adaptation of the right ventricle to an increased afterload in the chronically volume overloaded heart. Ann Thorac Surg. 82:989–895

Szabó G, Soós P, Heger U, Flechtenmacher C, Bahrle S, Zsengeller Z, Szabo C, Hagl S (2005) Poly (ADP-ribose) polymerase inhibition attenuates biventricular reperfusion injury after orthotopic heart transplantation. Eur J Cardiothorac Surg. 27:226–234

Ukkonen H, Saraste M, Akkila J, Knuuti MJ, Karanko M, Iida H, Lehikoinen P, Nagren K, Lehtonen L, Voipio-Pulkki LM (2000) Myocardial efficiency during levosimendan infusion in congestive heart failure. Clin Pharmacol Ther 68:522–531

Vincent JL, Carlier E, Pinsky MR, Goldstein J, Naeije R, Lejeune P, Brimioulle S, Leclerc JL, Kahn RJ, Primo G (1992) Prostaglandin E1 infusion for right ventricular failure after cardiac transplantation. J Thorac Cardiovasc Surg 103:33–39

Visner MC, Arentzen CE, O'Conner MJ, Larson EV, Anderson RW (1983) Alterations in left ventricular three-dimensional dynamic geometry and systolic function during acute right ventricular hypertension in the conscious dog. Circulation 67:353–365

Wanthy P, Pagnamenta A, Vassili F, Nacija R, Brimioulle S (2004) Right ventricular adaptation to pulmonary hypertension: an interspecies comparison. Am J Physiol 286:H1441–H1447

Protection of the Failing Heart

Bruno K. Podesser, Karola Trescher, and Wolfgang Dietl

7.1 Background and Definition

In the developed world, heart failure (HF) is the only cardiovascular disease that is steadily increasing. Both in Europe and the United States about five million people live with the diagnosis of HF, and about 400,000 patients are newly diagnosed every year. Several epidemiological and demographic factors contribute to this trend (Hunt et al. 2005). (a) The development of HF goes parallel with the rise in life expectancy. HF is clearly a disease of the elderly because 80% of the patients admitted to hospital with the diagnosis of HF are older than 65 years (Katz and Konstam 2008). (b) Improved treatment regimens of acute myocardial infarction (MI) increase survival. Consequently, the survivors are more likely to develop HF due to postMI remodelling later in their life (Opie 2003). (c) A general increase in pharmacological and non-pharmacological treatment modalities heightens the number of patients living with HF and/or reaching later stages of HF.

According to the ACC/AHA guidelines (Hunt et al. 2005), HF is defined as a clinical syndrome characterized by specific symptoms (dyspnea and fatigue) in the medical history and signs (edema, rales) on the physical examination. It is a complex clinical syndrome that can result from any structural or functional cardiac disorder that impairs the ability of the ventricle to fill with or eject blood. Coronary artery disease, hypertension, valve disease and dilated cardiomyopathy are the most frequent causes of HF in Europe and North America. In about 30% of the patients affected, a genetic disorder is the underlying cause of HF. The clinical syndrome can be triggered by disorders of the pericardium, myocardium, endocardium, or great vessels; the majority of patients, however, suffer from heart failure symptoms due to an impaired LV function (Hunt et al. 2005).

B.K. Podesser (✉), K. Trescher, and W. Dietl
Department of Cardiac Surgery, Landesklinikum St. Pölten, Propst Führerstr. 4, 3100 St. Pölten, Austria
The Ludwig Boltzmann Cluster for Cardiovascular Research, Medical University of Vienna, Vienna, Austria
e-mail: bruno.podesser@meduniwien.ac.at

7.2
The Surgeon's Challenge

The increasing incidence of HF has direct consequences for the everyday business of a cardiac surgeon. Besides cardiac transplantation, cardiac surgeons are confronted with chronic HF patients in two situations: (1) during conventional revascularization and valve surgery in patients with reduced LV function and (2) in so-called "heart failure" surgery like ventricular restoration surgery or ventricular assist devices. Myocardial protection is essential in all these surgical procedures to reduce operative mortality and to improve long-term outcome. Protection strategies have to meet the special needs of failing ventricles, which result from their pathophysiological characteristics. In this chapter, we will discuss the different ways how HF develops, and describe the consequences of HF on the myocardium as well as the vascular system, including the activation of the neurohumoral response. We will try to provide evidence that revascularization or correction of underlying valve pathology improves outcome in patients with HF. Finally we will identify potential therapeutic regimens to improve perioperative myocardial protection in patients with HF.

7.3
Development of HF

7.3.1
LaPlaces Law

Every insult to the heart induces adaptive and maladaptive responses of both the heart itself and the whole circulation to maintain cardiac function. Anatomically, there is a characteristic change in cardiac geometry and structure seen as either concentric hypertrophy (as a result of pressure overload) or eccentric hypertrophy (due to volume overload, to regional wall motion abnormality or dilated cardiomyopathy). With the progression of disease, the ventricular chamber changes from an elliptical to a spherical shape. This different anatomical shape is accompanied by alterations of contractile state, metabolic state, vascular resistance, oxygen demand and energy metabolism. In the beginning, most of these changes are an attempt to maintain normal cardiac function as seen in the state of compensated hypertrophy where they normally precede the onset of clinical symptoms. In the long run, however, they become maladaptive and result in progressive remodelling with ventricular dilation (Katz and Konstam 2008).

Due to the changes in ventricular geometry, failing hearts have increased regional myocardial work with consequent increase in oxygen demand while higher vascular resistance decreases vascular flow. This results in a mismatch of oxygen demand and supply. Increase of LV chamber diameter and change from an elliptical to a spherical shape leads to an increase in wall tension according to the law of LaPlace:

$$\text{Wall Stress} = \frac{\text{LV Pressure} \times \text{LV Radius}}{\text{Wall Thickness}}$$

7.3.2
Pressure and Volume Overload

In pressure overload, typically seen in patients with aortic valve stenosis or severe systemic hypertension, LV pressure developed by the myocardium must increase to overcome the resistance to the ejection of blood. Thereby, as LV pressure rises, wall tension increases and the transmural force tends to dilate the ventricle. As an adaptive mechanism, the myocardium hypertrophies in a concentric way to reduce wall stress by increasing wall thickness. Initially, increased wall stress can be normalized, but this compensation has a cost resulting in impaired diastolic function and higher susceptibility to ischemia. The thickened myocardium is characterized by an increase in stiffness, impaired relaxation and decreased early diastolic filling.

In case of volume overload, such as in aortic or mitral regurgitation, volume load of the ventricle increases the size of the LV cavity causing a rise in wall stress. Adaptively, the myocardium develops eccentric hypertrophy and wall thickness rises to reduce wall stress – to a lesser extent, however, than in concentric hypertrophy (Opie 2003). Compensated hypertrophy progresses to HF when increased radius and wall stress cannot be overcome by further increase of wall thickness.

The mechanisms behind the progression from compensation to decompensation are not fully understood – a major problem, and probably the driving force, might be the imbalance of oxygen supply. Repeated phases of ischemia and the activation of the local neuro-humoral response – especially of angiotensin II and aldosterone – lead to fibrosis by collagen formation and cause irreversible damage of myocardial structure. Enhanced fibrosis of the ventricle further raises myocardial stiffness and causes a disproportionally high increase of wall tension, which increases oxygen demand and aggravates the imbalance in oxygen demand and supply, which further enhances fibrosis.

7.4
Consequences of HF

7.4.1
Vascular Dysfunction

Another pathophysiological issue in HF is vascular dysfunction (VD), which impairs both systemic and myocardial perfusion (Fang and Marwick 2002; Bauersachs and Widder 2008). It is difficult to distinguish whether VD is an etiological agent and/or an epiphenomenon: VD due to systemic adaptive response to an impaired cardiac function interacts with VD as a result of comorbidities such as diabetes, hypertension or renal failure.

Consequently, progressive impairment of vascular function is a vicious circle. The clinical implications of VD are diverse: on the one hand it can be used to monitor HF therapy because flow mediated dilation of the radial and brachial arteries correlate inversely with mortality in HF patients (Fischer et al. 2005; Katz and Konstam 2008). On the other hand, VD can be a target for adjuncts to cardioplegia to enhance myocardial protection by improving endothelial protection and function.

According to current knowledge, the endothelium is an active organ releasing vasoconstrictive and vasodilative substances and is a target of circulating neurotransmitters, hormones, and physiologic stimuli. Vascular tone itself is regulated by endothelium-derived factors like nitric oxide (NO), prostacyclin and endothelium-derived hyperpolarizing factor. Dysfunction of the coronary and systemic vessels is caused by an imbalance of constrictive and dilative factors.

7.4.2
Neurohumoral Defense Reaction

In HF, several factors contributing to endothelial dysfunction could be identified with the major determinant being reduced bioavailability of NO (Bauersachs and Widder 2008). The hemodynamic abnormalities associated with reduced LV pump function lead to a neurohumoral response as "defense reaction" aimed to maintain systemic blood pressure (Katz et al. 2005). This reaction is very similar to the "physiologic" reaction seen during exercise or hemorrhage but it becomes pathological because of its duration – in HF it normally persists for a lifetime. The mediators of this neurohumoral reaction lead to vasoconstriction.

7.4.2.1
The Renin-Angiotensin-Aldosterone System

One of the major players in neurohumoral activation is the renin-angiotensin-aldosterone system (RAAS). Increased levels of angiotensin II in both the heart and the vessel wall increase formation of reactive oxygen species in the vasculature, which is at least partially mediated by aldosterone generated from both the adrenal glands and a local aldosterone system within the myocardium and the vessel wall. Reactive oxygen species lead to the reduction of NO bioavailability by reacting rapidly with NO and forming peroxynitrite. In addition to that, the activation of RAAS leads to an enhanced breakdown of bradykinin, which consequently reduces NO release, prostacyclin and prostglandin E2 (Opie 2003; Katz et al. 2005).

7.4.2.2
The Endothelin System

Another key factor activated during neurohumoral defense is the strong vasoconstrictor endothelin (ET) and especially its isoform ET-1. The effects of ET-1 are mediated by two receptor subtypes: ET_A receptors induce vasoconstriction and cellular proliferation, and are mainly located in the medial smooth muscle cell layers of blood vessels, and atrial and ventricular myocardium (Hosoda et al. 1991). ET_B receptors are located on endothelial cells and to some extent on vascular smooth muscle cells and macrophages. Activation of the ET_B receptor leads to the release of NO and prostacyclin (Ogawa et al. 1991). It is known that ET_A-receptor density is enhanced in chronic heart failure and that there is a massive release of ET-1 after ischemia/reperfusion from the injured tissue. Via activation of the ET_A receptor ET-1 plays an important role in vascular dysfunction during HF and after acute ischemia/reperfusion injury (Pernow and Wang 1997; Benigni and Remuzzi 1999). Experimental studies using both selective ET_A (Gonon et al. 2000; Gourine et al. 2001), and unselective ET_A/ET_B (Wang et al. 1995; Gonon et al. 2000) receptor blockers demonstrated a close relationship between the endothelin system and NO and suggest that the protective effect of endothelin receptor blockade in ischemia/reperfusion injury is mediated by enhancing the bioavailability of NO.

7.4.2.3
Systemic and Local Inflammation

Finally, an important part of the neurohumoral response is the systemic and local inflammatory reaction associated with the progression of HF (Katz et al. 2005). Similar to the hemodynamic defense reaction, inflammatory mediators may be beneficial during the initial development of HF, such as in infarct healing or the initiation of hypertrophy, but they become detrimental when they persist. Besides their participation in the heart's adaptive and maladaptive growth response or cell damage, cytokines contribute to vascular dysfunction especially via generation of oxidative stress. Particularly tumor necrosis factor (TNF)-α is elevated in the plasma of HF patients (Seta et al. 1996) and its level correlates with the severeness of endothelial dysfunction. It could be demostrated that TNF-α downregulates NO production (Yoshizumi et al. 1993; Agnoletti et al. 1999).

7.4.3
Additional Factors Affecting NO Bioavailability, Myocardial Perfusion and Contractility

7.4.3.1
Reduction of Shear Stress

The reduction of shear stress on the luminal surface of the endothelium as a consequence of impaired LV function leads to reduced bioavailable NO; hence, shear stress is the most important physiological stimulus for NO generation. Endothelial dysfunction results in an increase in vascular resistance and impairs myocardial perfusion. In addition to endothelial dysfunction several other factors contribute to a further impairment of coronary flow and myocardial blood supply.

7.4.3.2
Geometrical Changes of the Ventricle

Both concentric and eccentric hypertrophy increase the length of the coronary artery segments penetrating the wall originating from the large vessels located in the epicardium. As stated above, according to the law of La Place, wall stress increases as diameter increases; therefore, subendocardial regions in particular are underperfused. Additionally, diffusion of metabolic substrates and oxygen is reduced by a decreased capillary density and increased intercapillary distance. This leads to a mismatch between blood supply and demand of the failing myocardium in general. As a consequence, an imbalance between energy production and consumption can be seen in failing hearts – termed as energy starvation. In biopsies of failing myocardium, a reduced content of high-energy phosphates (ATP, ADP, AMP, and phosphocreatine) can be found. As mitochondrial energy production is impaired in the failing heart due to mitochondrial damage and gene abnormalities. The failing heart resembles the type of energy production of the fetal heart. The particular pathogenic mechanism of reduced high-energy levels is still not fully understood. Its consequence, however, is that the increased energy demand of the failing, working myocardium cannot be sufficiently met.

7.5
Evidence that Revascularization in Patients with HF and Coronary Artery Disease is Useful

Left ventricular dysfunction can be defined as ischemic cardiomyopathy with left ventricular ejection fraction of less than 35%, and coronary artery disease (CAD) defined angiographically as 70% narrowing of one or more coronary arteries. Although there are clear indications (class I) for revascularization in patients with heart failure, these are limited to patients with demonstrable angina and significant CAD (Eagle et al. 2004). The management of patients with ischemic cardiomyopathy without angina remains challenging mostly because of the paucity of data from randomized controlled studies.

7.5.1
Theoretical Rationale Behind Revascularization

The most commonly proposed mechanism by which revascularization may improve outcome in patients with ischemic left ventricular dysfunction has been the recruitment of hibernating or stunned myocardium in an effort to improve overall myocardial contractility. In support of this has been the suggestion that 60% of patients with ischemic cardiomyopathy have viable myocardium (Bax et al. 2004). Hibernation has been described as a downregulation of contractile function due to chronic reduction in myocardial perfusion or coronary flow reserve. The myocardium, although functionally non-contractile, is metabolically active. Most of the energy utilized by the ventricle is expended in contractile work, with oxygen requirements for contractility far exceeding those needed for myocyte survival, and thus contractility decreases to the point that is sustainable by oxygen availability. The demonstration of metabolism implies the presence of viable myocardium with contractile potential upon restoration of blood flow. Revascularization potentially resuscitates dormant viable myocardium and results in the recruitment of contractile reserve, thereby improving contractility, wall motion abnormalities, pump function, and symptoms, and serves to protect previously functioning myocardium from further ischemia. The demonstration of viability in failing ventricles is, therefore, particulary important in selecting patients who will benefit from revascularization, and in predicting the extent of benefit from revascularization (Bell et al. 1992; Bax et al. 2005). Conversely, completeness of revascularization is vital in patients with left ventricular dysfunction (Bell et al. 1992). However, one should note that viable myocardial segments may not always improve after revascularization for reasons that include severe cellular damage, extensively remodelled and dilated ventricles, subendocardial scar, the duration of hibernation, incomplete revascularization, ischemic damage during revascularization resulting in the transition of viable myocardium into scar tissue, and graft occlusion or restenosis (Bell et al. 1992; Bax et al. 2005).

Stunned myocardium is defined as a state of transient ischemic contractile dysfunction due to a reversible (short) ischemic event. When blood flow is restored, function recovers completely after time. The mechanisms involved include calcium overload, the generation of oxygen-derived free radicals, excitation–contraction uncoupling as a result of sarcoplasmic reticulum dysfunction, insufficient energy production, impaired myocardial perfusion, and decreased myofilament sensitivity to calcium.

Additional mechanisms of benefit in patients receiving late reperfusion therapy include a reduction of ventricular remodelling, diminished ventricular instability reducing the incidence of arrhythmias, and the provision of collaterals to other territories in the event of further coronary artery occlusion (Centurión 2007). In addition to myocardial recruitment, revascularization can prevent further functional decline and reduce the risk of sudden death independent of functional improvement (Samady et al. 1999).

7.5.2
Coronary Artery Bypass Graft Surgery Versus Medical Therapy

The role of coronary artery bypass graft (CABG) surgery in patients with ischemic cardiomyopathy is based entirely on observational data. There are no currently published randomized controlled trials in patients with ischemic cardiomyopathy and predominant symptoms of HF. What has been demonstrated is that CABG surgery is feasible in selected patients suffering from ischemic cardiomyopathy with short-term mortality that is probably higher than in patients with normal left ventricular function. The reported operative mortality has varied tremendously (5–30%) depending on the severity of left ventricular dysfunction and the co-morbidities (Phillips et al. 2007). In addition, CABG surgery has been shown to improve HF symptoms in 60–90% of patients (Baker et al. 1994). Surprisingly, some have suggested that operative mortality did not depend on concomitant procedures such as mitral valve surgery or ventricular remodelling (Fedoruk et al. 2007).

In a large retrospective study comparing CABG with medical management of ischemic cardiomyopathy, O'Connor et al. (O'Connor et al. 2002) were able to show that, after adjusting for preoperative differences, patients undergoing revascularization had better 1, 5, and 10-year survival rates and that these findings were independent of the presence of angina. Similar findings have been duplicated from the Duke Database suggesting a significant survival benefit of CABG in patients with CAD and low ejection fraction compared with medical management (Smith et al. 2006).

7.5.3
CABG Versus PCI

Although PCI has become the predominant treatment for angina, no data or guidelines exist for patients with ischemic cardiomyopathy without angina (Phillips et al. 2007). Some old registry data demonstrate a poor outcome, a significant risk of emergeny CABG (18%), and a high risk of acute closure of the treated vessel (8%) (Holmes et al. 1993). The recent APPROACH trail included 2,538 patients with diagnosed HF and CAD. CABG showed the best survival compared to PCI (Tsuyuki et al. 2006). Similarly, some large registry data on patients with CAD and low ejection fraction appear to favour CABG over PCI (Hannan et al. 2005).

7.5.4
Viability Testing

The detection of viable myocardium is based on the identification of preserved metabolism by positron emission tomography, cell membrane integrity by thallium-201 or technetium-99 m single-photon emission computed tomography, as well as maintained contractility by dobutamine stress echocardiography or magnetic resonance imaging, tissue doppler imaging and strain rate imaging (Bax et al. 2004; Chareonthaitawee et al. 2005).

Several retrospective studies and meta-analyses have consistently shown improved survival in patients with ischemic but viable myocardium who subsequently underwent revascularization (Allman et al. 2002; Bourque et al. 2003a, b). The results of the various pooled analyses are stratified in four areas of clinical interest: recovery of regional function, recovery of global left ventricular function, improvement of symptoms and exercise capacity, and prognosis. The A meta-analysis of Allman et al. (Allman et al. 2002) demonstrated an 80% reduction in annual mortality when patients with ischemic but viable myocardium underwent surgery compared with medical therapy. In contrast, in those without demonstrable viability, the mortality rates were similar. Carluccio and associates (Carluccio et al. 2006) showed that left ventricular systolic dysfunction in the presence of hibernation leads to left ventricular remodelling. Revascularization in this scenario results in reverse remodelling with a reduction in left ventricular end diastolic volume and left ventricular end systolic volume, a reduction in left ventricular sphericity, and an increase in left ventricular ejection fraction.

Limitations of the aforementioned retrospective studies include selection bias, evolution of imaging and surgical techniques over time, and suboptimal medical therapy in earlier series, leading to misinterpretation of the data, and disparate recommendations for diagnostic testing and revascularization in these patients. Non-invasive imaging to detect myocardial viability thus currently constitutes a class IIa recommendation in patients with HF and known CAD. Viability testing aids decision-making in patients without angina, borderline coronary anatomy, or significant co-morbidities (Phillips et al. 2007). It is important to note that there appears to be tremendous variability between institutions depending on the availability and experience with these techniques, making any guidelines difficult to generalize.

In summary, there seems to be no question that revascularization is superior to medical therapy in patients with ischemic cardiomyopathy. When it comes to the choice of method of revascularization, most clinicians tend to approach each patient individually. Besides favoring CAGB, one must include the number of co-morbidities favoring PCI and the completeness of revascularization favoring CABG (Chareonthaitawee et al. 2005). Finally, whenever valvular lesions or ventricular aneurysms are present, these lesions can only be addressed by surgery (Fedoruk et al. 2007). Viability testing is vital for the decision-making, planning and prognosis in these patients. Hopefully, in the near future, data from randomized control studies such as the currently conducted STICH trial (Surgical Treatment for IsChemic Heart failure), assigning patients with predominantly heart failure symptoms randomly to surgery versus medical management, will clarify the role of CABG and lead to clearer guidelines.

7.6
Evidence that High Risk Valvular Surgery in Patients with HF Improves Outcome

7.6.1
Aortic Stenosis and Severely Reduced LV Function

Aortic valve replacement is possible in patients with severe aortic stenosis (AS) and HF. Preoperatively, one should try to identify the presence or absence of ventricular dysfunction, using dobutamine echocardiography. It is then possible to differentiate between those patients with severe AS, left ventricular dysfunction and a low transvalvular gradient with irreversible myocardial damage versus those with reversible myocardial dysfunction (Monin et al. 2001). Thus, aortic valve area is determined in two different flow states (baseline and stress). Those patients with flow-dependent AS will demonstrate a decrease in valve area with the increased flow caused by the enhanced inotropic mediated contractile state, and in these patients the transvalvular gradient will increase. This group of patients is more likely to benefit from AV replacement as the depressed contractility is due to increased afterload (afterload mismatch).

Only a few studies are available that specifically looked at patients with severe AS and LV dysfunction. Powell and colleagues (Powell et al. 2000) reported an operative mortality of 18%, with prior myocardial infarction being a risk factor for perioperative mortality, and

Table 1 Summary of clinical studies investigating the outcome of aortic valve replacement for patients with severe left ventricular dysfunction

Author	Year	n	EF (%)	Operative mortalitiy	5-years survival
Bonow	1985	50	37	0	63%
Acar	1996	46	<40	6.5	84%
Klodas	1997	128	NR	7.8	72%
Chaliki	2002	43	35	14	72%
Rothenburger	2003	20	<30	NR	74%

NR not recorded

it is suggested to avoid AV replacement in these patients. Also, high mortality rates have been reported by others (Table 1) of between 7 and 21%, but with improved functional capacity in most survivors. Long-term survival, when available, was comparable at 5 years to that of cardiac transplantation. Based on these reports and the beneficial effects on long-term survival, it is a general consensus that patients with severe AS and LV dysfunction, in whom contractile reserve can be documented, should undergo AV replacement.

7.6.2
Aortic Regurgitation and Severely Reduced LV Function

Improper coaptation of the aortic valve leaflets results in regurgitant blood flow during diastole, leading to both volume and pressure overload. The underlying pathologies are degenerative and/or calcific disease, rheumatic disease, endocarditis, hypertension, connective tissue diseases such as Marfan's syndrome, and traumatic injuries. The common final pathway is eccentric hypertrophy and myocardial fibrosis due to chronic underperfusion resulting either from increased wall stress or diminished diastolic coronary perfusion leading to progressive symptoms of HF.

The natural history of patients with chronic aortic regurgitation (AR) and reduced EF and/or NYHA III/IV symptoms under medical treatment is extremely poor with a 5-year survival between 20 and 66% (Dujardin et al. 1999). In the current AHA guidelines for these patients there are no special recommendations. More generally, AVR is recommended in patients with AR when they become symptomatic or if they are asymptomatic but show signs of ventricular deterioration, reduction of EF, a diastolic diameter approaching 75 mm or an end-systolic diameter approaching 55 mm. From the scarce sources in the literature, there is a consensus that AVR can be performed even in patients with severely reduced LV function and AR, providing an acceptable operative mortality of 8–15% leading to a 5-year survival of about 70%. Although operative mortality in this special cohort is doubled compared to patients with normal LV function, the 5-year survival is similar to the outcome of cardiac transplantation. Therefore, the replacement of the valve is still considered to be the first-line treatment whereas cardiac transplantation is a valuable option, if replacement fails.

7.6.3
Mitral Valve Surgery and Severely Reduced LV Function

Secondary or functional mitral valve regurgitation worsens symptoms and prognosis in patients with left ventricular dysfunction of both ischemic and non-ischemic etiology. Volume overload resulting from mitral valve regurgitation leads to ventricular dilatation and dysfunction, which subsequently leads to further regurgitation and annular dilatation. Thus, a vicious cycle is perpetuated whereby ventricular dilatation potentiates mitral regurgitation and mitral regurgitation potentiates ventricular dilatation.

Surgical repair of mitral regurgitation has been introduced successfully by Bolling et al. (Bolling et al. 1995). By eliminating the positive feedback of mitral regurgitation, it was suggested that this would reduce ventricular volume and allow the ventricle to recover. It is important to note that this surgical approach has to be performed at an early stage before irreversible dysfunction occurs. Most importantly, valve repair rather than replacement has to be chosen because only repair guarantees preservation of the subvalvular apparatus and thereby preserves ventricular shape and geometry, decreases wall stress and improves systolic and diastolic function (Cohn et al. 1995; Kouris et al. 2005). In addition, mortality and outcome data of mitral valve repair according to the principles of Carpentier (Carpentier 1983) have been proven to be superior in preserving geometric integrity compared to replacement. In most instances, functional regurgitation is the consequence of insufficient coaptation of the mitral valve leaflets resulting in a central jet. The underlying pathologies are ventricular enlargement as described above, annular dilatation, loss of systolic contraction, and papillary muscle dysfunction. The surgical correction aims to overcome the ventricular or subvalvular defect by a valvular correction, namely the implantation of a rigid or semi-rigid ring to increase the surface of coaptation to 7 mm and to stabilize annular dilatation. In more complex pathologies, more complex repair procedures can be applied (Carpentier 1983).

The study by Bolling and coworkers (Bolling et al. 1995) was the first to report the outcome of remodelling mitral annuloplasty with a flexible posterior ring in 16 patients with severe CHF and mitral regurgitation. Functional capacity was improved in all patients, ejection fraction rose from 16 to 25% and regurgitant volume was significantly reduced. Most importantly, it was demonstrated that a major corrective surgery could be performed safely in patients with severely depressed LV function. From the current literature, we know that survival rates after 5 years are about 70%. Interestingly, when the subvalvular apparatus is preserved during mitral valve replacement similar results were also obtained by others (David et al. 1995; Rothenburger et al. 2002). In conclusion, functional mitral regurgitation is commonly observed in patients with severe left ventricular dysfunction regardless of etiology. The presence of even mild regurgitation is associated with poor long-term prognosis. Early and intermittent results of annuloplasty result in partial reversal of LV remodelling and symptomatic improvement.

7.7 Potential Therapeutic Regimens To Improve Perioperative Myocardial Protection in Patients with HF

The ultimate goal of myocardial protection is reducing demand and maintaining supply of total energy. Content of high-energy phosphates in myocardial biopsies, taken at the end of ischemia, is an important and representative marker for the quality of myocardial protection i.e. cardioplegic strategies. Impaired myocardial perfusion due to ventricular and/or vascular remodelling leads to an inhomogenous distribution of cardioplegia to different regions of the heart. This is especially true for the subendocardial region, leading to inferior protection of the heart, which then might aggravate energy starvation.

7.7.1 Optimizing Delivery of Cardioplegia

In recent experimental studies, the differences in subendocardial flow were investigated in failing and control hearts in the beating and arrested state. Failing hearts showed a lower overall subendocardial flow compared to controls that could be increased only when the failing heart was arrested (Athanasuleas et al. 2001). A consecutive paper from the same group (Kassab et al. 2006) showed that pulsatile application of cardioplegia significantly improved subendocardial blood flow in failing hearts. Delivery of cardioplegia in a pulsatile fashion could be a new option for homogeneous delivery of cardioplegia, which demands further clinical evaluation.

7.7.2 Optimizing Temperature of Cardioplegia

The possible enhanced protective role of warm (normothermic) blood versus cold blood cardioplegia is controversial. The study from Emory University (Martin et al. 1994) described the largest series of patients comparing either continuous warm blood cardioplegia with systemic normothermia or intermittent cold, oxygenated crystalloid cardioplegia with systemic hypothermia in patients receiving elective CABG. Aortic cross-clamp time was significantly longer with warm cardioplegia, due to the reduced visibility in the continuously perfused hearts. Myocardial injury was similar but neurological complications were significantly higher in the warm group. A subsequent study (Rashid et al. 1995) compared two groups of patients operated by the same surgeon. The patients had significantly reduced LV function and were randomized to receive either moderate hypothermic cardiopulmonary bypass and antegrade cold-blood cardioplegia followed by intermittent retrograde cold blood cardioplegia. The second group of patients had normothermic cardiopulmonary bypass with continuous infusion of retrograde warm-blood cardioplegia. Again, there was no significant difference in outcome between the two groups.

Perioperative mortality and myocardial infarction was not significantly different between groups. The only major difference was that 88% of the patients in warm cardioplegia groups had spontaneous restoration of sinus rhythm as compared to 49% in the cold cardioplegia group ($p < 0.001$).

In our own institution, we compared normothermic cardiopulmonary bypass with antegrade and retrograde intermittent warm-blood cardioplegia to moderate hypothermic cardiopulmonary bypass with antegrade and retrograde intermittent cold-blood cardioplegia in all adult cardiac patients. Similar to Rashid's study, we did not see any difference in myocardial or neurologic injury but a significantly higher rate of spontaneous restoration of sinus rhythm in the warm group (79%) as compared to 45% in the cold group (unpublished data).

The safety of warm cardioplegic regimens is also underlined by data from donor hearts treated with warm-blood cardioplegia. The results of warm retrograde blood cardioplegia reperfusion led to improved initial recovery of transplanted hearts (Carrier et al. 1996). Similarly, in pediatric cardiac surgery the results from a retrospective analysis of more than 200 cases revealed that intermittent warm blood cardioplegia during prolonged aortic cross-clamp time is safe (Durandy et al. 2008) Finally, the information gained from hypertrophied hearts, undergoing aortic valve replacement, with myocardial protection of cold antegrade induction alone or in combination with a terminal warm-blood cardioplegia (hot-shot) is helpful (Ascione et al. 2008). The hot-shot did not add any additional benefit to antegrade cold-blood cardioplegia in preventing myocardial injury in these 36 randomized patients with LV hypertrophy. Nevertheless, the hot-shot reduced ischemic stress in the right ventricle by significantly increasing ATP content by 20 min of reperfusion (opening of the aortic cross clamp).

7.7.3
Cardioplegia Beyond Myocardial Protection: The Need of Endothelial Protection

Cardioplegic solutions have been developed to protect myocardial cells against ischemia and consecutive reperfusion. However, during recent years the endothelium has been identified to be the first site of injury. Ischemia/reperfusion leads to a decrease in NO concentration leading to the no- or low-reflow phenomenon, which has been described as "endothelial stunning" (Mizuno et al. 1997). This can lead to "myocardial stunning", a temporary reduction in myocardial function. However, in failing hearts with almost no reserve, this temporary dysfunction can lead to serious functional impairment with the need for increased inotropic support, prolonged operation time and intensive care stay or increased mortality.

Therefore, we have recently been examining pharmacologic additives to cardioplegia that can overcome the critical phase of ischemia and early reperfusion by either donating NO directly or by increasing the availability of NO. In an experimental model of ischemic heart failure by coronary ligation in the adult male rat, we (Podesser et al. 2002) have studied NO donors such as ACE-inhibitors and ET_A-receptor blockers. The first group of drugs block the degradation of bradykinin (thereby increasing NO levels) whereas the latter selectively block endothelin A receptors (thereby acting as a vasodilator, leaving NO-releasing endothelin B receptors untouched) (Trescher et al. 2009). When administered with blood cardioplegia during ischemia, the ACE-inhibitor quinaprilat was able to increase postischemic recovery of cardiac output, external heart work, coronary flow and the myocardial content of high-energy phosphates. Left ventricular enddiastolic pressure as a surrogate of diastolic function was significantly decreased, when quinaprilat was administered during ischemia (Fig. 1). Additionally, the ultrastructural evaluation revealed significant protection at the level of the mitochondria in the treatment group.

In contrast, when quinaprilat was administered only during reperfusion, these results were diminished, indicating the importance of starting protection at the time of ischemia.

Similarly, in the same model of ischemic cardiomyopathy with severely reduced cardiac function the selective ET_A-receptor blocker TBC-3214Na administered with blood cardioplegia during ischemia led to improved postischemic recovery of hemodynamic and metabolic parameters (Fig. 2). When chronically treated with the same drug, hearts also showed improved functional recovery but coronary flow recovery did not differ from controls, indicating the importance of acute treatment in these failing hearts (Trescher et al. 2009).

Finally, again in the same experimental model, we have tested a new crystalloid cardioplegic solution that has been developed from the original HTK solution, commonly known as Bretschneider's cardioplegic solution (Custodiol®, Dr. Köhler Chemie, Germany). In contrast to the original solution, modifications have been made by including the iron chelation binders, LK-614 and deferoxamine. Additionally, histidine was partially replaced by N-α-acetyl-L-histidine to address the problem of histidine-induced iron-dependent toxicity. When compared with the original HTK, the new HTKn46 shows improved myocardial protection with respect to functional outcome and metabolism (unpublished data).

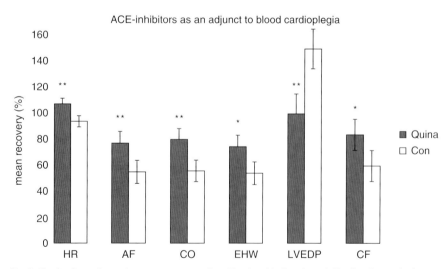

Fig. 1 Ex vivo hemodynamic measurements after 60 min of ischemia and 45 min of reperfusion on the red cell perfused isolated working heart. Mean recovery (%) of preischemic baseline values of heart rate (HR), aortic flow (AF), cardiac output (CO), external heart work (EHW), left ventricular enddiastolic pressure (LVEDP) and coronary flow (CF) of hearts treated with quinaprilat (*dark squares*) versus control (*open squares*). *p < 0.05 and **p < 0.01 versus control; All data are presented as mean ± SEM. Modified according to Podesser et al. (2002)

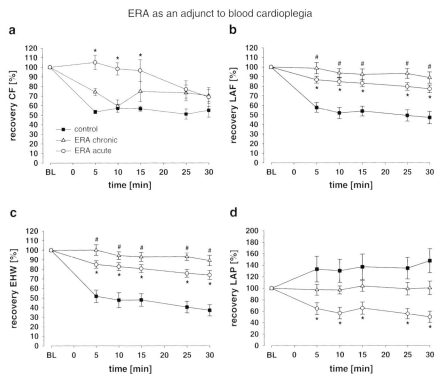

Fig. 2 Ex vivo hemodynamic measurements after 60 min of ischemia on the red cell perfused isolated working heart. Evaluation of the ETA-receptor antagonist TBC-3214Na administered as adjunct to cardioplegia (ERA acute) and during the development of HF (ERA chronic), respectively, versus Control. Data of the reperfusion period are presented as recovery values (percentage of baseline). (**a**) Recovery of Coronary Flow ERA acute versus both ERA chronic and Control groups; *$p < 0.01$; (BL = Baseline). (**b**) Recovery of Cardiac Output ERA acute versus Control group, *$p < 0.01$; ERA chronic versus Control group; #$p < 0.01$. (**c**) Recovery of External Heart Work (Cardiac Output × LV systolic pressure). ERA acute versus Control group, *$p < 0.01$; ERA chronic versus Control group; #$p < 0.01$. (**d**) Recovery of diastolic Left Atrial Pressure *$p < 0.01$ ERA acute versus Control group. All data are presented as mean ± SEM. Modified according to Trescher et al. (2009)

In summary, the possibility to improve cardioplegic solutions by NO-donating compounds is now well established in experimental studies, but the clinical efficacy has yet to be determined.

7.7.4 Mechanical Considerations

Besides careful patient selection, optimisation of cardioplegic delivery mode and temperature, it is appropriate to comment on mechanical support. The prophylactic use of the intraaortic balloon pump (IABP) has been advocated, especially by the Yale group

(Elefteriades et al. 1993). They reported their results in 83 patients with ejection fractions of less than 30%, who underwent CABG. The IABP was placed therapeutically in 19% of these patients and prophylactically in 43%, resulting in a total usage of IABP in 62% of patients with reduced LV function. Hospital mortality was 8.4%, but was 3.3% in patient, who did not require admission to the intensive care unit prior to surgery. In 3 patients, vascular complications occurred, with one of these patients requiring a limb resection. However, it was concluded that the early use of IABP prior to anesthesia and surgery improved outcome and survival in this high-risk group (Elefteriades et al. 1993).

7.7.5
Perioperative Conditioning of the Heart

Recently, a new drug, the calcium sensitizer levosimendan, has caught the attention of cardiac anaesthesiologists and surgeons. Initially used by cardiologists in acute decompensated heart failure (Slawsky et al. 2000), this drug has anti-ischemic and vasodilatory effects mediated via the opening of sarcolemmal and mitochondrial ATP-sensitive potassium channels (Du Toit et al. 1999). These properties suggest a potential application in the clinical situation where cardioprotection would be beneficial, such as cardiac surgery. In a study that randomised 106 patients undergoing elective CABG either to levosimendan or placebo prior to initiation of bypass (Tritapepe et al. 2009), the intubation time and length of stay on the ICU were significantly reduced, as was the postoperative serum levels for troponin I, and the cardiac index was higher in the levosimendan group.

In patients with reduced LV function, Eriksson and coworkers (Eriksson et al. 2009) were able to show, in 60 patients undergoing CABG in a randomised, placebo-controled study, that levosimendan significantly enhanced primary weaning from bypass compared to placebo. The need for additional inotropic and mechanical support was reduced. These beneficial effects of levosimendan were shown (Yilmaz et al. 2009) to occur on both the left and right ventricles when compared to dobutamine. In 40 consecutive patients with acute decompensated systolic heart failure with severely impaired right ventricular function, the effects were evaluated by echocardiography after the infusion of levosimendan or dobutamine; ejection fraction improved and systolic pulmonary artery pressure decreased significantly with both treatments but longitudinal systolic function of the tricuspid annulus improved significantly better in patients with levosimendan compared to dobutamine. Furthermore, urine output improved in the levosimendan treated patients, providing evidence that this new drug offers more beneficial effects compared to dobutamine in these specific patients.

Because the effects of levosimendan are long lasting, the conditioning can be started some days before surgery. In this case, close hemodynamic monitoring should guarantee an optimal success and less vasodilation during the surgical procedure that, in some cases, may require counter-regulatory vasoconstrictors. However, in patients with reduced LV function and aortic stenosis, the preoperative loading can be dangerous and should be avoided, due either to a decrease in afterload with a consecutive decrease in coronary perfusion pressure, or because an increase in contractility can lead to a critical aortic stenosis and acute decompensation.

7.8
Conclusion

HF is the common final pathway of different heart diseases. The number of patients diagnosed with heart failure is constantly increasing and represents a challenge for cardiologists and cardiac surgeons. The latter are confronted with patients with severely reduced pump function that require operations on their heart valves or coronary arteries. To keep the operative risk low, one has to understand the pathophysiologic background in order to take special precautions. Independent of pressure or volume overload, representing the classic prototypes that induce ventricular remodelling, it is the Law of LaPlace that helps in the understanding of the correlation between wall thickness, radius and pressure. The bottom line is that the heart tries to keep the wall stress constant as long as possible, (1) to perform the pressure-volume work with the highest possible degree of efficacy and the lowest energy consumption and (2) to guarantee optimal myocardial perfusion during diastole. The rationale for revascularization and valve operations in patients with severely reduced LV function is discussed. Finally, possible ways to support the heart during cardiac surgery are presented. These include changes in the delivery of cardioplegia using pulsatile perfusion. The temperature of cardioplegia can be modified and vasodilative substances such as NO donors can be used to improve postischemic recovery. Prophylactic use of IABP is another asset to reduce or bridge postoperative myocardial dysfunction. The preoperative conditioning by levosimendan is stressed as a valuable alternative. Although some of the proposed solutions have only been used preclinically, the given armamentarium should provide cardiac surgeons with tools that allow them to operate on patients with reduced cardiac function at an acceptable operative risk.

References

Agnoletti L, Curello S, Bachetti T, Malacarne F, Gaia G, Comini L, Volterrani M, Bonetti P, Parrinello G, Cadei M, Grigolato PG, Ferrari R (1999) Serum from patients with severe heart failure downregulates eNOS and is proapoptotic: role of tumor necrosis factor-alpha. Circulation 100: 1983–1991

Allman KC, Shaw LJ, Hachamovitch R, Udelson JE (2002) Myocardial viability testing and impact of revascularization on prognosis in patients with coronary artery disease and left ventricular dysfunction: a meta-analysis. J Am Coll Cardiol 39: 1151–1158

Ascione R, Suleiman SM, Angelini GD (2008) Retrograde hot-shot cardioplegia in patients with left ventricular hypertrophy undergoing aortic valve replacement. Ann Thorac Surg 85: 454–458

Athanasuleas CL, Stanley AW, Buckberg GD, Dor V, DiDonato M, Blackstone EH (2001) Surgical anterior ventricular endocardial restoration (SAVER) in the dilated remodeled ventricle after anterior myocardial infarction. RESTORE group. Reconstructive Endoventricular Surgery, returning Torsion Original Radius Elliptical Shape to the LV. J Am Coll Cardiol 37: 1199–1209

Baker DW, Jones R, Hodges J, Massie BM, Konstam MA, Rose EA (1994) Management of heart failure. III. The role of revascularization in the treatment of patients with moderate or severe left ventricular systolic dysfunction. JAMA 272: 1528–1534

Bauersachs J, Widder JD (2008) Endothelial dysfunction in heart failure. Pharmacol Rep 60: 119–126

Bax JJ, Poldermans D, Elhendy A, Boersma E, van der Wall EE (2005) Assessment of myocardial viability by nuclear imaging techniques. Curr Cardiol Rep 7: 124–129

Bax JJ, van der Wall EE, Harbinson M (2004) Radionuclide techniques for the assessment of myocardial viability and hibernation. Heart 90 Suppl 5: v26–v33

Bell MR, Gersh BJ, Schaff HV, Holmes DR, Fisher LD, Alderman EL, Myers WO, Parsons LS, Reeder GS (1992) Effect of completeness of revascularization on long-term outcome of patients with three-vessel disease undergoing coronary artery bypass surgery. A report from the Coronary Artery Surgery Study (CASS) Registry. Circulation 86: 446–457

Benigni A, Remuzzi G (1999) Endothelin antagonists. Lancet 353: 133–138

Bolling SF, Deeb GM, Brunsting LA, Bach DS (1995) Early outcome of mitral valve reconstruction in patients with end-stage cardiomyopathy. J Thorac Cardiovasc Surg 109: 676–682; discussion 682–683

Bourque JM, Hasselblad V, Velazquez EJ, Borges-Neto S, O'connor CM (2003a) Revascularization in patients with coronary artery disease, left ventricular dysfunction, and viability: a meta-analysis. Am Heart J 146: 621–627

Bourque JM, Velazquez EJ, Borges-Neto S, Shaw LK, Whellan DJ, O'Connor CM (2003b) Radionuclide viability testing: should it affect treatment strategy in patients with cardiomyopathy and significant coronary artery disease? Am Heart J 145: 758–767

Carluccio E, Biagioli P, Alunni G, Murrone A, Giombolini C, Ragni T, Marino PN, Reboldi G, Ambrosio G (2006) Patients with hibernating myocardium show altered left ventricular volumes and shape, which revert after revascularization: evidence that dyssynergy might directly induce cardiac remodeling. J Am Coll Cardiol 47: 969–977

Carpentier A (1983) Cardiac valve surgery–the "French correction". J Thorac Cardiovasc Surg 86: 323–337

Carrier M, Leung TK, Solymoss BC, Cartier R, Leclerc Y, Pelletier LC (1996) Clinical trial of retrograde warm blood reperfusion versus standard cold topical irrigation of transplanted hearts. Ann Thorac Surg 61: 1310–4; discussion 1314–1315

Centurión OA (2007) The open artery hypothesis: beneficial effects and long-term prognostic importance of patency of the infarct-related coronary artery. Angiology 58: 34–44

Chareonthaitawee P, Gersh BJ, Araoz PA, Gibbons RJ (2005) Revascularization in severe left ventricular dysfunction: the role of viability testing. J Am Coll Cardiol 46: 567–574

Cohn LH, Kowalker W, Bhatia S, DiSesa VJ, St John-Sutton M, Shemin RJ, Collins JJ (1995) Comparative morbidity of mitral valve repair versus replacement for mitral regurgitation with and without coronary artery disease. 1988. Updated in 1995. Ann Thorac Surg 60: 1452–1453

David TE, Armstrong S, Sun Z (1995) Left ventricular function after mitral valve surgery. J Heart Valve Dis 4 Suppl 2: S175–S180

Du Toit EF, Muller CA, McCarthy J, Opie LH (1999) Levosimendan: effects of a calcium sensitizer on function and arrhythmias and cyclic nucleotide levels during ischemia/reperfusion in the Langendorff-perfused guinea pig heart. J Pharmacol Exp Ther 290: 505–514

Dujardin KS, Enriquez-Sarano M, Schaff HV, Bailey KR, Seward JB, Tajik AJ (1999) Mortality and morbidity of aortic regurgitation in clinical practice. A long-term follow-up study. Circulation 99: 1851–1857

Durandy YD, Younes M, Mahut B (2008) Pediatric warm open heart surgery and prolonged cross-clamp time. Ann Thorac Surg 86: 1941–1947

Eagle KA, Guyton RA, Davidoff R, Edwards FH, Ewy GA, Gardner TJ, Hart JC, Herrmann HC, Hillis LD, Hutter AM, Lytle BW, Marlow RA, Nugent WC, Orszulak TA, Antman EM, Smith SC, Alpert JS, Anderson JL, Faxon DP, Fuster V, Gibbons RJ, Gregoratos G, Halperin JL, Hiratzka LF, Hunt SA, Jacobs AK, Ornato JP (2004) ACC/AHA 2004 guideline update for coronary artery bypass graft surgery: summary article. A report of the American College of

Cardiology/American Heart Association Task Force on Practice Guidelines (Committee to Update the 1999 Guidelines for Coronary Artery Bypass Graft Surgery). J Am Coll Cardiol 44: e213–e310

Elefteriades JA, Tolis G, Levi E, Mills LK, Zaret BL (1993) Coronary artery bypass grafting in severe left ventricular dysfunction: excellent survival with improved ejection fraction and functional state. J Am Coll Cardiol 22: 1411–1417

Eriksson HI, Jalonen JR, Heikkinen LO, Kivikko M, Laine M, Leino KA, Kuitunen AH, Kuttila KT, Peräkylä TK, Sarapohja T, Suojaranta-Ylinen RT, Valtonen M, Salmenperä MT (2009) Levosimendan facilitates weaning from cardiopulmonary bypass in patients undergoing coronary artery bypass grafting with impaired left ventricular function. Ann Thorac Surg 87: 448–454

Fang ZY, Marwick TH (2002) Vascular dysfunction and heart failure: epiphenomenon or etiologic agent? Am Heart J 143: 383–390

Feduruk LM, Tribble CG, Kern JA, Peeler BB, Kron IL (2007) Predicting operative mortality after surgery for ischemic cardiomyopathy. Ann Thorac Surg 83: 2029–2035, discussion 2035

Fischer D, Rossa S, Landmesser U, Spiekermann S, Engberding N, Hornig B, Drexler H (2005) Endothelial dysfunction in patients with chronic heart failure is independently associated with increased incidence of hospitalization, cardiac transplantation, or death. Eur Heart J 26: 65–69

Gonon AT, Gourine AV, Pernow J (2000) Cardioprotection from ischemia and reperfusion injury by an endothelin A-receptor antagonist in relation to nitric oxide production. J Cardiovasc Pharmacol 36: 405–412

Gourine AV, Gonon AT, Pernow J (2001) Involvement of nitric oxide in cardioprotective effect of endothelin receptor antagonist during ischemia-reperfusion. Am J Physiol Heart Circ Physiol 280: H1105–H1112

Hannan EL, Racz MJ, Walford G, Jones RH, Ryan TJ, Bennett E, Culliford AT, Isom OW, Gold JP, Rose EA (2005) Long-term outcomes of coronary-artery bypass grafting versus stent implantation. N Engl J Med 352: 2174–2183

Holmes DR, Detre KM, Williams DO, Kent KM, King SB, Yeh W, Steenkiste A (1993) Long-term outcome of patients with depressed left ventricular function undergoing percutaneous transluminal coronary angioplasty. The NHLBI PTCA Registry. Circulation 87: 21–29

Hosoda K, Nakao K, Hiroshi-Arai Suga S, Ogawa Y, Mukoyama M, Shirakami G, Saito Y, Nakanishi S, Imura H (1991) Cloning and expression of human endothelin-1 receptor cDNA. FEBS Lett 287: 23–26

Hunt SA, Abraham WT, Chin MH, Feldman AM, Francis GS, Ganiats TG, Jessup M, Konstam MA, Mancini DM, Michl K, Oates JA, Rahko PS, Silver MA, Stevenson LW, Yancy CW, Antman EM, Smith SCJ, Adams CD, Anderson JL, Faxon DP, Fuster V, Halperin JL, Hiratzka LF, Jacobs AK, Nishimura R, Ornato JP, Page RL, Riegel B (2005) ACC/AHA 2005 Guideline Update for the Diagnosis and Management of Chronic Heart Failure in the Adult: a report of the American College of Cardiology/American Heart Association Task Force on Practice Guidelines (Writing Committee to Update the 2001 Guidelines for the Evaluation and Management of Heart Failure): developed in collaboration with the American College of Chest Physicians and the International Society for Heart and Lung Transplantation: endorsed by the Heart Rhythm Society. Circulation 112: e154–e235

Kassab GS, Kostelec M, Buckberg GD, Covell J, Sadeghi A, Hoffman JI (2006) Myocardial protection in the failing heart: II. Effect of pulsatile cardioplegic perfusion under simulated left ventricular restoration. J Thorac Cardiovasc Surg 132: 884–890

Katz AM, Konstam MA (2008) Heart failure: pathophysiology, molecular biology, and clinical management (Heart Failure: Pathophysiology, Molec Biol & Clin Mgt). Lippincott Williams & Wilkins

Katz SD, Hryniewicz K, Hrljac I, Balidemaj K, Dimayuga C, Hudaihed A, Yasskiy A (2005) Vascular endothelial dysfunction and mortality risk in patients with chronic heart failure. Circulation 111: 310–314

Kouris N, Ikonomidis I, Kontogianni D, Smith P, Nihoyannopoulos P (2005) Mitral valve repair versus replacement for isolated non-ischemic mitral regurgitation in patients with preoperative left ventricular dysfunction. A long-term follow-up echocardiography study. Eur J Echocardiogr: 6: 435–442

Martin T, Craver J, Gott J, Weintraub W, Ramsay J, Mora C, Guyton R (1994) Prospective, randomized trial of retrograde warm blood cardioplegia: myocardial benefit and neurologic threat. Ann Thorac Surg 57: 298 http://ats.ctsnetjournals.org/cgi/content/abstract/57/2/298

Mizuno A, Baretti R, Buckberg GD, Young HH, Vinten-Johansen J, Ma XL, Ignarro LJ (1997) Endothelial stunning and myocyte recovery after reperfusion of jeopardized muscle: a role of L-arginine blood cardioplegia. J Thorac Cardiovasc Surg 113: 379–389

Monin JL, Monchi M, Gest V, Duval-Moulin AM, Dubois-Rande JL, Gueret P (2001) Aortic stenosis with severe left ventricular dysfunction and low transvalvular pressure gradients: risk stratification by low-dose dobutamine echocardiography. J Am Coll Cardiol 37: 2101–2107

O'Connor CM, Velazquez EJ, Gardner LH, Smith PK, Newman MF, Landolfo KP, Lee KL, Califf RM, Jones RH (2002) Comparison of coronary artery bypass grafting versus medical therapy on long-term outcome in patients with ischemic cardiomyopathy (a 25-year experience from the Duke Cardiovascular Disease Databank). Am J Cardiol 90: 101–107

Ogawa Y, Nakao K, Arai H, Nakagawa O, Hosoda K, Suga S, Nakanishi S, Imura H (1991) Molecular cloning of a non-isopeptide-selective human endothelin receptor. Biochem Biophys Res Commun 178: 248–255

Opie LH (2003) Heart physiology: From cell to circulation. Lippincott Williams & Wilkins, Philadelphia

Pernow J, Wang QD (1997) Endothelin in myocardial ischaemia and reperfusion. Cardiovasc Res 33: 518–526

Phillips HR, O'Connor CM, Rogers J (2007) Revascularization for heart failure. Am Heart J 153: 65–73

Podesser BK, Schirnhofer J, Bernecker OY, Kröner A, Franz M, Semsroth S, Fellner B, Neumüller J, Hallström S, Wolner E (2002) Optimizing ischemia/reperfusion in the failing rat heart–improved myocardial protection with acute ACE inhibition. Circulation 106: I277–I283

Powell DE, Tunick PA, Rosenzweig BP, Freedberg RS, Katz ES, Applebaum RM, Perez JL, Kronzon I (2000) Aortic valve replacement in patients with aortic stenosis and severe left ventricular dysfunction. Arch Intern Med 160: 1337–1341

Rashid A, Jackson M, Page RD, Desmond MJ, Fabri BM (1995) Continuous warm versus intermittent cold blood cardioplegia for coronary bypass surgery in patients with left ventricular dysfunction. Eur J Cardiothorac Surg 9: 405–408

Rothenburger M, Rukosujew A, Hammel D, Dorenkamp A, Schmidt C, Schmid C, Wichter T, Scheld HH (2002) Mitral valve surgery in patients with poor left ventricular function. Thorac Cardiovasc Surg 50: 351–354

Samady H, Elefteriades JA, Abbott BG, Mattera JA, McPherson CA, Wackers FJ (1999) Failure to improve left ventricular function after coronary revascularization for ischemic cardiomyopathy is not associated with worse outcome. Circulation 100: 1298–1304

Seta Y, Shan K, Bozkurt B, Oral H, Mann DL (1996) Basic mechanisms in heart failure: the cytokine hypothesis. J Card Fail 2: 243–249

Slawsky MT, Colucci WS, Gottlieb SS, Greenberg BH, Haeusslein E, Hare J, Hutchins S, Leier CV, LeJemtel TH, Loh E, Nicklas J, Ogilby D, Singh BN, Smith W (2000) Acute hemodynamic and clinical effects of levosimendan in patients with severe heart failure. Study Investigators. Circulation 102: 2222–2227

Smith PK, Califf RM, Tuttle RH, Shaw LK, Lee KL, Delong ER, Lilly RE, Sketch MH, Peterson ED, Jones RH (2006) Selection of surgical or percutaneous coronary intervention provides differential longevity benefit. Ann Thorac Surg 82: 1420–1428, discussion 1428–1429

Trescher K, Bauer M, Dietl W, Hallström S, Wick N, Wolfsberger M, Ullrich R, Jürgens G, Wolner E, Podesser BK (2009) Improved myocardial protection in the failing heart by selective endothelin-A receptor blockade. J Thorac Cardiovasc Surg 137: 1005–1011, 1011e1

Tritapepe L, De Santis V, Vitale D, Guarracino F, Pellegrini F, Pietropaoli P, Singer M (2009) Levosimendan pre-treatment improves outcomes in patients undergoing coronary artery bypass graft surgery. Br J Anaesth 102: 198–204

Tsuyuki RT, Shrive FM, Galbraith PD, Knudtson ML, Graham MM, Investigators APPROACH (2006) Revascularization in patients with heart failure. CMAJ: Canadian Medical Association Journal = journal de l'Association medicale canadienne 175: 361–365

Wang QD, Li XS, Pernow J (1995) The nonpeptide endothelin receptor antagonist bosentan enhances myocardial recovery and endothelial function during reperfusion of the ischemic rat heart. J Cardiovasc Pharmacol 26 Suppl 3: S445–S447

Yilmaz MB, Yontar C, Erdem A, Karadas F, Yalta K, Turgut OO, Yilmaz A, Tandogan I (2009) Comparative effects of levosimendan and dobutamine on right ventricular function in patients with biventricular heart failure. Heart Vessels 24: 16–21

Yoshizumi M, Perrella MA, Burnett JCJ, Lee ME (1993) Tumor necrosis factor downregulates an endothelial nitric oxide synthase mRNA by shortening its half-life. Circ Res 73: 205–209

Protection During Heart Transplantation

Allanah Barker and Stephen Large

8.1
Background: Heart Transplantation in the Current Era

Heart transplantation is now the best treatment for patients with severe and refractory end-stage cardiac failure (*American Heart Association* stage D) (Hunt et al. 2005). It improves both patient survival and quality of life. However, this therapy is threatened by the increasing scarcity of suitable human donor hearts. In 1995, 4,399 heart transplants were reported worldwide to ISHLT (Taylor et al. 2007) Over a 10-year period, this number has fallen by 30% to 3,095. The fall in the UK has been more dramatic, reducing by 74% in the last 10 years (393 in 1997 to 101 on 2007) (UK Transplant activity report 2008), and numbers are expected to continue to decrease.

The year on year fall in number of cardiothoracic transplants in the UK is directly related to the number of donor organs available (Fig. 1). The number of cardiac failure patients referred for heart transplant has not decreased, but centres like ours balance the number of patients placed onto the list to match donor supply. Donor organ shortage is probably the major challenge facing intra-thoracic organ transplantation.

Remuneration for donor hospitals, and government targets for increasing the number of donors referred from each intensive care unit, have played a central role in increasing the number of organs available for transplant in North America, who continue to transplant a steady number of hearts per year. Countries like the US have different donor population from European countries. For instance, the USA continues to gather young donors from trauma (Organ Procurement and Transplantation Network data 2009) and is less affected by donor shortages than the UK. In one way the fall in available donors is good news, with lower death rates following improved public health measures (eg: compulsory wearing of seat belts), and improved neurosurgical strategies for intracranial hypertension. However, from a transplant perspective, these changes have led to the use of older donors who often have co-morbidities such as hypertension and coronary artery disease.

As the number of donor organs fall, all offers are precious. It is clear from the work of several researchers that optimal donor management during donor heart retrieval improves

---

A. Barker and S. Large (✉)
Papworth Everard, Cambridge, CB3 8RE, United Kingdom
e-mail: stephen.large@papworth.nhs.uk

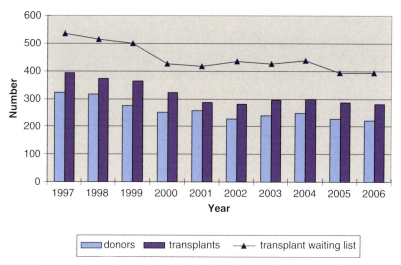

Fig. 1 UK Transplant data on the number of Cardiothoracic Organ donors, transplants and patients on the active transplant waiting list from 1997 to 2006. http://www.uktransplant.org.uk/ukt/i/g/statistics/yearly07. The number of donors available for heart, heart/lung and lung transplantation has fallen in the last 10 years with a corresponding decrease in number of transplants performed. Although the number of patients who could benefit from transplantation is increasing, the scarcity of donors means that transplant centres manage their waiting list so that the number of patients placed on the list matches donor supply

recipient outcomes (Taylor et al. 2007), and improving donor management may also salvage organs that might otherwise go unused.

8.2
Minimising Myocardial Damage

Minimisation of myocardial damage begins around the point of brain death and continues throughout organ retrieval, transport, and on into the post-operative period (Fig. 2). It is clear that there are many opportunities for the donor heart to be damaged and a corresponding number of chances for the transplant team to protect, or even improve, the myocardium.

There is no doubt that cardiac function is profoundly affected by brain death (Baroldi et al. 1997; Galinanes and Hearse 1994; Novitzky et al. 1984; Shivalkar et al. 1993). Organ dysfunction may be the product of humoral and/or neural responses to brain death. During the procurement of the donor heart the first step is an assessment of quality in terms of the organ's appropriateness for transplantation. Initial assessment of cardiac function may suggest that it is inadequate, but previous work suggests that cardiac dysfunction in the brain-dead donor may be temporary (Szabo et al. 1999). Quite what leads to cardiac dysfunction after brain death remains uncertain. It could be the result of direct myocardial injury, or the dysfunction may be due to more reversible insults such as coronary perfusion

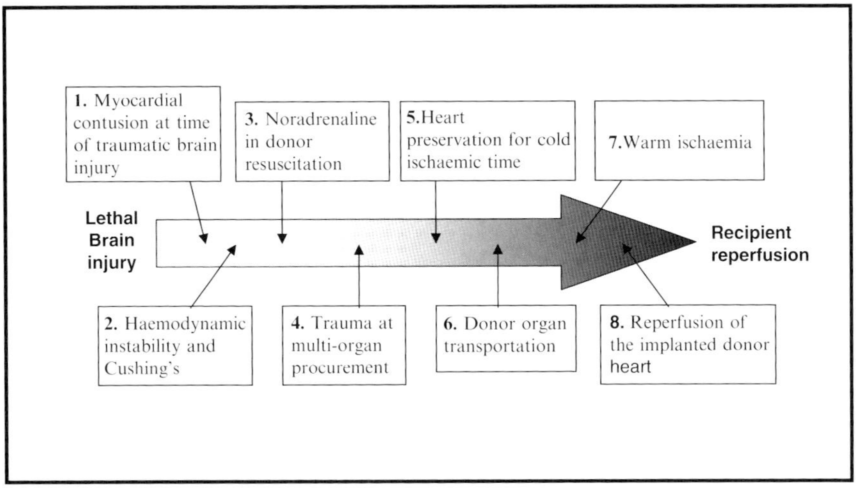

8 Protection During Heart Transplantation

```
┌─────────────────┐  ┌──────────────┐  ┌──────────────────┐  ┌──────────────┐
│ 1. Myocardial   │  │3. Noradrenaline│ │5. Heart          │  │7. Warm ischaemia│
│ contusion at time│  │in donor        │ │preservation for cold│                │
│ of traumatic brain│ │resuscitation   │ │ischaemic time    │  │              │
│ injury          │  │              │  │                  │  │              │
└─────────────────┘  └──────────────┘  └──────────────────┘  └──────────────┘
```

Lethal Brain injury →→→→→→→→→→→→→→→→→→→→→→→→→→→→→ Recipient reperfusion

```
┌─────────────────┐  ┌──────────────┐  ┌──────────────┐  ┌──────────────────┐
│ 2. Haemodynamic │  │4. Trauma at  │  │6. Donor organ│  │8. Reperfusion of │
│ instability and │  │multi-organ   │  │transportation│  │the implanted donor│
│ Cushing's       │  │procurement   │  │              │  │heart             │
└─────────────────┘  └──────────────┘  └──────────────┘  └──────────────────┘
```

Fig. 2 Minimising damage to the donor heart. A timeline identifying points of potential cardiac damage in the donor heart between brain death and recipient reperfusion: There are multiple points throughout the process of heart transplantation where cardiac damage may occur. Protection strategies should ideally be implemented in the donor management and during organ procurement, continue throughout organ transport and on into transplantation and the post-operative period

abnormalities and alteration in loading conditions (Novitzky et al. 1984; Shivalkar et al. 1993; Szabo et al. 1999, 2000). These observations suggest that organs discarded on the basis of apparent poor function in the donor may in fact be suitable for transplantation.

8.2.1
Brainstem Death and Donor Organ Injury

It is appropriate to provide details for the sequence of possible injury to the donor heart in Fig. 2:

8.2.1.1
Myocardial Contusion at the Time of Brain Injury

In trauma cases, there is probably little that can be done to minimise damage to the heart if myocardial contusions were sustained during the lethal primary insult.

8.2.1.2
Haemodynamic Instability and Cushing Response

Several research groups have shown that brain stem dead organ donors have profoundly upset cardiac function (Baroldi et al. 1997; Galinanes and Hearse 1994; Novitzky et al. 1984; Shivalkar et al. 1993; Szabo et al. 1999, 2000). The humoral response to brain death is characterised by a marked rise in circulating catecholamines – a "catecholamine storm". Resulting myocardial ischaemia is one factor implicated in the impairment of cardiac function observed following brainstem death (Halejcio-Delophont et al. 1998). The physiological response to the "catecholamine storm" is dilatation of the right ventricle, reduction of contractility and loss of contractile reserve (Satchithanada et al. 2001). Recently, investigators have attempted to elaborate on the mechanisms responsible for brain death related cardiac dysfunction. Szabo and colleagues explored the role of altered loading conditions and coronary perfusion in brain death associated cardiac dysfunction (Szabo et al. 2000; Szabo et al. 1999) concluding that cardiac dysfunction may be temporary. With this in mind there may be ways to improve donor organ function.

(a) First a measurement of cardiac function is made. Many transplant units use a pulmonary artery floatation catheter (PAFC) to assess the heart. Empirically accepted parameters are summarized in Table 1. These data are obtained in the setting of the profound humoral and neural disturbances that accompany brainstem death in the human organ donor.

(b) Optimisation of donor heart function involves in-vivo resuscitation of organs in the human donor. The time from brain-stem death to organ retrieval can often be more than 24 h, during which time the organs are exposed to the hostile neural and humoral environment of the brain dead donor. The extent of the success of donor organ resuscitation is monitored by the results of further PAFC measurements, but up to 20% of donors may be lost due to haemodynamic instability (Ojeda-Rivero et al. 2002). Optimal donor management with hormonal therapy (tri-iodothyronine and vasopressin) (Wheeldon et al. 1994), limiting the use of inotropic support and proper fluid management can make the difference between transplanting organs, and losing donors. In addition, respiratory problems (atelectasis or lobar collapse, retained secretions, misplaced endo-tracheal tube), metabolic upset (hyperglycaemia, hypoxia, acidosis, anaemia) and imbalance of circulating space and circulating volume are responsible for making donor hearts unusable. An approach to management of these issues is summarized in Table 2.

8.2.1.3
Noradrenaline in Donor Resuscitation

There is evidence to suggest that noradrenaline may be harmful to the human brain stem dead donor heart. Stoica and colleagues (Stoica et al. 2004) demonstrated that the combination of brain death and noradrenaline is detrimental to right ventricular systolic

Table 1 Summary of empirically acceptable pulmonary artery flotation catheter (PAFC) values (wheeldon et al.)

PAFC measure	Empirical acceptable range
C.I.	≥ 2.1 L min^{-1}.M$^{2-1}$
SVRI	400–700 units.M$^{2-1}$
PAWP	≤ 10 mm Hg
Catecholamine drive	< equivalent dopamine @ 5 μg Kg^{-1} min^{-1}

8 Protection During Heart Transplantation

Table 2 Summary of steps to resuscitate the human brain stem donor heart

System	Action
Respiratory	
Atelectasis/lobar collapse	Bronchoscopy
Retained secretions	Bronchoscopy
Metabolic	
Acidosis	Correct
Hyperglycaemia	Insulin infusion
Anaemia	Blood transfusion
Hypovolaemia	Colloid transfusion
Cardio-vascular	
Reduce inotrope	Normalise circulating volume
Low SVR	
Noradrenaline infusion	ADH infusion
Low CI	Replace with ADH
High filling pressures	Normalise filling pressures
	Reduce pressors, blood let
Hormonal	
Tri-iodothyronine infusion	4–6 ng.ml^{-1}.min^{-1}.
ADH	3 μg.min^{-1}.
Insulin & dextrose	15 Units insulin + 50 ml 50% dextrose

function. Ideally noradrenaline infusion should be weaned off and, if needed, should be replaced with appropriate colloid and ADH to support the circulation.

8.2.1.4
Trauma at Multi-Organ Procurement

The multi-organ procurement procedure is a huge operation and may involve many surgical teams. From time to time the heart may be damaged (with an inexperienced team opening the chest, or error over inferior vena cava harvesting). Attention to detail in coordinating arrival at the donor hospital and during the multiple procedures will minimise this risk. If the heart is unstable in terms of rhythm or function it is wise to regard this as a relative contraindication to procurement.

8.2.1.5
Heart Preservation During the Cold Ischaemic Period

This is divided into two steps, the cessation of heart action (primary cardioplegia) and safe storage for transportation:

Primary cardioplegia: A solution is given to arrest the cardiac rhythm; it is usually cold in order to limit the amount of energy spent on cardiac contraction and basal metabolic function. Many different solutions have been developed, and are broadly split into extracellular and intracellular. University of Wisconsin (UW) solution is an example of an intracellular composition. It was developed in the 1980s for abdominal organs, but is also safe for 4–6 h of cardiac preservation (Stringham et al. 1992). Extracellular solutions include the widely used St. Thomas' solutions, which were widely used in the past, and continue to be to a lesser extent, as crystalloid cardioplegia, and are also suitable for donor heart preservation. Histidine-Typtophan-Ketoglutarate (HTK) solution is similar to St Thomas' solutions and is particularly popular in Europe. HTK and Celsior solutions were developed specifically for solid organ preservation in conjunction with myocardial metabolism, rather than adapted from abdominal retrieval solutions (like UW) (Stoica et al. 2001). Most units now use Celsior, an extra-cellular-like electrolyte solution containing substrate that promotes anaerobic metabolism and limits calcium overload (Menasche et al. 1994).

8.2.1.6
Safe Storage for Transportation

Once explanted, the heart is usually carried in bags of cold isotonic saline (2 l/bag) so that it floats to avoid frostbite. Heart transplantation inevitably has longer ischaemic times than most cardiac surgery procedures. Length of cold ischaemic time has considerable impact

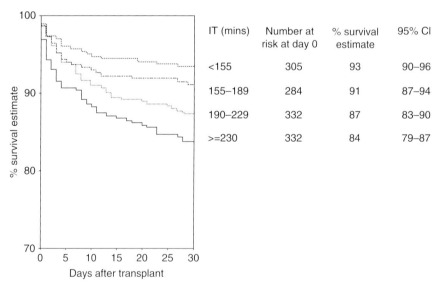

Fig. 3 The effect of cold ischaemic time on actuarial recipient survival post cardiac transplantation: Prolonged ischaemic time has a detrimental effect on survival post cardiac transplant. Data from the UK Transplant Cardiothoracic Advisory Group, taken from their 2007 report. *IT* Ischaemic Time. Ref: UK Transplant Cardiothoracic Advisory Group: The influence of ischaemia time on the outcome of heart transplantation. Summer 2007

8 Protection During Heart Transplantation

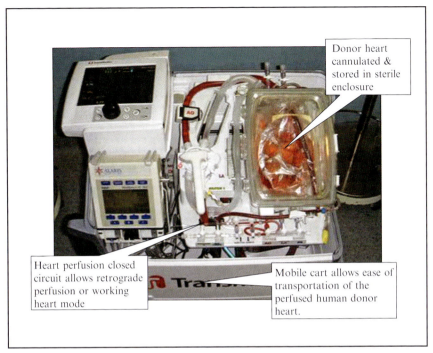

Fig. 4 A commercially manufactured continuous donor heart perfusion device: The donor heart is cannulated onto the ex-vivo perfusion rig at the donor hospital site. Normothermic oxygenated blood perfusate is continuously circulated around the heart to maintain coronary perfusion throughout organ transport. The transportation is more physiologically "normal" then cold storage and therefore theoretically superior. The device also allows observation of cardiac function outside the donor environment

on graft function in the longer term (Fig. 3), so every attempt should be made to minimise ischaemic time. A safe total ischaemic time of <4 h is widely accepted.

There have been several attempts over time to preserve the heart using continuous coronary perfusion. Such systems hope to extend the *reasonable* cold ischaemic time to permit extended travel time, or timelier surgical implantation. In the 1980s micro-perfusion appeared to be helpful with these aims in animal models, but it did not translate clinically (Wicomb et al. 1984). More recently, continuous warm perfusion storage is being re-visited, with clinical trials to look at the extent of preservation, and explore the possibilities for ex-vivo donor heart resuscitation (Fig. 4).

8.2.1.7
Warm Ischaemic Time

Once out of storage, there is substantial risk of myocardial damage during the implantation of the heart. Sewing the heart in requires four suture lines; the donor and recipient left and right atria, followed by pulmonary arteries and finally the aorta (five suture lines if you do a bicaval anastomosis on the right atrium). Work by Stoica and colleagues (2003) has demonstrated the consumption of energy stores during this time. They described an unpredictable course of energy replenishment during reperfusion, with a pattern of outcome paralleling risk to donor heart function and life of recipient. Traditionally the time taken for implantation involves ischaemia and warming of the heart. To minimise this "warm ischaemia", cold heart jackets, and starting the implant with the aortic anastomosis are strategies that have been described to shorten the danger period.

8.2.1.8
Reperfusion of the Implanted Donor Heart

As the donor heart is reperfused, it is at risk from ischaemia-reperfusion injury. Immediate reperfusion injury manifests on a scale of severity – some hearts require increased inotropic support for the first few days, whereas others suffer severe primary graft dysfunction and fail to wean from cardiopulmonary bypass without mechanical circulatory support (usually BiVAD or ECMO in these catastrophic circumstances).

Reperfusion injury has also been linked to increased rates of rejection and accelerated allograft coronary disease in the longer term, perhaps through endothelial damage at the time of reperfusion (Labarrere et al. 1994).

Several mechanisms for reperfusion injury have been described (Yellon and Hausenloy 2007). There has been a great deal written on the alteration of the conditions of myocardial reperfusion in order to limit reperfusion related ischaemic heart damage. Low pressure reperfusion with mild hypothermia is probably the most well adopted technique.

Despite much interest in ischaemic pre-conditioning, the strategy appears to have little effect on the donor heart (Kharbanda et al. 2002; Kloner et al. 2002).

8.3
Results: Outcome of Cardiac Transplantation

Cardiac allograft transplantation improves both quality of life and life expectancy, with 50% survival at 10 years overall, and 50% at 13 years if recipients survive the first year (Taylor et al. 2007). The 20% mortality at 1 year (Taylor et al. 2007), reflects the surgical, immediate post op, and immunosupressant risks associated with this procedure.

One of the main purposes of optimising protection strategies in the pre-implantation heart is to avoid primary graft dysfunction. Although there is no official definition of Primary Graft Dysfunction (PGD) in heart transplantation, it is recognised as the need for either mechanical circulatory support or high dose inotropic infusions to separate the patient from cardiopulmonary bypass (Lima et al. 2006). If need for prolonged inotropic support is added to the PGD definition, PGD rates of around 30% are reported (Collins et al. 2008; Taylor et al. 2007). Although PGD is probably multifactorial, reperfusion injury appears to play a large role (Yellon and Hausenloy 2007).

8.4
Conclusion: Future Perspectives

There is evidence to suggest that the attenuation of brain-stem death related myocardial damage can be diminished by β-receptor blockade. (Ojeda-Rivero et al. 2002). However, it is likely that treatment with β-blockers will be begun after brain-stem death, in much the same way as hormonal treatment is currently used, rather than starting treatment prior to brain death as described in the experimental animal studies on this subject. It seems unlikely that ethical opinion will ever permit treatment of a patient who is likely to suffer brain-stem damage from rising intra-cranial pressure prior to brain death. Indeed more aggressive neurosurgical management may now prevent brain damage by carrying out cranial flap elevation. This development is likely to reduce the incidence of brain stem damage, which is good news overall but will lead to an inevitable further reduction of available human donor hearts. In the presence of further falls in the number of brain-stem dead donors, it may be that non-heart beating heart donation becomes a reality. Early laboratory evidence suggests that non-heart beating donor hearts may be superior to the traditional human donor heart as they will avoid the peri-brain death cardiac damage associated with brain-stem death (personal communication).

With new strategies for continuous coronary perfusion during donor organ transportation, there may be a future where ischaemia, both cold and warm is abolished. Such programmes could perhaps be extended to allow ex-vivo resuscitation of donor hearts that would otherwise be discarded, and in this way may help to realise maximal use of all human donor hearts that are offered for transplantation.

8.5
Summary

The number of patients who could benefit from a heart transplant is increasing, while the number of donors is static, and even decreasing in some countries, although average donor age is on the increase (Taylor et al. 2007). Donors therefore require careful management so that no transplantable organs are wasted.

Heart transplantation has some of the longest ischaemic times of any cardiac surgical procedure. There are multiple opportunities to minimise myocardial damage throughout the process, and an equal number of steps where protection strategies may fail.

Protection strategies should begin around the point of brain death and continue throughout organ retrieval, transport, and on into the post-operative period:

- Brain-death causes haemodynamic instability and impairment of myocardial function, which may or may not be transient. To assess which organs are transplantable, pulmonary artery flotation catheter measurements are used to assess and guide donor management, and hormonal therapy given to improve cardiac function. Noradrenaline has been linked to right ventricular dysfunction and should be weaned off or replaced with vasopressin as soon as possible.

- Despite best efforts, around half of the hearts assessed by retrieval teams are unsuitable for transplant.
- Increased length of cold ischaemic time has been directly linked to poorer outcomes post transplant. Although most donor hearts are stored in cold saline for transport, continuous perfusion systems are now commercially available and continue to be assessed. It is widely accepted that <4 h cold ischaemic time is "safe".
- Reperfusion injury can result in the need for mechanical support and/or high dose inotropic support. Low pressure reperfusion with mild hypothermia may minimise risk of this type of injury. Ischaemic pre-conditioning may also have a role, but is not yet well proven.

Without an increase in donors it is likely that transplant numbers will continue to fall. Potential strategies for increasing the donor pool include resuscitation of donor organs, perhaps with ex-vivo perfusion systems, better management of intra-cranial pressure, and possibly the use of non-heart beating donors.

References

Baroldi, G., Di Pasquale, G., Silver, M. D., Pinelli, G., Lusa, A. M., & Fineschi, V. (1997). Type and extent of myocardial injury related to brain damage and its significance in heart transplantation: a morphometric study. *J Heart Lung Transplant, 16*(10), 994–1000.

Collins, J.M., Moainie, L.S., Griffith, P.B., & Poston, S.R. (2008). Preserving and evaluating hearts with ex vivo machine perfusion: an avenue to improve early graft performance and expand the donor pool. *Eur J Cardiothorac Surg, 34*(2), 318–325.

Galinanes, M., & Hearse, J.D. (1994). Brain-death-induced cardiac contractile dysfunction: studies of possible neurohormonal and blood-borne mediators. *J Mol Cell Cardiol, 26*(4), 481–498.

Halejcio-Delophont, P., Siaghy, M.E., Devaux, Y., Ungureanu-Longrois, D., Richoux, P.J., Beck, B., et al. (1998). Increase in myocardial interstitial adenosine and net lactate production in brain-dead pigs: an in vivo microdialysis study. *Transplantation, 66*(10), 1278–1284.

Hunt A.S., W.A., Chin H.M.,Feldman M.A., Francis G.S., Ganiats T.G., Jessup M., Konstam M.A., Mancini D.M., Michl K.,Oates J.A., Rahko P.S., Silver M.A., Stevenson L.W., Yancy C.W., Antman E.M., Smith S.C. Jr, Adams C.D., Anderson J.L., Faxon D.P., Fuster V., Halperin J.L., Hiratzka L.F. ,Jacobs A.K., Nishimura R,Ornato JP,Page RL,Riegel B (2005). ACC/AHA 2005 Guideline Update for the Diagnosis and Management of Chronic Heart Failure in the Adult: a report of the American College of Cardiology/American Heart Association Task Force on Practice Guidelines (Writing Committee to Update the 2001 Guidelines for the Evaluation and Management of Heart Failure): developed in collaboration with the American College of Chest Physicians and the International Society for Heart and Lung Transplantation: endorsed by the Heart Rhythm Society.,American College of Cardiology,American Heart Association Task Force on Practice Guidelines,American College of Chest Physicians,International Society for Heart and Lung Transplantation,Heart Rhythm [Journal Article, Practice Guideline,Research Support, N.I.H., Extramural,Research Support, Non-U.S. Gov't,Research Support, U.S. Gov't, P.H.S.]. *Circulation, Sep 2005, is. 112/,*(12(e154-235)), 1524–4539.

Kharbanda, K.R., Mortensen, M.U., White, A.P., Kristiansen, B.S., Schmidt, R.M., Hoschtitzky, A. J., et al. (2002). Transient limb ischemia induces remote ischemic preconditioning in vivo. *Circulation, 106*(23), 2881–2883.

Kloner, A.R., Speakman, T.M., & Przyklenk, K. (2002). Ischemic preconditioning: a plea for rationally targeted clinical trials. *Cardiovasc Res, 55*(3), 526–533.

Labarrere, A.C., Pitts, D., Halbrook, H., & Faulk, P.W. (1994). Tissue plasminogen activator, plasminogen activator inhibitor-1, and fibrin as indexes of clinical course in cardiac allograft recipients. An immunocytochemical study. *Circulation, 89*(4), 1599–1608.

Lima, B., Rajagopal, K., Petersen, P.R., Shah, S.A., Soule, B., Felker, M.G., et al. (2006). Marginal cardiac allografts do not have increased primary graft dysfunction in alternate list transplantation. *Circulation, 114*(1 suppl), I-27–32.

Menasche, P., Termignon, L.J., Pradier, F., Grousset, C., Mouas, C., Alberici, G., et al. (1994). Experimental evaluation of Celsior, a new heart preservation solution. *Eur J Cardiothorac Surg, 8*(4), 207–213.

Novitzky, D., Wicomb, N.W., & Cooper, K.D. C. (1984). Electrocardiographic, hemodynamic & endocrine changes occurring during experimental brain death in the Chacma baboon. *J Heart Transplant, 4*(1), 63–69.

Ojeda-Rivero, R., Hernandez-Fernand, A., Dominguez-Roldan, M.J., Calderon, E., Ruiz, M., Lage, E., et al. (2002). Experimental treatment with beta blockers of hemodynamic and myocardial changes in organ donors. *Transplant Proc, 34*(1), 185–186.

Organ Procurement and Transplantation Network, D.U.partment of Health & Human Services, 2009. Data: Deceased Donors Recovered in the U.S. by Circumstance of Death : Donors Recovered : January 1, 1988 – May 31, 2009. http://optn.transplant.hrsa.gov

Satchithanada, D., Stoica, S., White, P., Charman, S., Luckraz, H., Schofield, P., et al. (2001). Systolic right ventricular dysfunction in good donor hearts – a normal finding? . *J Heart Lung Transplant, 20*(2), 243.

Shivalkar, B., Van Loon, J., Wieland, W., Tjandra-Maga, B.T., Borgers, M., Plets, C., et al. (1993). Variable effects of explosive or gradual increase of intracranial pressure on myocardial structure and function. *Circulation, 87*(1), 230–239.

Stoica, C.S., Satchithananda, K.D., Dunning, J., & Large, R.S. (2001). Two-decade analysis of cardiac storage for transplantation. *Eur J Cardiothorac Surg, 20*(4), 792–798.

Stoica, C.S., Satchithananda, K.D., Atkinson, C., White, A.P., Redington, N.A., Goddard, M., et al. (2003). The energy metabolism in the right and left ventricles of human donor hearts across transplantation. *Eur J Cardiothorac Surg, 23*(4), 503–512.

Stoica, C.S., Satchithananda, K.D., White, A.P., Parameshwar, J., Redington, N.A., & Large, R.S. (2004). Noradrenaline use in the human donor and relationship with load-independent right ventricular contractility. *Transplantation, 78*(8), 1193–1197.

Stringham, C.J., Southard, H.J., Hegge, J., Triemstra, L., Fields, L.B., & Belzer, O.F. (1992). Limitations of heart preservation by cold storage. *Transplantation, 53*(2), 287–294.

Szabo, G., Hackert, T., Sebening, C., Vahl, F.C., & Hagl, S. (1999). Modulation of coronary perfusion pressure can reverse cardiac dysfunction after brain death. *Ann Thorac Surg, 67*(1), 18–25; discussion 25–26.

Szabo, G., Hackert, T., Sebening, C., Melnitchuk, S., Vahl, F.C., & Hagl, S. (2000). Role of neural and humoral factors in hyperdynamic reaction and cardiac dysfunction following brain death. *J Heart Lung Transplant, 19*(7), 683–693.

Taylor, O.D., Edwards, B.L., Boucek, M.M., Trulock, P.E., Aurora, P., Christie, J., et al. (2007). Registry of the International Society for Heart and Lung Transplantation: twenty-fourth official adult heart transplant report–2007. *J Heart Lung Transplant, 26*(8), 769–781.

UK Transplant activity report (2008) http://www.uktransplant.org.uk/ukt/statistics/transplant_activity_report/current_activity_reports/ukt/tx_activity_report_2008_uk_pp26-32.pdf.

Wheeldon, R.D., Potter, D.C., Jonas, M., Wallwork, J., & Large, R.S. (1994). Using "unsuitable" hearts for transplantation. *Eur J Cardiothorac Surg, 8*(1), 7–9.

Wicomb, N.W., Cooper, K.D., Novitzky, D., & Barnard, N.C. (1984). Cardiac transplantation following storage of the donor heart by a portable hypothermic perfusion system. *Ann Thorac Surg, 37*(3), 243–248.

Yellon, M.D., & Hausenloy, D.J. (2007). Myocardial reperfusion injury. *N Engl J Med, 357*(11), 1121–1135.

Part IV
New Approaches and Technologies

The Endothelium As Target for Interventions 9

Seth Hallström and Bruno K. Podesser

Abbreviations

ACE	angiotensin converting enzyme
BH_4	(6R)-5,6,7,8-tetrahydrobiopterin
eNOS	endothelial nitric oxide synthase
I/R	ischemia/reperfusion
iNOS	inducible NO synthase
nNOS	neuronal NO synthase
NO	nitric oxide
O_2^-	superoxide
SOD	superoxide dismutase.

9.1
Introduction

Cardiovascular research has recognized rather late that the endothelium of the heart is an important organ that locally regulates coronary perfusion and cardiac function by paracrine secretion of NO and vasoactive peptides (Linz et al. 1992). Therefore, cardioplegic solutions in general and storage solutions in cardiac transplantation in particular, are now

S. Hallström
Institute of Physiological Chemistry, Center of Physiological Medicine, Medical University of Graz, Graz, Austria

B.K. Podesser (✉)
The Ludwig Boltzmann Cluster for Cardiovascular Research, Medical University of Vienna, Vienna, Austria
Department of Cardiac Surgery, Landesklinikum St. Pölten, Propst Führerstr. 4, 3100, St. Pölten, Austria
e-mail: bruno.podesser@meduniwien.ac.at

critically discussed with respect to preservation of both the integrity and function of myocytes and endothelial cells.

This chapter will focus on the role of the endothelium in cardioplegic arrest. The maintenance of NO homeostasis is a complex field and, in the case of cardioplegia, directly related to prevention of ischemia/reperfusion damage as well as a functioning endothelial NO–synthase (eNOS). Strategies for additives to cardioplegic solutions include calcium antagonists, scavengers of superoxide and indirect and direct supplementation of NO. After cardioplegic arrest and storage, initial reperfusion is a critical step. Better organ preservation with improved cardioplegic solutions, focusing on both myocytes and endothelial cells, are of major interest. Also the first step of many, leading to successful heart transplantation, is adequate organ preservation ensuring maintenance of organ viability and function. Therefore, the major challenge is to minimize pathologic damage and impairment of function because during procurement, storage, and implantation the heart is always exposed to I/R.

Consequently, an imbalance in NO production, NO availability or increased NO degradation on the one hand, and increased endothelin production or reduced degradation on the other hand, leads to vasoconstriction. In contrast, NO-overproduction seen in acute organ rejection or during septic shock leads to vasoplegia. Therefore, it is fair to say that NO homeostasis is the prerequisite for physiologic blood pressure and flow conditions. The action of NO in vascular and cardiovascular regulation is not limited to its vasodilatation properties. NO inhibits platelet aggregation, reduces oxygen consumption, has lusotropic potential, influences directly or indirectly myocardial contractility, scavenges superoxide (antioxidant properties), prevents leukocyte adhesion and is an antiproliferative and anti-inflammatory mediator. However, it is little appreciated that routine cardiac surgery or cardiologic interventions lead to a serious temporary or persistent disturbance in NO homeostasis. The clinical consequences of persistent impairment of NO activity and increased radical oxygen species activity lead to "endothelial dysfunction" and ultimately to "myocardial dysfunction": no- or low-reflow phenomenon and temporary reduction of myocardial pump function. However, cardioplegic solutions have been primarily designed to protect the myocytes from ischemia and subsequent reperfusion (Bretschneider et al. 1975; Braimbridge et al. 1977; Buckberg 1979; Southard 1995). Therefore, this chapter will briefly address ways in which cardioplegia, ischemia/reperfusion and NO influence endothelial function and dysfunction (Fig. 1).

9.2
NO Pathway

NO is constitutively produced under physiologic conditions by the two isoenzymes eNOS (endothelial NO synthase, NOS-3) and nNOS (neuronal NO synthase, NOS-1) that are both calcium and calmodulin dependent, and a third enzyme, iNOS (inducible NO synthase, NOS-2) which is independent of the calcium–calmodulin pathway and not expressed under physiologic circumstances in the endothelium (Balligand and Cannon 1997).

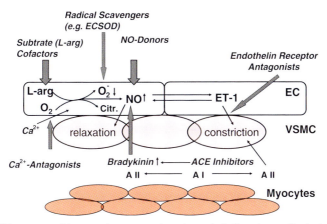

Fig. 1 *Possible routes of intervention concerning the endothelium in cardioplegia.* Following reperfusion after cardioplegia the levels of nitric oxide (NO) are decreased mainly due to "uncoupling" of eNOS, which leads to enhanced level of superoxide (O_2^-). This results in increased vascular tone due to reduced bioavailability of NO and therefore reduced relaxation as well as enhanced production of the vasoconstrictors endothelin-1 (ET-1) and angiotensin II (A II). This reperfusion injury can be attenuated by enhancing the levels of bioavailable NO with substrates/cofactors of eNOS, NO-donors (feedback inhibition and prevention of "uncoupling"), bradykinin, blocking ET-I receptors, blocking the receptors (AT-I) or production (ACE-inhibitors) of angiotensin II and free radical scavengers of superoxide such as extracellar superoxide dismutase (ECSOD). Calcium antagonists on the other hand can counteract the initial Ca^{2+} increase at the onset of ischemia and prevent eNOS stimulation. The enhanced (normalized) levels of bioavailable NO can attenuate/prevent inflammation by inhibiting the activation of the pro-inflammatory transcription factor nuclear factor kappa B (NFκB) and cell adhesion molecules. As a consequence, a decreased expression of pro-inflammatory cytokines and reduced leukocyte (neutrophil) adhesion occurs. The figure illustrates the possible routes of intervention. Fig. 1 is modified from Podesser and Hallström (2007)

Within the cardiovascular system eNOS is the most important isoform. eNOS is a Ca^{2+}-, NADPH-, flavin- and biopterin-dependent enzyme which utilizes the guanido nitrogen atom of L-arginine and incorporates molecular oxygen to generate NO and L-citrulline (Wu 2002). Thus, NO is concerned with the regulation of vascular tone by inducing relaxation of vascular smooth muscle cells through stimulation of the enzyme soluble guanylyl cyclase. Activation of soluble guanylate cyclase leads to conversion of magnesium guanosine 3′, 5′-triphosphate (Mg–ATP) to the second messenger cyclic 3′, 5′-monophosphate guanosine (cGMP), which stimulates two cGMP-dependent protein kinases (PKG I and PKG II) (Kojda and Kottenberg 1999). PKG I is the major kinase mediating vasodilatation and inhibition of platelet aggregation. PKG I acts via a phosphorylation of phospholamban and a phosphorylation of the 1, 4, 5-inositoltriphosphate- (IP3)-receptor associated cGMP kinase substrate. The activity of cGMP is terminated by a rapid conversion to GMP, catalyzed by various phosphodiesterases (Gewaltig and Kojda 2002; Moncada et al. 1991).

9.2.1
NO Mediated Effects

Produced by endothelial cells, NO is responsible for the following actions:

- Vasodilatation (Ignarro et al. 1987)
- Inhibition of platelet aggregation (Azuma et al. 1986; Kalinowski et al. 2002; Radomski et al. 1987)
- Reduction of oxygen consumption (Recchia et al. 1999; Loke et al. 1999)
- Lusitropy (an increase in cardiac compliance) (Paulus and Shah 1999) and therefore
- A direct or indirect mediated increase in myocardial contractility (Kanai et al. 1997; Brady et al. 1993)
- Scavenging of superoxide (antioxidant properties)
- Prevention of leukocyte (neutrophil) adhesion
- Reduction of proliferation and inflammation

9.3
Endothelium Dysfunction During I/R

Re-establishing blood flow to ischemic tissues or organs (reperfusion) is an essential step in many surgical procedures (Korthuis et al. 1985) including reperfusion after cardioplegic arrest or transplantation. However, reperfusion, especially after prolonged ischemia, leads to changes in vasomotility and an increase in microvascular permeability causing tissue reperfusion oedema (Sternbergh et al. 1993). These are constant features of I/R injury. The consequences of such an injury are frequently massive oedema formation and tissue destruction (Baue 1992; Grace 1994). Constitutive eNOS plays a fundamental role in the pathogenesis of I/R injury. The onset of ischemia leads to elevated intracellular calcium ion concentrations mediated by increased levels of catecholamines. These increased calcium ion concentrations activate eNOS (enhanced generation of NO). I/R injury can be initiated (Huk et al. 1997; Hallström et al. 2002) by a massive burst of NO production (measured in vivo with a porphyrinic-based microsensor (Malinski and Taha 1992)) after onset of ischemia, which depletes local L-arginine and/or tetrahydrobiopterin concentrations, followed by high production of superoxide (O_2^-) after reperfusion and consequently high production of peroxynitrite. It has become clear from studies with purified eNOS that, under substrate or cofactor depletion, the enzyme may become "uncoupled". In such an uncoupled state, electrons are rather diverted to molecular oxygen rather than to L-arginine, resulting in production of superoxide (Vasquez-Vivar et al. 1998; Xia and Zweier 1997) and consequently high production of peroxynitrite. Although the mechanisms underlying endothelial dysfunction are likely to be multi-factorial, it is important to note that increased production of oxygen-derived free radicals by an uncoupled eNOS markedly contributes to this phenomenon (Münzel et al. 2005).

The formation of excessive local peroxynitrite concentrations and consequent cleavage products during the initial phase of reperfusion is deleterious. Three of these cleavage products (hydroxyl free radical, nitrogen dioxide free radical, and nitronium cation) are among the most reactive and damaging species and may be major contributors to the severe I/R damage (Huk et al. 1997). The pathophysiologic settings mentioned above are associated with endothelial dysfunction. In cardiac transplantation I/R, hypothermia and atherosclerosis are of particular interest. The first two pathologic conditions contribute to endothelial dysfunction during and shortly after transplantation. Atherosclerosis of the coronary arteries of the transplanted organ, to some extent being a result of the endothelial dysfunction set by hypothermia and I/R, is one of the leading causes for deaths years after transplantation and is directly related to the time of ischemia of the allograft (Valantine 2003; Weis and Cooke 2003).

The immediate consequences of I/R and hypothermia are endothelial dysfunction: vasoconstriction due to decreased NO production or bioavailability and dominance of endothelins, a group of vasoactive peptides, produced by the endothelium (Laude et al. 2001; Gourine et al. 2001). This leads to no-reflow and finally to organ failure. In the heart, this temporary failure is called "myocardial stunning". The term myocardial stunning as it is used by many authors is characterized as a mechanical dysfunction that persists after reperfusion despite the absence of irreversible damage and despite restoration of normal or near-normal coronary blood flow. This implies that this is a postischemic dysfunction that is fully reversible, no matter how severe or prolonged, and that the dysfunction is not caused by a primary deficit of myocardial perfusion (Bolli 1990).

9.4
Clinical State-of-the-Art to Preserve the Heart During Cardiac Surgery and Transplantation

Currently, the vast majority of heart operations are performed on the arrested heart. The concept of cardiac arrest has been developed by the demands of cardiac surgeons to replace a calcified, stenotic valve or to perform a perfect anastomosis on the coronary arteries. However, uncoupling the heart from its natural source of oxygen and fuel (carbohydrates and fatty acids) leads to I/R damage and ultimately to myocardial infarction.

Therefore, strategies were developed to protect against this necessary uncoupling since the start of cardiac surgery (Shumway et al. 1959; Melrose et al. 1955). The common goal is the reduction of myocardial oxygen consumption either by hypothermia or by uncoupling of cardiac contraction. The former is based on experimental data that show that reduction of myocardial temperature from 37°C to 22°C reduces oxygen consumption by 90% (Buckberg et al. 1977). The latter is based on the fact that 60–70% of cardiac energy goes into contraction. Depolarization or hyperpolarization by K^+, Mg^+ or Na^+ containing cardioplegic solutions induces cardiac arrest even under normothermic conditions (Bretschneider et al. 1975; Braimbridge et al. 1977). Currently, either of these two techniques is the gold standard of myocardial protection for cardiac arrest. In general, cardiac surgery temperature can vary from cold to tepid or normothermia, according to the patients special needs and the surgeons preferences (Guru et al. 2006).

Depending on the concentration of Na^+, two types of cardioplegic solutions can be distinguished: intra- and extracellular solutions (Podesser et al. 1996). In Europe, the clinically most relevant intracellular solution is Bretschneiders HTK solution with a Na^+ concentration of 15 mmol/L compared to the extracellular solutions such as St. Thomas' cardioplegia (Na^+ 117 mmol/L) or blood cardioplegia according to Buckberg (Na^+ 120 mmol/L). HTK is also widely accepted as a storage solution for cardiac transplantation, together with Celsior, a solution designed to combine the general principles of hypothermic organ preservation specific to the heart with the possibilities to use it also during initial donor arrest, post-storage graft re-implantation and early reperfusion (Perrault et al. 2001).

Whenever the aortic root is not only clamped but also dissected and the heart is arrested and excised for organ procurement, it has to be stored. Again, these storage solutions have been designed as cardioplegic solutions for myocyte preservation only. Current clinical routine allows 4–5 h maximum for organ procurement, transport and beginning of reperfusion (Jahania et al. 1999). Experiments conducted with isolated porcine coronary endothelial cells to investigate the effect of cold ischemic storage of these cells in University of Wisconsin solution, another storage solution, mainly used for visceral organs in the US, have shown that a significant decrease in eNOS activity was seen after storage for more than 6 h. There was no significant decrease in cells subjected to cold ischemic storage for 1 h only (Redondo et al. 2000).

However, with an increase in the average life span, cardiac surgeons face an older population of patients who will be undergoing coronary bypass surgery, valve replacement and reconstruction as well as transplantation. This cohort of patients is more likely to have impaired endothelial function. Consequently, new strategies have to be developed to maintain operative mortality and morbidity at acceptable levels.

9.5
The Endothelium as Target for Interventions

9.5.1
Drugs Influencing NO Homeostasis

9.5.1.1
Radical Scavengers

Scavenging of superoxide may increase NO bioavailability. Indeed, in the past 3 decades much work has been performed to use superoxide dismutase (SOD) as a therapeutic agent. Most efforts focused on cytosolic SOD, although it is not normally found in extracellular sites. Despite some success in experimental studies there has been little success in clinical applications. The variable effects of cytosolic SOD may be related to the limited cell penetration of the exogenous applied cytosolic enzyme (Table 1).

New approaches focus on therapeutic equivalents of extracellular SOD (ECSOD), which is electrostatically bound to heparan sulfate proteoglycans in the glycocalyx of various cell types (e.g., endothelial cells). The ECSOD is the major SOD in extracellular

Table 1 Additives to cardioplegic solutions influencing NO homeostasis (relevant experimental and clinical studies)

Additives	Results	References
Radical scavengers	ECSOD type C is cardioprotective in isolated cold-arrested rat hearts; human chimeric SOD improves myocardial preservation in the rabbit heart	Sjöquist et al. (1991), Hatori et al. (1992), Nelson et al. (2002)
Calcium antagonists	Diltiazem protects lipid fraction within the cell membrane against the toxic effects of free oxygen radicals	Koller et al. (1989),
	diltiazem reduces infarct size and protects against reperfusion injury	Kröner et al. (2002), Tadokoro et al. (1996), Klein et al. (1984)
ACE inhibitors	Quinaprilat improves postischemic systolic and diastolic function, coronary perfusion and energy phosphates in the healthy rabbit and the failing rat heart undergoing I/R	Korn et al. (2002), Podesser et al. (2002),
	captopril and TCV-116 reduce chronic allograft rejection	Furukawa et al. (1996)
Bradykinin	Bradykinin preconditioning improves postischemic left ventricular and microvascular function	Feng et al. (2000), Feng et al. (2006)
Endothelin receptor antagonists	Bosentan preserves endothelial and cardiac contractile function during I/R in isolated rat and mouse hearts via a NO-mediated mechanism	Gonon et al. (2004),
	TBC-3214Na improves postischemic systolic and diastolic function, in the failing rat heart undergoing I/R	Trescher et al. (2006)
Substrates and cofactors of eNOS	L-arginine cardioplegia supplementation reduces troponin T and CK-MB levels in CABG	Carrier et al. (2002), Kiziltepe et al. (2004), Colagrande et al. (2006),
	L-arginine reduces cytokine release and wedge pressure in CABG	Yamashiro et al. (2003)
	BH$_4$ is cardioprotective in cold rat heart preservation	
NO-releasing compounds	S-nitrosoglutathione monoethyl ester shows protective effects during cardioplegic arrest in isolated rat hearts	Konorev et al. (1996),
	S-NO-HSA improves functional and metabolic outcome after cold organ storage in the isolated rabbit heart (6 h) and in orthotopically transplanted pig hearts (4 h)	Semsroth et al. (2005), Gottardi et al. (2004)

ECSOD extracellular super oxide dismutase, *I/R* ischemia/reperfusion, *TCV-116* selective angiotensin II receptor blocker, *TBC-3214Na* selective endothelin A receptor blocker, *CKMB* creatinine kinase-myocardial band, *CABG* coronary artery bypass grafting, *BH$_4$* (6R)-5,6,7,8-tetrahydrobiopterin, *S-NO-HSA* S-NO-human serum albumin fluids. Extracellular SOD has a highly hydrophilic, positively charged, carboxyl terminal that imparts a high heparin affinity, and allows the enzyme to be bound to heparin sulfate proteoglycans on the endothelial surface (Sandstrom et al. 1992). Recombinant human ECSOD type C has been shown to have cardioprotective effects in isolated rat heart subjected to I/R (Sjöquist et al. 1991) as well as in isolated cold-arrested rat hearts (Hatori et al. 1992). More recently, a human chimeric SOD, a product of a fusion gene encoding a mutant manganese SOD and the carboxy terminal 26-amino acid tail from ECSOD, has been shown to improve myocardial preservation of isolated rabbit hearts subjected to warm and cold ischemia (Nelson et al. 2002).

9.5.1.2
Calcium Antagonists

A number of studies have reported that administration of diltiazem prior to or during I/R reduces infarct size and protects against reperfusion injury (Tadokoro et al. 1996; Klein et al. 1984; Seitelberger et al. 1994). The beneficial effects of diltiazem on ischemic myocardium are generally thought to be due to coronary artery vasodilatation and a decrease of heart rate as well as cardiac contractility (Ferrari and Visioli 1991). The net result of these effects is a reduction in the imbalance between oxygen supply and demand in acutely ischemic myocardium, through a simultaneous increase in collateral blood flow (mediated by coronary vasodilatation) and a reduction in oxygen consumption (secondary to a decrease in heart rate, contractility and afterload).

It has become apparent that free oxygen radical generation and calcium overload contribute to the development of reperfusion injury (Hess and Manson 1984; Ferrari (1996)). We, and others, have shown that calcium antagonists appear to protect the lipid fraction within the cell membrane against the toxic effects of free oxygen radicals (Koller and Bergmann 1989; Kröner et al. 2002). Lipid peroxidation is considered a major mechanism of oxygen radical toxicity, thereby altering membrane permeability (Hess and Manson 1984; Ambrosio et al. 1991). Calcium antagonists, administered prior to ischemia, may help maintain NO homeostasis by preventing activation of eNOS and thereby prevent "uncoupling".

9.5.1.3
ACE Inhibitors and Bradykinin

There have been numerous experimental (Kitakaze et al. 1995; Zahler et al. 1999; Korn et al. 2002) and clinical reports (The GISSI-3 APPI study Group 1996; Lazar et al. 1998) on the beneficial action of ACE inhibitors in the setting of I/R. The concept behind the use of ACE inhibitors is well understood: ACE is also known as kininase II. This dual enzymatic position explains its dual action; on the one hand the conversion of angiotensin I (AT I) to angiotensin II is blocked, leading directly to vasorelaxation, and on the other hand the breakdown of bradykinin is blocked, leading to an increase in NO with consequent vasodilatation (Hartman 1995). The cardioprotective effect of ACE inhibitors could be abolished by the presence of icatibant (HOE 140), a specific bradykinin-B2 receptor antagonist (Linz et al. 1992).

Similarly, both captopril and lisinopril were able to enhance sub-threshold preconditioning by augmenting bradykinin levels, an effect also eliminated by icatibant. (Morris and Yellon 1997). However, the ability of ACE inhibitors to confer protection in the absence of a preconditioning stimulus is more controversial (Baxter and Ebrahim 2002). Experimental studies have used bradykinin-preconditioning prior to ischemic arrest with cold crystalloid cardioplegia (Feng et al. 2005; Feng et al. 2006). In the cardiovascular system, the action of bradykinin is vasodilatation, mediated in several vascular beds by the release of NO and prostacyclin (Hatta et al. 1997; Wirth et al. 1997). Pretreating the heart with bradykinin before crystalloid cardioplegic ischemia significantly improved postischemic left ventricular and microvascular function, suggesting that pharmacological bradykinin may be an important addition to our current methods of myocardial and microvascular protection with hyperkalemic cardioplegia (Feng et al. 2000).

In two recent studies, we have shown that pre-ischemic ACE-inhibition can significantly improve myocardial function in the healthy and in the failing heart undergoing I/R when compared to cardioplegia alone. The treated hearts showed an improvement in postischemic systolic and diastolic function, coronary perfusion as well as higher levels of high-energy phosphates (Korn et al. 2002; Podesser et al. 2002). The direct use of ACE-inhibitors in the setting of heart transplantation is rare. The effect of captopril and a selective angiotensin II (AT II) receptor blocker in a murine model of graft atherosclerosis have been reported (Furukawa et al. 1996). Both the ACE-inhibitor and the AT II receptor blocker were able to reduce chronic allograft rejection compared to controls.

9.5.1.4
Endothelin Receptor Antagonists

Another endothelium-derived substance is the potent vasoconstrictor endothelin 1 (Yanagisawa et al. 1988). Endothelin 1 (ET-1) mediates vasoconstriction by binding to the endothelin type A and B receptors located on the smooth muscle cells. ET-1 may also mediate NO-dependent vasodilatation by activation of the endothelin type B receptor located on the vascular endothelium (Arai et al. 1990; de Nucci et al. 1988; Sakurai et al. 1990). NO not only counteracts the vasoconstrictor effect (Kourembanas et al. 1991) but also inhibits the release of ET-1 from endothelial cells (Boulanger and Lüscher 1990). The production and release of ET-1 is increased during ischemia and contributes to I/R-injury. Selective ET_A and mixed ET_A/ET_B receptor agonists have been shown to be cardioprotective in I/R. For instance the dual ET_A/ET_B receptor agonist bosentan has been shown to preserve endothelial and cardiac contractile function during I/R in isolated rat and mouse hearts via a mechanism dependent on endothelial NO production (Gonon et al. 2004).

Similarly, we (Trescher et al. 2006) have studied the selective ET_A-receptor blocker TBC1421 as an adjunct to blood cardioplegia in healthy and failing rat hearts in the setting of acute and chronic ischemia. Interestingly, cardiac function was preserved in both the acute and the chronic treatment group, whereas preservation of coronary relaxation was seen only in the acute group. These additional cardioprotective effects of ET receptor blockers are especially important, as chronic treatment with ET receptor blockers is currently only used in the clinical situation of severe pulmonary hypertension.

9.5.2
Substrates and Cofactors of eNOS

9.5.2.1
L-Arginine

The most widely investigated additive to cardioplegia concerning NO homeostasis is L-arginine. The NOS substrate L-arginine has been reported to be effective as a supplement to cardioplegia in a dose range between 2 and 5 mmol/L in numerous experimental studies. The critical timing of L-arginine in cardioplegic arrest and reperfusion seems to be important. It has been shown in isolated working rat hearts, that L-arginine given during initial reperfusion is deleterious to recovery of myocardial function; however, given prior to cardioplegic arrest it exerts its beneficial effects (Engelman et al. 1996). Furthermore, different effects of L-arginine after cardioplegic arrest under moderate and deep hypothermia in isolated working rat hearts, have been reported (Amrani et al. 1997). In this study, L-arginine as an additive to St Thomas' No 1 cardioplegic solution was effective only after moderate hypothermic ischemia (1 h; 20°C) and not after deep hypothermic ischemia (4 h; 4°C). Temperature therefore seams to be another important factor. The different approaches include supplementation of L-arginine during warm blood cardioplegia (Hayashida et al. 2000), supplementation of L-arginine directly to different cardioplegic solutions prior to short (Amrani et al. 1997) and long-term ischemia in isolated working rat hearts (Desrois et al. 2000), or in a heterotopic rat heart transplantation model (Caus et al. 2003).

In a recent study on cardiac allograft preservation in an orthotropic cardiac transplant pig model using intermittent perfusion of donor shed blood supplemented with L-arginine, the question of dose is addressed. The low dose group (L-arginine: 2.5 mmol/L) showed a greater ability to wean off cardiopulmonary bypass, had an improved recovery of left ventricular function and a decreased release of inflammatory cytokines compared to control. In contrast, the high dose group (L-arginine: 5.0 mmol/L) resulted in severe endothelial injury in terms of uniform ischemic contracture and no recovery of ventricular function after 5 h of global ischemia (Ramzy et al. 2005).

Recent clinical studies using L-arginine as an additive to cardioplegia demonstrated efficacy in reducing postoperative troponin T and creatine kinase-myocardial band (CK-MB) levels in coronary bypass graft operations (Carrier et al. 2002; Kiziltepe et al. 2004). A more recent study (Colagrande et al. 2006) also showed significantly reduced cytokine release (interleukin (IL)-6) and myocardial damage (troponin T) in coronary artery bypass patients due to L-arginine cardioplegia supplementation. Wedge pressure as a clinical surrogate for ventricular volume load and intensive care unit stay was also significantly reduced in the treatment group. Common to all these studies was that high doses (7.5 g) of L-arginine were added to the initial 500 mL of cardioplegic solution

(Carrier et al. 2002; Colagrande et al. 2006), with best results obtained when warm (33°C) cardioplegia was infused. Lower doses were safe but inefficient (Carrier et al. 1998). According to the results from experimental studies, all the above clinical approaches were performed using addition of L-arginine to cardioplegia prior to reperfusion.

9.5.2.2
Cofactors of eNOS

Tetrahydrobiopterin (BH_4) is an absolute cofactor required for NO synthase and is thus a critical determinant of NO production. Activation of purified eNOS in the presence of suboptimal levels of BH_4 results in uncoupling. The concomitant addition of L-arginine and tetrahydrobiopterin abolishes superoxide generation by eNOS (Vasquez-Vivar et al. 1998).

Furthermore, in human aortic endothelial cells exposed to prolonged stretching, inhibition of BH_4 synthesis has been shown to stimulate superoxide production (Hishikawa and Lüscher 1997). Effects of BH_4 (20 µmol/L) supplementation have been studied in an in vitro human ventricular heart cell model of simulated I/R. Cellular injury, as assessed by means of trypan blue uptake, was significantly prevented (Verma et al. 2002). Very recently, the cardioprotective effects of BH_4 in cold heart preservation (4°C) have been demonstrated (Yamashiro et al. 2003); BH_4 improved the contractile and metabolic abnormalities in the reperfused cold preserved rat hearts that were subjected to normothermic ischemia. Additionally, BH_4 significantly attenuated ischemic contracture and restored the perfusate levels of nitrite plus nitrate. The cardioprotective effect of BH_4 implies that it could be a novel therapeutic option. Although not discussed, it is known that BH_4 is a very unstable compound, which is rapidly oxidized to dihydrobiopterin. Therefore, the compound in solution is presumably dihydrobiopterin, which is converted intracellularly to BH_4 by dihydrobiopterin reductase with NADPH. This possibility has previously been suggested (Hasegawa et al. 2005).

9.5.3
NO-Releasing Compounds

In models of myocardial I/R injury, damage can also be reduced by addition of exogenous NO either as authentic NO gas (Johnson et al. 1991), or NO donating compounds (Siegfried et al. 1992; Bilinska et al. 1996). Similarly, in the setting of organ transplantation, improved organ function has been observed when exogenous NO donating agents have been included in the hypothermic storage solution in a heart model (Pinsky et al. 1994). Exogenous NO exhibits a negative feedback on the production of NO by eNOS (product inhibition of the enzyme; Griscavage et al. 1995) and thereby can prevent uncoupling of the enzyme in I/R. NO donors used in storage solutions to date have been glyceryl trinitrate (Bhabra et al. 1997), sodium nitroprusside (Yamashita et al. 1996) and diazeniumdiolates (Du et al. 1998). For the NO donor sodium nitroprusside (SNP), a molecule of NO is complexed with iron metal, forming the square bipyramidal complex with five cyanide anions. Interactions of SNP with reducing agents lead to the formation of NO. In the vascular system, NO release by SNP requires the presence of vascular tissue (Bates et al. 1991; Marks et al. 1995). NO formation from SNP is accompanied by cyanide release (Bates et al. 1991), which can be toxic to the vascular cells. It has also been reported that SNP could be involved in the formation of superoxide anions and, consequently, peroxynitrite. Due to these toxic effects of SNP, different metallonitrosyl complexes have recently been developed as NO delivery agents such as nitrosyl ruthenium complexes (Wang et al. 2000; Sauaia et al. 2003; Oliveira et al. 2004; Bonventura et al. 2004). These agents have not, however, been used as drug additives to cardioplegic solutions thus far.

A new class of compounds with special features are S-nitrosothiols. Low molecular weight S-nitrosothiols such as S-nitrosoglutathione and S-nitrosocysteine have a short half-life in a range of a few seconds, whereas high molecular weight S-nitrosothiols such as S-nitrosoalbumin show a more prolonged half-life of 15–20 min in vivo (Hallström et al. 2002). Various compounds have been developed and examined: S-nitroso-N-acetyl-DL-penicillamine induces late preconditioning against myocardial stunning and infarction in conscious rabbits (Takano et al. 1998); S-nitrosoglutathione monoethyl ester has protective effects in isolated rat hearts during cardioplegic ischemic arrest (Konorev et al. 1996); S-nitrosoglutathione inhibits platelet activity during coronary angioplasty (Langford et al. 1994) and suppresses increased NOS activity after canine cardiopulmonary bypass (Mayers et al. 1999). In addition, studies have shown that synthetic compounds such as furoxans require thiols for their thiol-mediated generation of NO (Feelisch et al. 1992).

Concerning NO homeostasis and cardioplegia, we are currently working with a new NO-Donor, S-nitroso human serum albumin (S-NO-HSA). This special high molecular weight S-nitrosothiol has an exact equimolar S-nitrosation and high S-nitrosograde due to a defined preprocessing (Hallström et al. 2002). In an experimental setting of 2 h of hindlimb ischemia and reperfusion, we (Hallström et al. 2002) showed that a supplementation of NO with S-NO-HSA prior to ischemia or prior to reperfusion preserves the function of eNOS, stabilizes the basal production of NO, decreases production of reactive oxygen species, and therefore has beneficial effects in reduction of I/R injury. In a second study (Semsroth et al. 2005), simulating clinical cold organ procurement and storage, hearts were reperfused after 6 h of ischemia on an isolated, erythrocyte-perfused working heart model. We could not only show a statistical significant beneficial hemodynamic and metabolic effect of S-NO-HSA compared to control but also compared to supplementation with L-arginine. In a third group of experiments, orthotopically transplanted pig hearts underwent 4 h of ischemia followed by 3 h of reperfusion. We (Dworschak et al. 2004; Gottardi et al. 2004) observed beneficial hemodynamic and metabolic effects of S-NO-HSA compared to control. Finally, we (Hallström et al. 2008) recently showed that even in unprotected, warm ischemia S-NO-HSA given prior to ischemia and during ischemia and reperfusion leads to a significant improvement of cardiac functional recovery and improved preservation of high-energy phosphates. In Figs. 2, 3, and 4 we have included data from these experiments.

9 The Endothelium As Target for Interventions

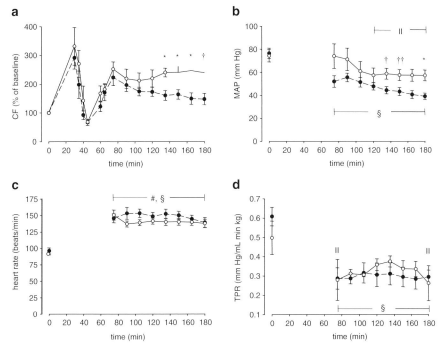

Fig. 2 *Postischemic recovery of hemodynamics in pig.* Post-ischemic recovery of hemodynamic parameters in pig hearts treated with either human serum albumin (HSA) as control, or S-NO-HSA in an I/R model of unprotected warm ischemia. Panel (**a**): time course of coronary flow expressed as percent recovery from baseline values, Panel (**b**): mean arterial blood pressure, Panel (**c**): heart rate, and Panel (**d**) total peripheral resistance. *$P < 0.01$, †$P < 0.05$: S-NO-HSA group (-○-) vs. control group (HSA: --●--). §$P < 0.01$: Control group vs. baseline; ‖$P < 0.05$, #$P < 0.01$: S-NO-HSA group vs. baseline. Time course of coronary flow is expressed as recovery of preischemic baseline values of each individual animal in percent. Modified from Hallström et al. 2008

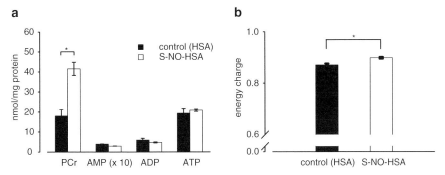

Fig. 3 *Postischemic recovery of high-energy phosphates in the pig.* High-energy phosphates in biopsies of the left ventricle from pig hearts treated with S-NO-HSA compared to control hearts (treated with HSA alone) in an I/R model of unprotected warm ischemia. Changes in PCr and adenine nucleotide levels (**a**) and energy charge (**b**) in S-NO-HSA vs. control group *$P < 0.01$ vs. control. The freeze-clamped biopsies were taken at the termination of the experiments. Modified from Hallström et al. 2008

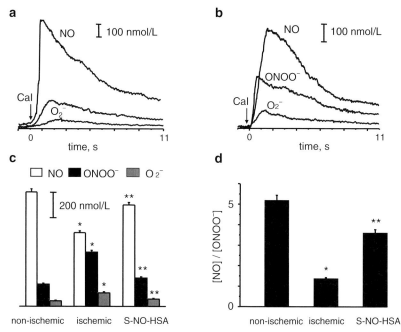

Fig. 4 *NO, O_2^- and $ONOO^-$ concentrations in the pig.* Typical amperograms showing changes of NO, O_2^- and $ONOO^-$ concentrations recorded in vitro after calciumionophore (CaI) stimulation with nanosensors in the myocardium of (**a**) non-ischemic recipient hearts obtained from an ongoing study of orthotropic heart transplantation, and (**b**) control ischemic heart. Non-ischemic heart biopsies ("baseline values"; n = 6) were from Peak NO, O_2^- and $ONOO^-$ concentrations in non-ischemic hearts, ischemic hearts (control group) and S-NO-HSA treated hearts; (**c**) control group vs. non-ischemic hearts *$P < 0.001$ and S-NO-HSA vs. control group **$P < 0.001$. The concentration ratio: [NO]/[ONOO$^-$] in non-ischemic hearts, ischemic (control) and S-NO-HSA treated hearts; (**d**) *$P < 0.001$ control group vs. non-ischemic hearts and S-NO-HSA vs. control group **$P < 0.001$. Modified from Hallström et al. 2008

9.6 Discussion

Supplementation of NO remains controversial, with many studies reporting both positive and negative effects. These differences might be caused by either different experimental settings, differences in NO donors or different methods of supplementation. A review by Bolli (Bolli 2001) concludes that endogenous and exogenous NO is beneficial in protecting the unstressed heart, that has not been acutely preconditioned against damage occurring during I/R. NO plays a critical bifunctional role in late preconditioning, a preconditioning phase that appears 12–24 h after an ischemic stimulus and persists for 72 h. In the latter situation, enhanced production of NO by eNOS is essential to trigger enhanced production of NO by iNOS that is required to mediate the anti-stunning and anti-infarct actions of late preconditioning.

The production of NO depends on a sufficient supply of its substrate L-arginine, and cofactors such as BH_4 (Vasquez-Vivar et al. 1998; Huk et al. 1997). A relative deficiency of L-arginine leads to an "uncoupling" of NOS activity with the production of superoxide anion instead of NO. It is important to note that if iNOS is expressed in vivo (e.g., in sepsis), being independent of calcium and calmodulin, there is a much higher production of NO. Therefore, iNOS is even more predisposed to deplete substrates and co-factors and to predominantly produce O_2^-. This circumstance might also explain the deleterious effects of iNOS induction in many experimental settings. An example of this may be found in a model of transgenic mice transfected with iNOS under the control of a cardiac specific promotor leading to cardiomyopathy, bradyarrhythmia and sudden cardiac death (Mungrue et al. 2002). Therefore, preservation of NO production during organ storage by either supplementation of L-arginine as the physiologic substrate of eNOS or supplementation of NO via the use of a NO-donor may be beneficial for the subsequent heart transplantation.

In a recent review (Bolli 2001) the role of NO in modulating the severity of I/R injury was examined; 73% of the reviewed studies showed that either endogenous or exogenous NO exerted beneficial effects on myocardial protection against infarction or stunning. have shown In a heterotopic rat heart transplant model (Caus et al. 2003), the addition of L-arginine to their storage solution for 3 h of ischemia had a highly significant beneficial effect on graft function during early reperfusion (1 h after aortic declamping).

Reduced NO bioavailability not only has effects on the endothelium but also on the sarcolemmal membrane of the cardiac myocytes (Xu et al. 2003). The sarcolemmal associated NOS isoforms, nNOS and eNOS, may serve to modulate oxidative stress during ischemia in cardiac muscle and thereby regulate the function of key membrane enzymes (including Na^+/K^+-ATPase) with the resultant prevention of calcium overload. Pretreatment with a NO-donor, NOC-7 (1-hydroxy-2-oxo-3-(N-3-methyl-aminopropyl)-3-methyl-l-triazene), markedly protected both sarcolemmal NOS isoforms as well as the function of the Na^+/K^+-ATPase during ischemia. The protection was also facilitated by the radical scavenging properties of NO released by NOC-7.

9.7
Summary

The vascular endothelium of the coronary arteries has been identified as the important organ that locally regulates coronary perfusion and cardiac function by paracrine secretion of nitric oxide (NO) and vasoactive peptides. NO is constitutively produced in endothelial cells by endothelial nitric oxide synthase (eNOS). NO derived from this enzyme exerts important biological functions including vasodilatation, scavenging of superoxide and inhibition of platelet aggregation. Routine cardiac surgery or cardiologic interventions lead to a serious temporary or persistent disturbance in NO homeostasis. The clinical consequences are "endothelial dysfunction", leading to "myocardial dysfunction": no- or low-reflow phenomenon and temporary reduction of myocardial pump function. Uncoupling of eNOS (one electron transfer to molecular oxygen, the second substrate of eNOS) during ischemia/reperfusion due to diminished availability of L-arginine and/or tetrahydrobiopterin is a major source of superoxide formation. Therefore maintenance of normal NO homeostasis seems to be an important factor protecting from ischemia/reperfusion (I/R) injury. Both, the clinical situations of cardioplegic arrest as well as hypothermic cardioplegic storage are followed by reperfusion. However, the current cardioplegic solutions used to arrest and/or store the heart, thereby reducing myocardial oxygen consumption and metabolism, are designed mainly to preserve myocytes and not endothelial cells. This chapter has dealt with special strategies to prevent endothelium dysfunction in the setting of cardioplegia using either additives that preserve NO homeostasis, substrates and cofactors of eNOS or NO-releasing compounds. In summary, protection of the endothelium and maintenance of NO homeostasis has been recognized as an important concept for myocardial protection and is currently being evaluated both experimentally and clinically.

Acknowledgement The authors thank the Ludwig Boltzmann Gesellschaft, 1010 Vienna, for the continuous support. The authors have reproduced parts and Fig. 1 of their contribution to *British Journal of Pharmacology* (Podesser and Hallström 2007) and panel parts of Figs. 2, 3, and 4 of the contribution to *Cardiovascular Research* (Hallström et al. 2008)

References

Ambrosio G, Flaherty JT, Duilio C, Tritto I, Santoro G, Elia PP, Condorelli M, Chiariello M (1991). Oxygen radicals generated at reflow induce peroxidation of membrane lipids in reperfused hearts. *J Clin Invest* **87**:2056–2066.

Amrani M, Gray CC, Smolenski RT, Goodwin AT, London A, Yacoub MH (1997). The effect of L-arginine on myocardial recovery after cardioplegic arrest and ischemia under moderate and deep hypothermia. *Circulation* **96**:II274–II279

Arai H, Hori S, Aramori I, Ohkubo H, Nakashini S (1990). Cloning and expression of a cDNA encoding an endothelin receptor. *Nature* **3458**:730–732.

Azuma H, Ishikawa M, Sekizaki S (1986) Endothelium–dependent inhibition of platelet aggregation. *Br J Pharmacol* **88**:411–415.

Balligand JL, Cannon PJ (1997). Nitric oxide synthases and cardiac muscle. *Arterioscler Thromb Vasc Biol* **17**:1846–1858

Bates JN, Baker MT, Guerra Jr R, Harrison DG (1991). Nitric oxide generation from nitroprusside by vascular tissue. Evidence that reduction of the nitroprusside anion and cyanide loss is required. *Biochem. Pharmacol* **42**:157–165.

Baue AE (1992). The horror autotoxicus and multiple-organ failure. Arch Surg; **127**:1451–1462.

Baxter GF, Ebrahim Z (2002). Role of bradykinin in preconditioning and protection of the ischemic myocardium. *Br J Pharmacol* **135**:843–854.

Bhabra MS, Hopkinson DN, Shaw TE, Hooper TL (1997). Attenuation of lung graft reperfusion injury by a nitric oxide donor. *J Thorac Cardiovasc Surg* **113**:327–334.

Bilinska M, Maczewski M, Beresewicz A (1996). Donors of nitric oxide mimic effects of ischemic preconditioning on perfusion induced arrhythmias in isolated rat hearts. *Mol Cell Biochem* **161**:265–271.

Bolli R (1990). Mechanism of myocardial "stunning". *Circulation* **82**:723–738.

Bolli R (2001). Cardioprotective function of inducible nitric oxide synthase and role of nitric oxide in myocardial ischemia and preconditioning: an overview of a decade of research. *J Mol Cell Cardiol* **33**:1897–1918.

Bonventura D, Oliveira FS, Tognioli V, Tedesco AC, da Silva RS (2004). A macrocyclic nitrosyl ruthenium complex is a NO donor that induces rat aorta relaxation. *Nitric oxide* **10**:83–91

Boulanger C, Lüscher TF (1990). Release of endothelin from the porcine aorta. Inhibition by endothelium-derived nitric oxide. *J Clin Invest* 85:597–590.

Brady AJ, Warren JB, Poole-Wilson PA, Williams TJ, Harding SE (1993). Nitric oxide attenuates cardiac myocyte contraction. *Am J Physiol* **265**: H176–H182.

Braimbridge MV, Chayen J, Bitensky L, Hearse DJ, Jynge P, Cankovic-Darracott S (1977). Cold cardioplegia or continous coronary perfusion? Report on preliminary clinical experience as assessed cytochemically. *J Thorac Cardiovasc Surg* **74**:900–906.

Bretschneider HJ, Hubner G, Knoll D, Lohr B, Nordbeck H, Spieckermann PG (1975). Myocardial resistance and tolerance to ischemia: physiological and biochemical basis. *J Cardiovasc Surg (Torino)* **16**:241–260.

Buckberg GD (1979). A proposed "solution" to the cardioplegic controversy. *J Thorac Cardiovasc Surg* **77**:803–815.

Buckberg GD, Brazier JR, Nelson RL, Goldstein SM, MyConnell DH, Cooper N (1977). Studies of the effects of hypothermia on regional myocardial blood flow and metabolism during cardiopulmonary bypass. III. Effects of temperature, time, and perfusion pressure in fibrillating hearts. *J Thorac Cardiovasc Surg* **73**:87–94.

Carrier M, Pellerin M, Perrault LP, Bouchard D, Page P, Searle N, Lavoie J (2002). Cardioplegic arrest with L-arginine improves myocardial protection: results of a prospective randomized clinical trial. *Ann Thoracic Surg* **73**:837–842.

Carrier M, Pellerin M, Page PL, Searle NR, Martineau R, Caron C, Solymoss BC, Pelletier LC (1998). Can L-arginine improve myocardial protection during cardioplegic arrest? Results of a phase I pilot study. *Ann Thorac Surg* **66**:108–112.

Caus T, Desrois M, Izquierdo M, Lan C, LeFur Y, Confort-Gouny S, Metras D, Clarke K, Cozzone PJ, Bernard M (2003). NOS substrate during cardioplegic arrest and cold storage decreases stunning after heart transplantation in a rat model. *J Heart Lung Transplant* **22**:184–191

Colagrande L, Formica F, Porta F, Martino A, Sangalli F, AvalLi L, Paolini G (2006). Reduced cytokines release and myocardial damage in coronary artery bypass patients due to L-arginine cardioplegia supplementation. *Ann Thoracic Surg* **81**:1256–1261.

De Nucci G, Gryglewski RJ, Warner TD, Vane JR (1988). Receptor-mediated release of endothelium-derived relaxing factor and prostacyclin from bovine aortic endothelial cells is coupled. *Proc Natl Acad Sci U S A* **85**:2334–2338.

Desrois M, Sciacky M, Lan C, Cozzone PJ, Bernard M (2000). L-arginine during long-term ischemia: effects on cardiac function, energetic metabolism and endothelial damage. *J Heart Lung Transplant* **19**:367–376.

Du ZY, Hicks M, Jansz P, Rainer S, Spratt P, Macdonald P (1998). The nitric oxide donor, diethylamine NONOate, enhances preservation of the donor rat heart. *J Heart Lung Transplant* **17**:1113–1120.

Dworschak M, Franz M, Hallström S, Semsroth S, Gasser H, Haisjackl M, Podesser BK, Malinski T (2004). S-Nitroso human serum albumin improves oxygen metabolism during early reperfusion after severe myocardial ischemia. *Pharmacol* **72**:106–112.

Engelman DT, Watanabe M, Maulik N, Engelman RM, Rousou JA, Flack JE 3rd, Deaton DW, Das DK (1996). Critical timing of nitric oxide supplementation in cardioplegic arrest and reperfusion. *Circulation* **94**(9 Suppl):II407–II411.

Feelisch M, Schonafinger K, Noack E (1992). Thiol-mediated generation of nitric oxide accounts for the vasodilator action of furoxans. *Biochem Pharmacol* **44**:1149–1157.

Feng J, Bianchi C, Sandmeyer JL, Sellke FW (2005). Bradykinin preconditioning improves the profile of cell survival proteins and limits apoptosis after cardioplegic arrest. *Circulation* **112**: I190–I195.

Feng J, Li JY, Rosenkranz ER (2000). Bradykinin protects the heart after cardioplegic ischemia via NO-dependent mechanisms. *Ann Thoracic Surg.* **70**:2119–2124

Feng J, Sellke ME, Ramlawi B, Boodhwani M, Clements R, Li J, Bianchi C, Sellke FW (2006). Bradykinin induces microvascular preconditioning through the opening of calcium-activated potassium channels. *Surgery* **140**:192–197.

Ferrari R (1996). The role of mitochondria in ischemic heart disease. *J Cardiovasc Pharmacol* **28**:1–10.

Ferrari R, Visioli O (1991). Protective effects of calcium antagonists against ischemia and reperfusion damage. *Drugs* **42**:14–26.

Furukawa Y, Matsumori A, Hirozane T, Sasayama S (1996). S. Angiotensin II receptor antagonist TCV-116 reduces graft coronary artery disease and preserves graft status in a murine model. A comparative study with captopril. *Circulation* **93**:333–339.

Gewaltig MT, Kojda G (2002). Vasoprotection by nitric oxide: mechanisms and therapeutic potential. *Cardiovasc Res* **55**:250–260.

Gonon AT, Erbas D, Bröijerson A, Valen G, Pernow J (2004). Nitric oxide mediates protective effect of endothelin receptor antagonism during myocardial ischemia and reperfusion. *Am J Physiol Heart Circ Physiol* **286**:H1767–H1774.

Gottardi R, Szerafin T, Semsroth S, Trescher K, Wolner E, Hallström S, Podesser BK. (2004). S-nitroso-human serum albumin improves organ preservation in orthotopic heart transplantation in the pig. *J Heart Lung Transplant* **23**:172 (abstract).

Gourine AV, Gonon AT, Pernow J (2001). Involvement of nitric oxide in cardioprotective effect of endothelin receptor antagonist during ischemia-reperfusion. *Am J Physiol Heart Circ Physiol* **280**:H1105–H1112.

Grace PA (1994). Ischemia-reperfusion injury. *Brit J Surg* **81**:637–647.

Griscavage JM, Hobbs AJ, Ignarro lJ (1995). Negative modulation of nitric oxide synthase by nitric oxide and nitroso compounds. *Adv Pharmacol* **34**:215–234.

Guru V, Omura J, Alghamdi AA, Weisel R, Fremes SE (2006). Is blood superior to crystalloid cardioplegia? A meta-analysis of randomized clinical trails. *Circulation* **114**:1331–1338.

Hallström S., Gasser H., Neumayer C., Fügl A., Nanobashvili J., Jakubowski A., Huk I., Schlag G., Malinski T (2002). S-nitroso human serum albumin treatment reduces ischemia/reperfusion injury in skeletal muscle via nitric oxide release. *Circulation* **105**:3032–3038.

Hallström S, Franz M, Gasser H, Vodrazka M, Semsroth S, Losert UM, Haisjackl M, Podesser BK, Malinski T (2008) S-nitroso human serum albumin reduces ischaemia/reperfusion injury in the pig heart after unprotected warm ischaemia. *Cardiovasc Res* **77**:506–514

Hartman JC (1995). The role of bradykinin and nitric oxide in the cardioprotective action of ACE inhibitors. Ann Thorac Surg **60**:789–792.

Hasegawa H, Sawabe K, Nakanishi N, Wakasugi OK (2005). Delivery of exogenous tetrahydrobiopterin (BH_4) to cells of target organs: role of salvage pathway and uptake of its precursor in effective elevation of tissue BH_4. *Mol Genet Metab* **86** (Suppl 1):2–10.

Hatori N, Sjöquist PO, Marklund SL, Pehrsson SK, Ryden L (1992). Effects of recombinant human extracellular- superoxide dismutase type-c on myocardial reperfusion injury in isolated cold-arrested rat hearts. *Free radical Biol Med* **13**:137–142.

Hatta E, Rubin LE, Seyedi N (1997). Bradykinin and cardioprotection: don't set your heart on it. *Pharmacol Res* **35**(6):531–536.

Hayashida N, Tomoeda H, Oda T, Tayama E, Chihara S, Akasu K, Kosuga T, Kai E, Aoyagi S (2000). Effects of supplemental L-arginine during warm blood cardioplegia. *Ann Thorac Cardiovasc Surg* **6**:27–33.

Hess ML, Manson NH (1984). Molecular oxygen: friend and foe. The role of the oxygen free radical system in the calcium paradox, the oxygen paradox and ischemia/reperfusion injury. *J Mol Cell Cardiol* **16**:969–985.

Hishikawa K, Lüscher TF (1997). Pulsatile stretch stimulates superoxide production in human aortic endothelial cells. *Circulation* **96**:3610–3616.

Huk I, Nanobashvili J, Neumayer C, Punz A, Mueller M, Afkhampour K, Mittlboeck M, Losert U, Polterauer P, Roth E, Patton S, Malinski T (1997). L-arginine treatment alters the kinetics of nitric oxide and superoxide release and reduces ischemia/reperfusion injury in skeletal muscle. *Circulation* **96**:667–675.

Ignarro LJ, Buga GM, Wood KS, Byrns RE, Chaudhuri G (1987). Endothelium-derived relaxing factor produced and released from artery and vein is nitric oxide. *Proc Natl Acad Sci USA* **84** (24):9265–9269.

Jahania MS, Sanchez JA, Narayan P, Lasley RD, Mentzer RM Jr (1999). Heart preservation for transplantation: principles and strategies. *Ann Thorac Surg* **68**:1983–1987.

Johnson G 3rd, Tsao PS, Lefer AM (1991). Cardioprotective effects of authentic nitric oxide in myocardial ischemia with reperfusion. *Crit Care Med* **19**:244–252.

Kalinowski L, Matys T, Chabielska E, Buczko W, Malinski T (2002). Angiotensin II AT1 receptor antagonists inhibit platelet adhesion and aggregation by nitric oxide release. *Hypertension* **40**:521–527.

Kanai AJ, Mesaros S, Finkel MS, Oddis CV, Birder LA, Malinski T (1997). Beta-adrenergic regulation of constitutive nitric oxide synthase in cardiac myocytes. *Am J Physiol* **273**: C1371–C1377.

Kitakaze M, Minamino T, Node K, Komamura K, Shinozaki Y, Mori H, Kosaka H, Inoue M, Hori M, Kamada T (1995). Beneficial effects of inhibition of angiotensin-concerting enzyme on ischemic myocardium during coronary hypoperfusion in dogs. *Circulation* **92** (4):950–961.

Kiziltepe U, Tunctan B, Eyileten ZB, Sirlak M, Arikbuku M, Tasoz R, Uysalel A, Ozyurda U (2004). Efficiency of L-arginine enriched cardioplegia and non-cardioplegic reperfusion in ischemic hearts. *Int J Cardiol* **97**:93–100.

Klein HH, Schubothe M, Nebendahl K, Kreuzer H (1984). The effects of two different diltiazem treatments on infarct size in ischemic reperfused porcine hearts. *Circulation* **69**:1000–1005.

Kojda G, Kottenberg K (1999). Regulation of basal myocardial function by NO. *Cardiovasc Res* **41**:514–523.

Koller PT, Bergmann SR (1989). Reduction of lipid peroxidation in reperfused isolated hearts by diltiazem. *Circ Res* **65**:838–846.

Konorev EA, Joseph J, Tarpey MM, Kalyanaraman B (1996). The mechanism of cardioprotection by S-nitrosoglutathione monoethyl ester in rat isolated heart during cardioplegic ischaemic arrest. *Br J Pharmacol* **119**:511–518.

Korn P, Kröner A, Schirnhofer J, Hallström S, Bernecker O, Mallinger R, Franz M, Gasser H, Wolner E, Podesser BK (2002). Quinaprilar during cardioplegic arrest prevents ischemia-reperfusion injury. *J Thorac Cardiovasc Surg* **124**:352–360.

Korthuis RJ, Granger DN, Townsley MI, Taylor AE (1985). The role of oxygen – derived free radicals in ischemia induced increases in canine skeletal muscle vascular permeability. *Circ Res* **57**:599–609.

Kourembanas S, Marsden PA, McQuillan LP, Faller DV (1991) Hypoxia induces endothelin gene expression and secretion in cultured human endothelium. *J Clin Invest* **88**:1054–1057.

Kröner A, Seitelberger R, Schirnhofer J, Bernecker O, Mallinger R, Hallström S, Ploner M, Podesser BK (2002). Diltiazem during reperfusion preserves high-energy phosphates by protection of mitochondrial integrity. *Europ J Cardio-thorac Surg* **21**:224–231.

Langford EJ, Brown AS, Wainwright RJ, de Belder AJ, Thomas MR, Smith RE, Radomski MW, Matrin JF, Moncada S (1994). Inhibition of platelet activity by S-nitrosoglutathione during coronary angioplasty. *Lancet* **344**:1458–1460.

Laude K, Thuillez C, Richard V (2001). Coronary endothelial dysfunction after ischemia and reperfusion: a new therapeutic target? *Braz J Med Biol Res* **34**:1–7.

Lazar H, Volpe C, Bao Y, Rivers S, Vita JA, Keany JF Jr (1998). Beneficial effects of angiotensin-converting enzyme inhibitors during acute revascularization. *Ann Thorac Surg* **66**:487–492.

Linz W, Wiemer G, Schoelkens BA. (1992). ACE-inhibition induces NO-formation in cultured bovine endothelial cells and protects ischemic rat hearts. J Mol Cell Cardiol **24**:909–919.

Loke KE, McConnell PI, Tuzman JM, Shesely EG, Smith CJ, Stackpole CJ, Thompson CI, Kaley G, Wolin MS, Hintze TH (1999). Endogenous endothelial nitric oxide synthase-derived nitric oxide is a physiological regulator of myocardial oxygen consumption. *Circ Res* **84**:840–845.

Malinski T, Taha Z (1992). Nitric oxide release from a single cell measurement in situ by a porphyrinic based microsensor. *Nature* **358**:676–678.

Marks GS, McLaughlin BE, Jimmo, S.L., Poklewska-Koziell M, Brien JF, Nakatsu K (1995). Time-dependent increase in nitric oxide formation concurrent with vasodilation induced by sodium nitroprusside, 3-morpholinosydnonimine and S-nitroso-N-acetylpenicillamine but not by glyceryl trinitrate. *Drug Metab Dispos* **23**:1248–125.

Mayers I, Salas E, Hurst T, Johnson D, Radomski MW (1999). Increased nitric oxide synthase activity after canine cardiopulmonary bypass is suppressed by s-nitrosoglutathione. *J Thorac Cardiovasc Surg* **117**:1009–1016.

Melrose DG, Dreyer B, Bentall HH, Baker JB (1955). Elective cardiac arrest. *Lancet* **269**(6879): 21–22.

Moncada S, Palmer RM, Higgs EA (1991). Nitric oxide: phsiology, pathophsiology and pharmacology. *Pharmacol Rev* **43**:109–142.

Morris SD., Yellon, DM (1997). Angiotensin-converting enzyme inhibitors potentiate preconditioning through bradykinin B_2 receptor activation in human heart. *J Am Coll Cardiol* **29**:1559–1606.

Münzel T, Daiber A, Ullrich V, Mülsch A (2005). Vascular consequences of endothelial nitric oxide synthase uncoupling for the activity and expression of the soluble guanylyl cyclase and the cGMP-dependent protein kinase. *Arterioscl Thromb Vasc Biol* 1 **25**:1551–1557.

Mungrue IN, Gros R, You X, Pirani A, Azad A, Csont T (2002). Cardiomyocyte overexpression of iNOS in mice results in peroxynitrite generation, heart block, and sudden death. *J Clin Invest* **109**:735–743.

Nelson SK, Gao B, Bose S, Rizeq M, McCord JM (2002). A novel heparin-binding, human chimeric, superoxide dismutase improves myocardial preservation and protects from ischemia-reperfusion injury. *J Heart Lung Transplant* **21**:1296–1303.

Oliveira FS, Tognioli V., Pupo TT, Tedesco A.C., da Silva RS (2004). Nitrosyl ruthenium complex as nitric oxide delivery agent: synthesis characterization and photochemical properties. *Inorg Chem Commun* **7**:160–164.

Paulus WJ, Shah AM (1999). NO and cardiac diastolic function. *Cardiovasc Res* **43**:595–606.

Perrault LP, Nicker C, Desjardins N, Dumont E, Thai P, Carrier M (2001). Improved preservation of coronary endothelial function with Celsior compared with blood and crystalloid solutions in heart transplantation. *J Heart Lung Transplant*; **20**:549–558.

Pinsky DJ, Oz MC, Koga S, Taha Z, Broekman MJ, Marcus AJ, Liao H, Naka Y, Brett J, Cannon PJ, Nowygrod R, Malinski T, Stern DM (1994). Cardiac preservation is enhanced in a heterotopic rat transplant model by supplementing the nitric oxide pathway. *J Clin Invest* **93**:2291–2297.

Podesser, BK; Hallström, S (2007): Nitric oxide homeostasis as a target for drug additives to cardioplegia. Br J Pharmacol 151(7):930–940.

Podesser BK, Schirnhofer J, Bernecker OJ, Kröner A, Franz M, Semsroth S, Fellner B, Neumüller J, Hallström S, Wolner E (2002). Optimizing I/R-injury in the failing rat heart improved myocardial protection with acute ACE inhibition. *Circulation* **106**:1277–1283.

Podesser BK, Zegner M, Weisser J, Koci G, Kunold A, Hallström S, Mallinger R, Schima H, Wollenek G (1996). Vergleich dreier gängiger Kardioplegielösungen-Untersuchungen am isolierten Herz zur Myokardprotektion während Ischämie und Reperfusion. *Acta Chirurg Austriaca* **28**:17–28.

Radomski MW, Palmer RMJ, Moncada S (1987). Endogenous nitric oxide inhibits human platelet adhesion to vascular endothelium. *Lancet* **2**:1057–1058.

Ramzy D, RaoV, Mallidi H, Tumiati LC, Xu N, Miriuka S, Feindel CM (2005), Cardiac allograft preservation using donor-shed blood supplemented with L-arginine. *J Heart and Lung Transplant* **24**(10):1665–1672

Recchia FA, McConnell PI, Loke KE, Xu X, Ochoa M, Hintze TH (1999). Nitric oxide controls cardiac substrate utilization in the conscious dog. *Cardiovasc Res* **44**:325–332.

Redondo J, Manso AM, Pacheco ME, Hernandez L, Salaices M, Marin J (2000). Hypothermic storage of coronary endothelial cells reduces nitric oxide synthase activity and expression. Cryobiology **41**:292–300.

Sakurai T, Yanagisawa M, Takuwa Y, Miyazaki H, Kimura S, Goto K, Masaki T (1990). Cloning of a cDNA encoding a non-isopeptide-selective subtype of the endothelin receptor. *Nature* **348**:732–735.

Sandstrom J, Carlson L, Marklund SL, Edlund T (1992). The heparin binding domain of extra cellular superoxide dismutase-c and formation of varients with reduced heparin affinity. *J Biol Chem* **267**:18205–18209.

Sauaia MG, de Lima RG, Tedesco AC., da Silva RS (2003). Photoinduced NO release by visible light irradation from pyrazine-bridged nitrosyl ruthenium complexes. *J Am Chem Soc*;**125**: 14718–14719.

Seitelberger R, Hannes W, Gleichauf M, Keilich M, Christoph M, Fasol R (1994). Effects of diltiazem on perioperative ischemia, arrhythmias, and myocardial function in patients undergoing elective coronary bypass grafting. *J Thorac Cardiovasc Surg* **107**:811–821.

Semsroth S, Fellner B, Trescher T, Bernecker OY, Kalinowski L, Gasser H, Hallström S, Tadeusz Malinski T, Podesser BK (2005). S-Nitroso human serum albumin attenuates ischemia/reperfusion injury after prolonged cardioplegic arrest in isolated rabbit hearts. *J Heart Lung Transplant* **24**:2226–2234.

Shumway NE, Lower RR, Stofer RC (1959). Selective hypothermia of the heart in anoxic cardiac arrest. *Surg Gynecol Obstet* **109**:750–754.

Siegfried MR, Carey C, Ma XL, Lefer AM (1992). Beneficial effects of SPM-5185, a cysteine-containing NO donor in myocardial ischemia-reperfusion. *Am J Physiol* **263**:H771–H777.

Sjöquist PO, Carlson L, Jonason G, Marklund SL, Abrahamson T (1991). Cardioprotective effects of recombinant human extracellular- superoxide dismutase type C in rat isolated heart subjected to ischemia and reperfusion. *J Cardiovasc Pharmacol* **17**:678–683.

Southard JH (1995). Organ preservation. *Ann Rev Med* **46**:235–247.

Sternbergh WC, Makhoul RG, Adelman B (1993). Nitric oxide mediated endothelium dependent vasodilatation is selectively attenuated in the postischemic extremity. *Surgery* **114**:960–967.

Tadokoro H, Miyazaki A, Satomura K, Ryden L, Kaul S, Kar S, Corday E, Durury K (1996). Infarct size reduction with coronary venous retroinfusion of diltiazem in the acute occlusion/reperfusion porcine heart model. *J Cardiovasc Pharmacol* **28**:134–141.

Takano H, Tang XL, Qiu Y, Guo Y, French BA, Bolli R (1998). Nitric oxide donors induce late preconditioning against myocardial stunning and infarction in conscious rabbits via an antioxidant-sensitive mechanism. *Circ Res* **83**:73–84.

The GISSI-3 APPI study Group (1996). Early and six month outcome in patients with angina pectoris early after acute myocardial infarction (the GISSI-3 APPI study). *Am J Cardiol* **78**:1191–1197.

Trescher K, Bauer M, Dietl W, Gottardi R, Hallström S, Wick N, Wolner E, Podesser BK (2006). Improvement of cardioprotection by the selective endothelin-A-receptor antagonist TBC-3214Na: acute versus long-term blockade. *Interact Cardiovasc Thorac Surg* **5**: O55-I (Abstract).

Valantine HA (2003) Cardiac allograft vasculopathy: central role of endothelial injury leading to transplant "atheroma". *Transplantation* **76**:891–899.

Vasquez-Vivar J, Kalyanaraman B, Martasek P, Hogg N, Masters BS, Karoui H, Tordo P, Pritchard KA Jr (1998). Superoxide generation by endothelial nitric oxide synthase: the influence of cofactors. *Proc Natl Acad Sci USA* **95**:9220–9225.

Verma S, Maitland A, WEisel RD, Fedak PW, Pomroy NC, Li Sh, Mickle DA, Li RK, Rao V (2002). Novel cardioprotective effects of tetrahydrobiopterin after anoxia and reoxygenation: Identifying cellular targets for pharmacologic manipulation. *J Thorac Cardiovasc Surg* **123**:1074–1083.

Wang Y.X, Legzdins P., Poon J.S., Pang C.C (2000). Vasodilator effects of organotransition-metal nitrosyl complexes, novel nitric oxide donors. *J Cardiovascular Pharmacol* **35**:73–77.

Weis M, Cooke JP (2003). Cardiac allograft vasculopathy and dysregulation of the NO synthase pathway. *Arterioscler Thromb Vasc Biol* **23**:567–575.

Wirth KJ, Linz W, Weimer G, Schoelkens BA (1997). Kinins and cardioprotection. *Pharmacol Res* **35**:527–530.

Wu KK (2002). Regulation of endothelial nitric oxide synthase activity and gene expression. *Ann N Y Acad Sci* **962**:122–130.

Xia Y, Zweier JL (1997). Direct measurement of nitric oxide generation from nitric oxide synthase. *Proc Natl Acad Sci USA* **94**:12705–12710.

Xu KY, Kuppusamy SP, Wang JQ, Li H, Cui H, Dawson TM, Huang PL, Burnett Al, Kuppusamy P, Becker LC (2003) Nitric oxide protects cardiac sarcolemmal membrane enzyme function and ion active transport against ischemia-induced inactivation. *J Biol Chem* **278**:41798–41803.

Yamashiro S, Noguchi K, Kuniyoshi Y, Koya K, Sakanashi M (2003). Role of tetrahydrobiopterin on ischemia-reperfusion injury in isolated perfused rat hearts. *J Cardiovasc Surg* **44**:37–49

Yamashita M, Schmid RA, Ando K, Cooper JD, Patterson GA (1996). Nitroprusside ameliorates lung allograft injury. *Ann Thorac Surg* **62**:791–796.

Yanagisawa M, Kurihara H, Kimura S, Tomobe Y, Kobayashi M, Mitsui Y, Yazaki Y, Goto K, Masaki (1988). A novel potent vasoconstrictor peptide produced by vascular endothelial cells. *Nature* **332**:411–415.

Zahler S, Kupatt CH, Becker BF (1999). ACE inhibition attenuates cardiac cell damage and preserves release of NO in the postischemic heart. *Immunopharmacol* **44**:27–33.

Vascular Effects of Cardioplegic Arrest and Cardiopulmonary Bypass

10

Neel R. Sodha, Michael P. Robich, and Frank W. Sellke

10.1 Introduction

Cardiac surgery continues to depend on the use of hyperkalemic cardioplegia to arrest the heart for the vast majority of operations (Parolari et al. 2005). In addition to providing a quiescent heart on which to operate, the use of cardioplegia (CP) allows for a relatively bloodless operative field allowing a safe and successful operation. Myocardial protection strategies continue to improve, but cardiac surgery utilizing CP and cardiopulmonary bypass (CPB) is associated with significant systemic vascular dysfunction which can result in impairments to perfusion of the brain, myocardium, lungs, and other organs. The consequent altered perfusion may manifest as neurocognitive deficit, impairments in myocardial pump function secondary to coronary artery vasospasm or impaired coronary microcirculatory vasomotor function, persistent requirement for mechanical ventilatory support, systemic hypotension, and generalized edema secondary to increased vascular permeability.

The cause of vascular dysfunction after CP/CPB is multi-factorial, and involves the complex interaction between inflammatory mediators generated during the trauma of the incision, CPB, and alterations in endothelial function and vascular smooth muscle contractility. This chapter will outline some of these changes in vascular function that occur during cardiac surgery.

N.R. Sodha and M.P. Robich
Beth Israel Deaconess Medical Center, Harvard Medical School, Boston, MA 02215, USA
F.W. Sellke (✉)
Division of Cardiothoracic Surgery, Rhode Island Hospital and the Alpert Medical School of Brown University, APC 424, 593 Eddy Street, Providence, RI 02903, USA
Division of Cardiothoracic Surgery, Beth Israel Deaconess Medical Center, Harvard Medical School, Boston, MA 02215, USA
Brown Medical School, Division of Cardiothoracic Surgery, Rhode Island Hospital and The Miriam Hospital, 2 Dudley Street, MOC 500, Providence, RI 02905, USA
e-mail: fsellke@lifespan.org

10.2
Specific Mediators of Vasomotor Dysfunction

10.2.1
Nitric Oxide Synthase

Nitric oxide is synthesized in healthy endothelial cells via activation of a constitutive nitric oxide synthase (eNOS), and in a wide variety of other cell types such as activated endothelial cells, inflammatory cells and macrophages, cardiomyocytes, intestinal cells, and vascular smooth muscle cells by the inducible form of nitric oxide synthase (iNOS). eNOS is responsible for the endothelial production of NO via conversion of L-arginine to L-citrulline, initiating endothelial-dependent vasorelaxation through activation of guanylate cyclase, inhibition of leukocyte adhesion, and attenuation of platelet activation. eNOS also regulates tone in the vascular smooth muscle, and thus affects vasodilatory responses to many endogenous and pharmacologic agents (Beckman, Beckman et al. 1990).

Hyperkalemic cardioplegic arrest and ischemia-reperfusion alter endothelial structure and indices of endothelial function, most notably endothelial dependent vasorelaxation (Mankad et al. 1991; Cartier et al. 1993; Sellke et al. 1993a, b, c, d). The cause of this impairment in endothelial dependent relaxation is multi-factorial, with many studies demonstrating an impaired release of NO from eNOS after ischemic cardioplegic arrest (Engelman et al. 1995). When assessing eNOS activity via examination of endothelial dependent responses, this may occur due to changes in cell membrane potential (Engelman et al. 1995; He and Yang 1996), substrate cofactor depletion (Andrasi et al. 2003; Cakir et al. 2003), alterations in the concentration or compartmentalization of intracellular calcium (Cavallo et al. 1995; Meldrum et al. 1996), and injury to cell membranes, associated regulatory enzymes, or ion pumps (Sellke et al. 1993a). While impaired signal transduction and reduced agonist stimulated production of NO likely contributes to the reduced endothelial-dependent relaxation after cardioplegia, increased degradation or binding of NO through interactions with free radicals may decrease the bioavailability of NO to the vascular smooth muscle as well (Beckman et al. 1990). In addition, reperfusion after cardioplegic arrest may increase the breakdown of NO that occurs from increased oxidative stress secondary to the generation of oxygen-derived free radicals (Kukreja and Hess 1992). This may further impair synthesis of NO by exposure of the endothelium to fragments of activated complement (Stahl et al. 1995) (Friedman et al. 1995), activated neutrophils, and macrophages (Sellke et al. 1996).

In contrast to eNOS, the inducible form of NOS, or iNOS, is found in increasing quantities in the myocardium after cardioplegic arrest (de Vera et al. 1996; Tofukuji et al. 1998b), and to a lesser extent in other organs after CPB including the pulmonary vasculature (Sato et al. 2000; Hayashi et al. 2001), the mesenteric vasculature (Tofukuji et al. 2000), and brain (Mayers et al. 2003). Expression of cytokines, leukocyte adhesion, the large amounts of NO generated by iNOS under stressed local conditions can all lead to toxic and pro-inflammatory effects (Guzik et al. 2003). This is in part due to the excess spontaneous reaction of NO with the reactive oxygen radicals released under inflammatory or post-ischemic conditions by stressed endothelial cells and activated leukocytes resulting in formation of peroxynitrite, which may cause cell apoptosis, cell necrosis, and circulatory shock(Becker et al. 2000). Increased circulating levels of tumor necrosis factor-α (TNFα), interleukin (IL)-6, IL-8, and other cytokines liberated during CPB have also been shown to increase the expression of iNOS (de Vera et al. 1996; Downing and Edmunds 1992).

10.2.2
Endothelial Derived Hyperpolarizing Factor

Endothelial Derived Hyperpolarizing Factor (EDHF) refers to a group of signaling molecules, including epoxyeicosatrienoic acid (EET), H_2O_2, C-natriuretic peptide, as well as lipooxygenase metabolites (Feletou and Vanhoutte 2006). EDHF, which produces vasorelaxation at the level of the vascular smooth muscle, acts via hyperpolarizing the membrane potential. In vitro studies utilizing porcine coronary arteries indicate hyperkalemia induces impairments in vasorelaxation and endothelial dysfunction via a non-NO mediated pathway, specifically implicating EDHF signaling (He and Yang 1996). This signaling pathway seems to be particularly affected by the hyperkalemia utilized in cardioplegic arrest, whereas in vitro studies utilizing hyperpolarizing cardioplegic arrest have demonstrated preservation of EDHF mediated vasorelaxation (He et al. 2004).

10.2.3
Cyclooxygenase

Cyclooxygenase produces prostaglandins (PG) in a two-step conversion process from arachidonic acid (AA) (Needleman et al. 1986). Initially, cyclooxygenase converts AA to a cyclic endoperoxide (PGG_2) by the action of the constitutively expressed isoform of cyclooxygenase (COX-1) or the inducible isoform of cyclooxygenase, known as COX-2. PGG_2 is then cleaved via a peroxidase to yield endoperoxide (PGH_2). These short-lived products of AA metabolism by COX are then rapidly converted to prostaglandins (PGE_2, PGF_2, thromboxane A_2, PGI_2) by specific isomerase enzymes.

The expression of COX-2 (common in the endothelium of patients with coronary artery disease) is enhanced in the reperfusion phase following blood cardioplegia during coronary artery bypass graft surgery, while COX-1 expression remains relatively unchanged (Metais et al. 1999; Uotila et al. 2001). The release of prostaglandins such as thromboxane A_2 is stimulated which then activates the contractile response of coronary arterioles directly as a result of platelet activation or indirectly via other substances such as serotonin. The upregulation of COX-2 by CP/CPB also results in the generation of predominantly vasoconstrictive prostaglandins resulting in atrial and ventricular microvascular constriction (Sellke et al. 1993a, c; Metais et al. 1999; Metais et al. 2001). This enhanced response appears to be due to an increased production and release of contractile prostanoids since the response is inhibited in the presence of either indomethacin or the selective inhibitor of COX-2, NS398 (Metais et al. 1999). This may contribute to coronary spasm after cardiac surgery, which may contribute to myocardial ischemia and injury after surgery. In fact, continuous EKG monitoring detects asymptomatic EKG changes in a high proportion of patients after cardiac surgery. Furthermore, these inflammatory prostaglandin products can regulate vascular permeability in a manner similar to that of NO, in part through activation of tyrosine kinase receptors and mitogen activated protein (MAP) kinases (Parenti et al. 1998). The inducing factors leading to increased expression of COX-2 are most likely myocardial hypoxia and ischemia, which occurs during cardioplegic arrest as well as during the exposure of the myocardium and blood vessels to inflammatory cytokines. In contrast to iNOS, which is not regulated by agonist stimulation or by intracellular calcium concentration, there is evidence that COX-2 is regulated by agonists such as serotonin (Metais et al. 1999; Metais et al. 2001). Separating the effects of NO and PG when discussing changes in vasomotor activity and permeability during cardiac surgery remains difficult as they are often synergistic and complementary in their actions. In addition to coronary changes in COX-2 expression, experimental models utilizing rats undergoing CPB have demonstrated that COX-2 expression is significantly up-regulated in the cerebral cortex after CPB, a finding which may have clinical implications relating to neurocognitive function after cardiac surgery (Hindman et al. 2001). Increases in COX-2 mRNA and protein expression, but not COX-1, have been detected in the pulmonary vasculature after CPB, with concomitant increases in pulmonary microvascular vasoconstriction in response to serotonin. These increases in vasoconstrictive responses were partially inhibited by inhibition of COX-2 (Shafique et al. 1993; Sato et al. 2000). These findings implicate a contributory role of COX-2 expression for the increased pulmonary vascular resistance often observed after CPB.

10.2.4
Pro-Inflammatory Mediators

Cardioplegic arrest and reperfusion result in the generation of pro-inflammatory mediators and activation of complement which can directly injure the endothelium (Pinckard et al. 1975; Tofukuji et al. 1998b). The activation of the complement cascade after cardioplegic arrest has been shown to directly lead to endothelial cell death and dysfunction (Stahl et al. 1995), as well as increase the recruitment of inflammatory leukocytes (Chenoweth et al. 1981), resulting in additional damage to the endothelium from the release of free radicals, proteolytic enzymes, and inflammatory cytokines (Kawata et al. 1992a; Sellke et al. 1993a, b). Experimentally, endothelial and vascular smooth muscle dysfunction has been reduced with the administration of monoclonal antibodies prior to reperfusion (Kawata et al. 1992b; Tofukuji et al. 1998b), but this has yet to be demonstrated clinically.

10.2.5
Protein Kinase Pathways

Vascular dysfunction observed in the coronary and systemic circulation after CP/CPB relates in large part to the diminished vascular responsiveness to alpha-1 adrenergic agonists and similar vasopressor agents after cardiac surgery. These vascular alterations can range from diminished responsiveness to vasoconstricting pharmacologic agents to excess vasoconstriction and both culminate in insufficient tissue perfusion (Wang et al. 1994; de Vera et al. 1996; Wang et al. 1997). Protein Kinase C (PKC), and the downstream Mitogen Activated Protein Kinases (MAPK) are important in vascular signaling, especially with regard to maintaining vascular tone. The PKC family consists of 12 serine-threonine kinases, of which PKCα has been identified as the predominant isoform present in the human coronary and skeletal microcirculation (Sodha et al. 2007). Activation of the α-1 adrenoreceptor results in activation of Phospholipase C resulting in conversion of phosphoinositolphosphate-2 (PIP$_2$). This liberates 1,4,5-triphosphate (IP$_3$), diacylgylcerol (DAG) and calcium (Schubert and Mulvany 1999). DAG and calcium activate PKC, which can increase smooth muscle contraction directly through increased intracellular calcium (Martinez et al. 2000). This diminishes the activity of myosin light chain phosphatase (Somlyo and Somlyo 1994), or increasing myofilament sensitization to calcium, independent of increases in cytosolic calcium concentration (Hill et al. 1990). Activation of PKC may also cause activation of the MAPK ERK 1/2 (Hattori et al. 2001; Velarde et al. 2001). MAPK are serine-threonine kinases involved in vasomotor function and vascular permeability and can be found in endothelial cells and vascular smooth muscle (Khan et al. 2003a, b, c). Many factors have been shown to lead to MAPK activation, including ischemia, shear stress, and the presence of various vasoactive agents. The three major MAPK families implicated in cardiovascular signaling thus far include: the extracellular signal-regulated kinases (ERK), the c-Jun-NH$_2$-terminal protein kinases (JNK), and p38 kinase. Of the three, ERK 1/2 is thought to play the most significant role in postoperative vascular dysfunction, given it can regulate endothelial cell permeability/edema formation (Jaffee et al. 2000; Breslin et al. 2003), myogenic tone (Khan et al. 2003c) and contractile responses of microvessels to phenylephrine and vasopressin (Khan et al. 2007).

Postoperatively, the endogenous adrenergic stress response to CPB results in a release of vasoactive catecholamines, including norepinephrine and epinephrine(Hoar et al. 1980; Wallach et al. 1980), which act on α_1-adrenoreceptors. A sustained increase in circulating levels of catecholamines in vivo, or prolonged exposure to catecholamines in vitro results in subsequent loss of α_1-adrenoreceptor mediated vascular smooth muscle cell contraction, and diminished IP$_3$ turnover. This leads to decreased concentrations of DAG and calcium, both of which are required for conventional PKC activation (Lurie et al. 1985; Rosenbaum et al. 1986). The resulting lack of DAG and calcium may account for the decreases in PKC activity seen in coronary and skeletal microvessels after CP/CPB (Sodha et al. 2007). Decreases in PKC activity, which functions to activate MAPK, specifically ERK 1/2 (Hattori et al. 2001; Velarde et al. 2001), can lead to decreases in ERK 1/2 activity, as has been demonstrated after CP/CPB in the coronary and skeletal microcirculation (Khan et al. 2003a, b, c), culminating in impaired microvascular myogenic tone and vasoconstriction.

The vascular dysfunction induced by the effects of CP/CPB on kinase activity, are compounded by signal transduction mechanisms triggered by a broad range of inflammatory agents such as TNFα. TNFα is elevated after CP/CPB (Marano et al. 2000), and may lead to ERK 1/2 and MAPK activation. This in turn may induce IL-6 production (Hayashi et al. 2000) and lead to a cascade of inflammatory events that include leukocytosis, thrombosis, and lymphocyte activation (Van den Berghe 2000). In the pulmonary circulation, rapid induction of ERK 1/2 (Khan et al. 2003b) leads to enhanced vasoconstriction and likely contributes to the elevations in pulmonary vascular resistance commonly seen after CP/CPB. In the mesenteric microcirculation, key to the pathophysiology of mesenteric ischemia, ERK 1/2 activity and expression levels are markedly increased after CPB with significant augmentation of responses to phenylephrine (Khan et al. 2007).

10.2.6
Calcium

Cardioplegic arrest is associated with cellular depolarization, the influx of calcium through voltage dependent calcium channels, as well as the release of calcium from intracellular stores (Ruel et al. 2004). This influx of calcium may alter the sensitivity of the vascular smooth muscle, which is regulated by myosin light-chain kinase (MLK), whose activity is in turn regulated by calcium-calmodulin mediated phosphorylation. The end result of this sequence may lead to vascular smooth muscle spasm secondary to calcium overload (Pfitzer 2001). The addition of magnesium to cardioplegic solutions has been shown to reduce endothelial dysfunction (Tofukuji et al. 1997) and preserve agonist and myogenic induced vascular responses (Matsuda et al. 1999).

10.3
Clinical Perspective

The clinical manifestations of CP/CPB induced vascular dysfunction are significant and should not be underestimated. Surgeons and anesthesiologists often observe decreased basal vascular tone and decreased alpha-adrenergic microvascular responses in the peripheral vasculature. This may manifest as systemic hypotension, often necessitating the use of alpha-1 adrenergic or other vasopressor drugs to maintain adequate perfusion pressure (Tofukuji et al. 1998a, b; Khan et al. 2007). In the coronary circulation, impairments in smooth muscle contraction lead to decreased coronary vascular tone (Wang et al. 1995; Sodha et al. 2007), whereas decreased endothelial-mediated relaxation can lead to an increased propensity to spasm (Metais et al. 1999; Metais et al. 2001). The pulmonary circulation demonstrates increased microvascular contractile responses, which in addition to edema from increased endothelial permeability, result in increased pulmonary vascular resistance and shunting (Friedman et al. 1995; Sato et al. 2000). Similar increases in vasoconstrictor responses arise in the mesenteric microcirculation (Khan et al. 2007) predisposing to the development of mesenteric ischemia, particularly when vasoactive drugs are administered to regulate blood pressure after CPB (Allen et al. 1992).

Clinical interventions to limit the degree of vascular dysfunction have attempted to manipulate the previously described alterations after CP/CPB. The increased expression of COX-2 and enhanced contractile response of coronary arterioles to serotonin after CPB and cardioplegia (Metais et al. 1999; Metais et al. 2001) indicate the improvements in coronary bypass graft patency obtained from the perioperative administration of aspirin may not only derive from its effects on prevention of platelet aggregation and thrombus formation (Chesebro et al. 1982; Gavaghan et al. 1991; Mangano 2002), but also from the prevention of coronary spasm and preservation of microvascular flow as a result of COX-2 inhibition. However, some COX-2 inhibitors, but not all, have been implicated in a higher cardiovascular mortality. Thus, some clinical judgement needs to be made with the use of COX-2 inhibiting drugs.

Given the detrimental effects of hyperkalemia on EDHF-mediated coronary arterial and arteriolar vasorelaxation (He and Yang 1996; Yang et al. 2005), several investigators have attempted to limit this derangement by supplementing cardioplegic solutions with nicorandil (a K_{ATP} channel opener) (Yang et al. 2005), magnesium (Yang et al. 2002), and adenosine (Jakobsen et al. 2008). The pre-clinical studies utilizing nicorandil, magnesium, and adenosine to maintain EDHF-mediated vasorelaxation have been positive, but the benefit in the clinical setting has yet to be proven. The beneficial effects on the endothelium and vasculature of magnesium supplementation to cardioplegic solutions has been demonstrated and is used routinely in the clinical setting (Tsukube et al. 1994; Kronon et al. 1999; Matsuda et al. 1999). The advantages of blood over crystalloid cardioplegia has been demonstrated in animal models (Feng et al. 2005), and clinically in emergency or high-risk cases. This is likely due to the inhibitory effects of blood on oxygen-derived free radical generation, improved coronary endothelial oxygenation, enhanced buffering capacity from histidine and other blood proteins, and better preservation of the morphology of coronary endothelial cells (Sellke et al. 1993a, b, c; Sellke et al. 1996). The administration of glucocorticosteroids during CPB was thought to theoretically block the effects of inflammatory cytokines and the expression of iNOS and COX-2, but has not resulted in significant clinical benefit in most studies (Boscoe et al. 1983; Andersen et al. 1989). Attempts to improve the bioavailability of NO in the coronary circulation have led to multiple studies investigating the supplementation of L-arginine to cardioplegic solutions. These trials have demonstrated benefits to L-arginine supplementation, including reduced release of biochemical markers of myocardial damage (Carrier et al. 2002), reduced IL-2 receptor, IL-6, and TNFα expression (Colagrande et al. 2005), and better hemodynamic performance with shorter intensive care unit stays (Colagrande et al. 2006).

10.4
Conclusion

Cardioplegia and cardiopulmonary bypass are associated with changes in vascular function which can lead to significant derangements in end-organ perfusion. Central to these alterations are changes in expression of isoforms of nitric oxide synthase, increases in COX signaling, alterations in PKC and MAPK signaling, and changes in vascular permeability. Therapeutic interventions aimed at these targets have not resulted in clinically significant benefits to date, with the possible exception of aspirin therapy which may prevent coronary spasm and preserve microvascular flow and perhaps the use of blood cardioplegia for urgent cardiac surgical operations. Despite the dramatic degree of change in vascular physiology observed after cardiac surgery utilizing cardioplegic arrest and cardiopulmonary bypass, the vast majority of patients are able to undergo surgery safely

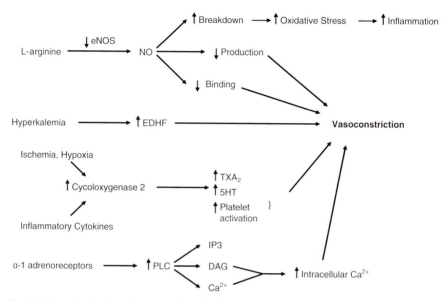

Fig. 1 Schematic drawing that summarizes the key pathways, most of which ultimately result in vasoconstriction. *5HT* serotonin, *DAG* diacylglycerol, *EDHF* endothelial derived hyperpolarizing factor, *eNOS* nitric oxide synthase, *NO* nitric oxide, *PLC* phospholipase C, *TXA₂* thromboxane A₂

without significant complication. Continued work in this area is needed in an effort to maximize the beneficial outcome of patients after cardiac surgery (Fig. 1).

References

Allen, K.B., A.A. Salam, et al. (1992). "Acute mesenteric ischemia after cardiopulmonary bypass". J Vasc Surg **16**(3): 391–5; discussion 395–396.

Andersen, L.W., L. Baek, et al. (1989). "Effect of methylprednisolone on endotoxemia and complement activation during cardiac surgery". J Cardiothorac Anesth **3**(5): 544–549.

Andrasi, T. B., P. Soos, et al. (2003). "L-arginine protects the mesenteric vascular circulation against cardiopulmonary bypass-induced vascular dysfunction". Surgery **134**(1): 72–79.

Becker, B.F., C. Kupatt, et al. (2000). "Reactive oxygen species and nitric oxide in myocardial ischemia and reperfusion". Z Kardiol **89**(Suppl 9): IX/88–91.

Beckman, J. S., T. W. Beckman, et al. (1990). "Apparent hydroxyl radical production by peroxynitrite: implications for endothelial injury from nitric oxide and superoxide". Proc Natl Acad Sci U S A **87**(4): 1620–1624.

Boscoe, M.J., V.M. Yewdall, et al. (1983). "Complement activation during cardiopulmonary bypass: quantitative study of effects of methylprednisolone and pulsatile flow". Br Med J (Clin Res Ed) **287**(6407): 1747–1750.

Breslin, J.W., P.J. Pappas, et al. (2003). "VEGF increases endothelial permeability by separate signaling pathways involving ERK-1/2 and nitric oxide". Am J Physiol Heart Circ Physiol **284**(1): H92–H100.

Cakir, O., A. Oruc, et al. (2003). "Does sodium nitroprusside reduce lung injury under cardiopulmonary bypass?" Eur J Cardiothorac Surg **23**(6): 1040–1045.

Carrier, M., M. Pellerin, et al. (2002). "Cardioplegic arrest with L-arginine improves myocardial protection: results of a prospective randomized clinical trial". Ann Thorac Surg **73**(3): 837–41.

Cartier, R., M. Pellerin, et al. (1993). "Effects of pressure and duration of hyperkalemic infusions on endothelial function". Ann Thorac Surg **55**(3): 700–705.

Cavallo, M. J., B. H. Dorman, et al. (1995). "Myocyte contractile responsiveness after hypothermic, hyperkalemic cardioplegic arrest. Disparity between exogenous calcium and beta-adrenergic stimulation". Anesthesiology **82**(4): 926–939.

Chenoweth, D. E., S. W. Cooper, et al. (1981). "Complement activation during cardiopulmonary bypass: evidence for generation of C3a and C5a anaphylatoxins". N Engl J Med **304**(9): 497–503.

Chesebro, J. H., I. P. Clements, et al. (1982). "A platelet-inhibitor-drug trial in coronary-artery bypass operations: benefit of perioperative dipyridamole and aspirin therapy on early postoperative vein-graft patency". N Engl J Med **307**(2): 73–78.

Colagrande, L., F. Formica, et al. (2005). "L-arginine effects on myocardial stress in cardiac surgery: preliminary results". Ital Heart J **6**(11): 904–910.

Colagrande, L., F. Formica, et al. (2006). "Reduced cytokines release and myocardial damage in coronary artery bypass patients due to L-arginine cardioplegia supplementation". Ann Thorac Surg **81**(4): 1256–1261.

de Vera, M. E., R. A. Shapiro, et al. (1996). "Transcriptional regulation of human inducible nitric oxide synthase (NOS2) gene by cytokines: initial analysis of the human NOS2 promoter." Proc Natl Acad Sci U S A **93**(3): 1054–1059.

Downing, S. W. and L. H. Edmunds, Jr. (1992). "Release of vasoactive substances during cardiopulmonary bypass." Ann Thorac Surg **54**(6): 1236–1243.

Engelman, D. T., M. Watanabe, et al. (1995). "Constitutive nitric oxide release is impaired after ischemia and reperfusion." J Thorac Cardiovasc Surg **110**(4 Pt 1): 1047–1053.

Feletou, M. and P. M. Vanhoutte (2006). "Endothelium-derived hyperpolarizing factor: where are we now?" Arterioscler Thromb Vasc Biol **26**(6): 1215–1225.

Feng, J., C. Bianchi, et al. (2005). "Molecular indices of apoptosis after intermittent blood and crystalloid cardioplegia." Circulation **112**(9 Suppl): I184–I189.

Friedman, M., S. Y. Wang, et al. (1995). "Altered beta-adrenergic and cholinergic pulmonary vascular responses after total cardiopulmonary bypass". J Appl Physiol **79**(6): 1998–2006.

Gavaghan, T. P., V. Gebski, et al. (1991). "Immediate postoperative aspirin improves vein graft patency early and late after coronary artery bypass graft surgery. A placebo-controlled, randomized study". Circulation **83**(5): 1526–1533.

Guzik, T. J., R. Korbut, et al. (2003). "Nitric oxide and superoxide in inflammation and immune regulation". J Physiol Pharmacol **54**(4): 469–487.

Hattori, Y., H. Kakishita, et al. (2001). "Glycated serum albumin-induced vascular smooth muscle cell proliferation through activation of the mitogen-activated protein kinase/extracellular signal-regulated kinase pathway by protein kinase C". Biochem Biophys Res Commun **281** (4): 891–896.

Hayashi, Y., Y. Sawa, et al. (2001). "Inducible nitric oxide production is an adaptation to cardiopulmonary bypass-induced inflammatory response". Ann Thorac Surg **72**(1): 149–155.

Hayashi, Y., Y. Sawa, et al. (2000). "P-selectin participates in cardiopulmonary bypass-induced inflammatory response in association with nitric oxide and peroxynitrite production". J Thorac Cardiovasc Surg **120**(3): 558–565.

He, G. W., Z. D. Ge, et al. (2004). "Electrophysiologic and mechanical evidence of superiority of hyperpolarizing versus depolarizing cardioplegia in protection of endothelium-derived hyperpolarizing factor-mediated endothelial function: a study in coronary resistance arteries." J Thorac Cardiovasc Surg **127**(6): 1773–1780.

He, G. W. and C. Q. Yang (1996). "Hyperkalemia alters endothelium-dependent relaxation through non-nitric oxide and noncyclooxygenase pathway: a mechanism for coronary dysfunction due to cardioplegia." Ann Thorac Surg **61**(5): 1394–1399.

Hill, M.A., J.C. Falcone, et al. (1990). "Evidence for protein kinase C involvement in arteriolar myogenic reactivity." Am J Physiol **259**(5 Pt 2): H1586–H1594.

Hindman, B.J., S.A. Moore, et al. (2001). "Brain expression of inducible cyclooxygenase 2 messenger RNA in rats undergoing cardiopulmonary bypass." Anesthesiology **95**(6): 1380–1388.

Hoar, P.F., J.G. Stone, et al. (1980). "Hemodynamic and adrenergic responses to anesthesia and operation for myocardial revascularization." J Thorac Cardiovasc Surg **80**(2): 242–248.

Jaffee, B.D., E.J. Manos, et al. (2000). "Inhibition of MAP kinase kinase (MEK) results in an anti-inflammatory response in vivo." Biochem Biophys Res Commun **268**(2): 647–651.

Jakobsen, O., T.A. Stenberg, et al. (2008). "Adenosine instead of supranormal potassium in cardioplegic solution preserves endothelium-derived hyperpolarization factor-dependent vasodilation." Eur J Cardiothorac Surg **33**(1): 18–24.

Kawata, H., M. Aoki, et al. (1992). "Effect of antibody to leukocyte adhesion molecule CD18 on recovery of neonatal lamb hearts after 2 hours of cold ischemia." Circulation **86**(5 Suppl): II364–II370.

Kawata, H., K. Sawatari, et al. (1992). "Evidence for the role of neutrophils in reperfusion injury after cold cardioplegic ischemia in neonatal lambs." J Thorac Cardiovasc Surg **103**(5): 908–17; discussion 917–918.

Khan, T.A., C. Bianchi, et al. (2003a). "Cardiopulmonary bypass reduces peripheral microvascular contractile function by inhibition of mitogen-activated protein kinase activity." Surgery **134**(2): 247–54.

Khan, T.A., C. Bianchi, et al. (2003b). "Activation of pulmonary mitogen-activated protein kinases during cardiopulmonary bypass." J Surg Res **115**(1): 56–62.

Khan, T.A., C. Bianchi, et al. (2007). "Differential effects on the mesenteric microcirculatory response to vasopressin and phenylephrine after cardiopulmonary bypass." J Thorac Cardiovasc Surg **133**(3): 682–688.

Khan, T.A., C. Bianchi, et al. (2003c). "Mitogen-activated protein kinase inhibition and cardioplegia-cardiopulmonary bypass reduce coronary myogenic tone." Circulation **108**(Suppl 1): II348–II353.

Kronon, M.T., B.S. Allen, et al. (1999). "Superiority of magnesium cardioplegia in neonatal myocardial protection." Ann Thorac Surg **68**(6): 2285–2291.

Kukreja, R. C. and M. L. Hess (1992). "The oxygen free radical system: from equations through membrane-protein interactions to cardiovascular injury and protection." Cardiovasc Res **26**(7): 641–655.

Lurie, K.G., G. Tsujimoto, et al. (1985). "Desensitization of alpha-1 adrenergic receptor-mediated vascular smooth muscle contraction." J Pharmacol Exp Ther **234**(1): 147–152.

Mangano, D. T. (2002). "Aspirin and mortality from coronary bypass surgery." N Engl J Med **347**(17): 1309–1317.

Mankad, P.S., A.H. Chester, et al. (1991). "Role of potassium concentration in cardioplegic solutions in mediating endothelial damage." Ann Thorac Surg **51**(1): 89–93.

Marano, C.W., L.A. Garulacan, et al. (2000). "Plasma concentrations of soluble tumor necrosis factor receptor I and tumor necrosis factor during cardiopulmonary bypass." Ann Thorac Surg **70**(4): 1313–1318.

Martinez, M.C., V. Randriamboavonjy, et al. (2000). "Involvement of protein kinase C, tyrosine kinases, and Rho kinase in Ca(2+) handling of human small arteries." Am J Physiol Heart Circ Physiol **279**(3): H1228–H1238.

Matsuda, N., M. Tofukuji, et al. (1999). "Coronary microvascular protection with mg^{2+}: effects on intracellular calcium regulation and vascular function." Am J Physiol **276**(4 Pt 2): H1124–H1130.

Mayers, I., T. Hurst, et al. (2003). "Increased matrix metalloproteinase activity after canine cardiopulmonary bypass is suppressed by a nitric oxide scavenger." J Thorac Cardiovasc Surg **125**(3): 661–668.

Meldrum, D.R., J.C. Cleveland, Jr., et al. (1996). "Cardiac surgical implications of calcium dyshomeostasis in the heart." Ann Thorac Surg **61**(4): 1273–1280.

Metais, C., C. Bianchi, et al. (2001). "Serotonin-induced human coronary microvascular contraction during acute myocardial ischemia is blocked by COX-2 inhibition." Basic Res Cardiol **96**(1): 59–67.

Metais, C., J. Li, et al. (1999). "Serotonin-induced coronary contraction increases after blood cardioplegia-reperfusion: role of COX-2 expression." Circulation **100**(19 Suppl): II328–II334.

Needleman, P., J. Turk, et al. (1986). "Arachidonic acid metabolism." Annu Rev Biochem **55**: 69–102.

Parenti, A., L. Morbidelli, et al. (1998). "Nitric oxide is an upstream signal of vascular endothelial growth factor-induced extracellular signal-regulated kinase1/2 activation in postcapillary endothelium." J Biol Chem **273**(7): 4220–4226.

Parolari, A., F. Alamanni, et al. (2005). "Meta-analysis of randomized trials comparing off-pump with on-pump coronary artery bypass graft patency." Ann Thorac Surg **80**(6): 2121–2125.

Pfitzer, G. (2001). "Invited review: regulation of myosin phosphorylation in smooth muscle." J Appl Physiol **91**(1): 497–503.

Pinckard, R.N., M.S. Olson, et al. (1975). "Consumption of classical complement components by heart subcellular membranes in vitro and in patients after acute myocardial infarction." J Clin Invest **56**(3): 740–750.

Rosenbaum, J.S., P. Zera, et al. (1986). "Desensitization of aortic smooth muscle contraction in rats harboring pheochromocytoma." J Pharmacol Exp Ther **238**(2): 396–400.

Ruel, M., T.A. Khan, et al. (2004). "Vasomotor dysfunction after cardiac surgery." Eur J Cardiothorac Surg **26**(5): 1002–1014.

Sato, K., J. Li, et al. (2000). "Increased pulmonary vascular contraction to serotonin after cardiopulmonary bypass: role of cyclooxygenase." J Surg Res **90**(2): 138–143.

Schubert, R. and M.J. Mulvany (1999). "The myogenic response: established facts and attractive hypotheses." Clin Sci (Lond) **96**(4): 313–326.

Sellke, F.W., E.M. Boyle, Jr., et al. (1996). "Endothelial cell injury in cardiovascular surgery: the pathophysiology of vasomotor dysfunction." Ann Thorac Surg **62**(4): 1222–1228.

Sellke, F.W., M. Friedman, et al. (1993a). "Mechanisms causing coronary microvascular dysfunction following crystalloid cardioplegia and reperfusion." Cardiovasc Res **27**(11): 1925–1932.

Sellke, F. W., T. Shafique, et al. (1993b). "Coronary endothelial injury after cardiopulmonary bypass and ischemic cardioplegia is mediated by oxygen-derived free radicals." Circulation **88**(5 Pt 2): II395–II400.

Sellke, F. W., T. Shafique, et al. (1993c). "Blood and albumin cardioplegia preserve endothelium-dependent microvascular responses." Ann Thorac Surg **55**(4): 977–985.

Sellke, F.W., T. Shafique, et al. (1993d). "Impaired endothelium-dependent coronary microvascular relaxation after cold potassium cardioplegia and reperfusion." J Thorac Cardiovasc Surg **105**(1): 52–58.

Shafique, T., R.G. Johnson, et al. (1993). "Altered pulmonary microvascular reactivity after total cardiopulmonary bypass." J Thorac Cardiovasc Surg **106**(3): 479–486.

Sodha, N.R., J. Feng, et al. (2007). "Protein kinase C alpha modulates microvascular reactivity in the human coronary and skeletal microcirculation." Surgery **142**(2): 243–252.

Somlyo, A.P. and A.V. Somlyo (1994). "Signal transduction and regulation in smooth muscle." Nature **372**(6503): 231–236.

Stahl, G.L., W.R. Reenstra, et al. (1995). "Complement-mediated loss of endothelium-dependent relaxation of porcine coronary arteries. Role of the terminal membrane attack complex." Circ Res **76**(4): 575–583.

Tofukuji, M., C. Metais, et al. (1998). "Myocardial VEGF expression after cardiopulmonary bypass and cardioplegia." Circulation **98**(19 Suppl): II242–6; discussion II247–II248.

Tofukuji, M., G.L. Stahl, et al. (1998). "Anti-C5a monoclonal antibody reduces cardiopulmonary bypass and cardioplegia-induced coronary endothelial dysfunction." J Thorac Cardiovasc Surg **116**(6): 1060–1068.

Tofukuji, M., G.L. Stahl, et al. (2000). "Mesenteric dysfunction after cardiopulmonary bypass: role of complement C5a." Ann Thorac Surg **69**(3): 799–807.

Tofukuji, M., A. Stamler, et al. (1997). "Effects of magnesium cardioplegia on regulation of the porcine coronary circulation." J Surg Res **69**(2): 233–239.

Tsukube, T., J.D. McCully, et al. (1994). "Magnesium cardioplegia reduces cytosolic and nuclear calcium and DNA fragmentation in the senescent myocardium." Ann Thorac Surg **58**(4): 1005–1011.

Uotila, P., A. Saraste, et al. (2001). "Stimulated expression of cyclooxygenase-2 in porcine heart after bypass circulation and cardioplegic arrest." Eur J Cardiothorac Surg **20**(5): 992–995.

Van den Berghe, G. (2000). "Novel insights into the neuroendocrinology of critical illness." Eur J Endocrinol **143**(1): 1–13.

Velarde, V., A.J. Jenkins, et al. (2001). "Activation of MAPK by modified low-density lipoproteins in vascular smooth muscle cells." J Appl Physiol **91**(3): 1412–1420.

Wallach, R., R.B. Karp, et al. (1980). "Pathogenesis of paroxysmal hypertension developing during and after coronary bypass surgery: a study of hemodynamic and humoral factors." Am J Cardiol **46**(4): 559–565.

Wang, S.Y., M. Friedman, et al. (1994). "Adrenergic regulation of coronary microcirculation after extracorporeal circulation and crystalloid cardioplegia." Am J Physiol **267**(6 Pt 2): H2462–H2470.

Wang, S.Y., M. Friedman, et al. (1995). "Adenosine triphosphate-sensitive K+ channels mediate postcardioplegia coronary hyperemia." J Thorac Cardiovasc Surg **110**(4 Pt 1): 1073–1082.

Wang, S.Y., A. Stamler, et al. (1997). "Decreased myogenic reactivity in skeletal muscle arterioles after hypothermic cardiopulmonary bypass." J Surg Res **69**(1): 40–44.

Yang, Q., Y.C. Liu, et al. (2002). "Protective effect of magnesium on the endothelial function mediated by endothelium-derived hyperpolarizing factor in coronary arteries during cardioplegic arrest in a porcine model." J Thorac Cardiovasc Surg **124**(2): 361–370.

Yang, Q., R.Z. Zhang, et al. (2005). "Release of nitric oxide and endothelium-derived hyperpolarizing factor (EDHF) in porcine coronary arteries exposed to hyperkalemia: effect of nicorandil." Ann Thorac Surg **79**(6): 2065–2071.

Oxygen Radical Scavengers

11

Jack A.T.C. Parker and Uwe Mehlhorn

11.1
Ischemia-Reperfusion Injury

The myocardium can tolerate only relatively short periods of total myocardial ischemia without myocardial cell death. Following short ischemic periods, ischemic damage is reversible by reperfusion. However, with increasing duration and severity of ischemia, the damage inflicted to cardiomyocytes following reperfusion becomes irreversible. The combined pathologic events in the myocardium that follow a critical period of ischemia and leading to either reversible or irreversible damage to both cardiomyocytes and cardiac microvasculature is known as ischemia-reperfusion injury (Goldhaber and Weiss 1992). Ischemia-reperfusion injury has several clinical manifestations. These include reperfusion arrhythmias, microvascular and endothelial injury, myocyte damage through myocardial stunning and ultimately cell death. Irreversible injury of the myocardium leading to cell death is characterized by a spectrum of apoptotic cellular ultrastructural changes such as membrane destruction, cell swelling, DNA degradation and cytolysis accompanied by the induction of an inflammatory reaction (Bolli and Marban 1999; Jeroudi and Hartley 1994; Vatner et al. 1993; Verma et al. 2002; Yellon and Baxter 2000). Myocardial stunning or postischemic dysfunction is the mechanical dysfunction that persists after reperfusion despite the absence of irreversible damage and despite restoration of normal or near-normal coronary flow (Bolli 1990, Bolli and Marban 1999). In conscious dogs, regional contractile function remained depressed for 3 and 6 h after 5 and 15 min of coronary occlusion (Verma et al. 2002). In such cases, the myocardium seems stunned and needs a certain period of time to recover function. As mentioned, ischemia-reperfusion injury can also lead to microvascular and endothelial damage resulting in vasoconstriction, platelet and leukocyte activation, increased oxidant production and increased fluid and protein extravasation (Carden and Granger 2000; Granger 1999; Verma et al. 2002). The vasoconstriction following reperfusion can limit adequate perfusion of myocardium; this is known as the "no reflow phenomenon". Evidence points to two possible explanations for myocardial ischemia-reperfusion injury: oxidative stress induced by reactive oxygen species (ROS)

J.A.T.C. Parker and U. Mehlhorn (✉)
Department of Cardiothoracic and Vascular Surgery, University of Mainz, Mainz, Germany
e-mail: uwe.mehlhorn@uni-mainz.de, jack.parker@ukmainz.de

and intracellular Ca^{2+} overload (Bolli and Marban 1999; Dhalla et al. 1996; Ferrari 1996; Griendling and Alexander 1997; Kaplan et al. 1997; Park and Lucchesi 1999) (see Fig. 1).

11.1.1
Reactive Oxygen Species

An important cause of reperfusion injury is the enhanced production of ROS in the formerly non-perfused, now reperfused myocardium. ROS are physiologic derivatives of the cellular oxygen metabolism. Examples of oxygen free radicals are superoxide (O_2^-), hydrogen peroxide (H_2O_2) and hydroxyl radical (OH^-). Superoxide dismutase converts superoxide (O_2^-) enzymically into hydrogen peroxide (H_2O_2). In biological tissues superoxide (O_2^-) can also be converted non-enzymically into hydrogen peroxide (H_2O_2) and singlet oxygen ($^1O_2$) (Steinbeck et al. 1993). Hydrogen peroxide (H_2O_2) can be converted into the hydroxyl radical (OH^-) in the presence of reduced transition metals (e.g. ferrous or cuprous ions (Dröge 2002). Alternatively, hydrogen peroxide may be converted into water by the enzymes catalase or glutathione peroxidase (see Fig. 2). Peroxynitrite ($ONOO^-$), which apart from its intermediate is itself not a free radical, is formed by a reaction between the radicales nitric oxide (NO) and superoxide anion mainly in the endothelium, myocytes and neutrophils (Pryor et al. 1995). ROS are therefore generated by the reduction of molecular oxygen, by enzymes such as xanthine oxidase, cytochrome oxidase, cyclooxygenase or by the oxidation of catecholamines. Physiologically, ROS function in both extra- and intracellular signaling pathways in small quantities. However, excessive formation of ROS can have cytotoxic effects on myocardial tissue. This can be due to leucocyte activation in ischemia-reperfusion injury and during cardiopulmonary bypass by contact of the blood with artificial surfaces. In addition, mitochondria are a primary source for intracellular ROS in cardiac myocytes (Narayan et al. 2001; Vanden Hoek et al. 1997) and increases in intracellular calcium during ischemia-reperfusion may adversely affect mitochondrial function, which leads to ROS production and release (Staat et al. 2005). Leukocyte activation and their sequestration into target organs is considered to be the main cause of capillary leakage and organ dysfunction (Carden and Granger 2000; Tanita et al. 1999). Neutrophil activation and accumulation by ROS-mediated endothelial release of platelet activating factor can be the source of more ROS production (Jordan et al. 1999). ROS produce damage by reacting with polyunsaturated fatty acids, resulting in the formation of lipid peroxides and hydroperoxides that damage the sarcolemma and impair the function of membrane-bound phospholipids and proteins. This process has been labeled as "oxidative stress". In addition, the intermediate of peroxynitrite can nitrate and hydroxylate phenolic compounds especially at tyrosine residues which in turn alter the activities of essential proteins and enzymes (Dhalla et al. 2000). Peroxynitrite can initiate lipid peroxidation and DNA fragmentation in the myocardium in addition to inducing depletion of antioxidants (Lin et al. 1997; Ma et al. 1997). In fact, various metabolic changes during ischemia reduce the endogenous antioxidant defense systems of cardiomyocytes. The main defense against mitochondrial ROS formation is the reduced glutathione/oxidized glutathione system, which is directly linked to the $NADPH:NADP^+$ ratio via the enzyme glutathione reductase.

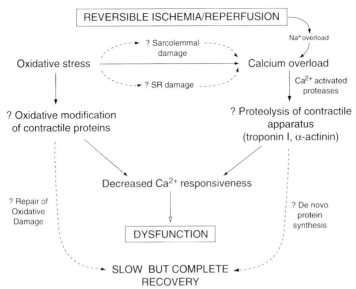

Fig. 1 Illustration of the proposed pathogenesis of postischemic myocardial dysfunction. This proposal integrates and reconciles different mechanisms into a unifying pathogenetic hypothesis. The central concepts of this proposal are that myocardial stunning is a myofilament disease, caused by impaired calcium responsiveness of contractile machinery of myocytes, and that this defect is the result of both oxidative stress and calcium overload. Transient reversible ischemia followed by reperfusion results in increased production of reactive oxygen species (ROS) and calcium overload. Oxidative stress resulting from ROS generation can lead to a decrease in calcium responsiveness of myofilaments either directly, by oxidative modification of contractile proteins (e.g., oxidation of critical thiol groups), or indirectly, by causing Ca^{2+} overload. There are at least two mechanisms whereby ROS can produce calcium overload: (1) ROS can promote sarcolemmal damage, with consequent loss of selective permeability, impairment of calcium-stimulated ATPase activity and calcium transport out of cell, and impairment of Na^+-K^+-ATPase activity with Na^+ overload; and (2) ROS can impair calcium-stimulated ATPase activity and calcium transport in the sarcoplasmic reticulum, resulting in decreased calcium sequestration and increased free cytosolic calcium. Reversible ischemia followed by reperfusion can also result in cellular calcium overload by ROS-independent mechanisms, such as cellular sodium overload due to inhibition of sarcolemmal Na^+-K^+-ATPase (caused by lack of ATP) and acidosis resulting in Na^+-H^+ exchange. Sodium overload would cause calcium overload via increased Na^+-Ca^{2+} exchange. Whatever its exact mechanism, an increase in free cytosolic calcium would activate a number of enzymes, including protein kinases, phospholipases, and other degradative enzymes, among which calcium-activated proteases are likely to be important. Activation of these proteases could lead to proteolysis of elements within the contractile apparatus (e.g., troponin I, α-actinin) and decreased calcium responsiveness of myofilaments. The slow but complete recovery characteristic of stunned myocardium could be the result of repair of oxidative damage and/or resynthesis of contractile proteins. This paradigm illustrates the fact that oxidative stress and calcium overload should not be viewed as mutually exclusive mechanisms of stunning, but rather as different components of the same pathophysiological process. (With kind permission from: The American Physiological Society; Bolli and Marban (1999))

Fig. 2 Pathways of reactive oxygen species (ROS) production and clearance. *GSH* glutathione, *GSSG* glutathione disulfide. (Used with kind permission from: The American physiological Society (Dröge (2002))

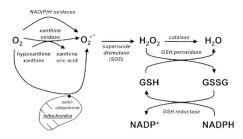

The depletion of glutathione levels increases ROS formation, oxidative stress and [Ca^{2+}] (Sharikabad et al. 2000; Verbunt and Van der Laarse 1997). Since NADPH is not formed during ischemia, the normal metabolic mechanism for regenerating reduced glutathione does not function and the endogenous defense is depressed (Mentzer et al. 2008). There is significant evidence that ROS are involved in mediating myocardial stunning (Obata et al. 1994; Sekili et al. 1993; Tang et al. 2002). It is recognized that mitochondria are a primary source of intracellular ROS in cardiomyocytes (Narayan et al. 2001; Tossios et al. 2003). ROS can attack thiol residues of numerous proteins such as the sarcoplasmic reticulum Ca^{2+}-ATP-ase, the ryanodine receptor, and contractile proteins (Sulakhe et al. 1997; Sun et al. 1996; Xu et al. 1997). This may explain why myofibrils isolated from in vivo reperfused stunned but not ischemic myocardium exhibit reduced Ca^{2+} sensitivity (Kawakami and Okabe 1998) (see Fig. 2). Direct measurement of short-lived free radicals in patients is difficult because of the transient nature of these species. Actually, most studies use indirect methods to measure free radical activity, for instance by measuring lipid peroxidation products. Direct measurement can be done with help of the electron spin trap technique (Garlick et al. 1987).

11.1.2
Reactive Nitrogen Species

The nitric oxide (NO) radical is produced by the oxidation of one of the terminal guanido-nitrogen atoms of L-Arginine (Palmer et al. 1988). This process is catalyzed by the enzyme nitric oxide synthase (NOS). NO can be converted to various other reactive nitrogen species such as nitrosonium cation (NO^+), nitroxyl anion (NO^-) or peroxynitrite ($ONOO^-$) (Stamler et al. 1992). The NADPH:$NADP^+$ ratio is a primary determinant of the redox state of the cell, and there is evidence that redox state plays a key role in determining the bioactivity and redox state of NO (Dröge 2002; Gow and Ischiropoulos 2001). In addition, possibly NOS itself can generate superoxide anion in the absence of its cofactors, such as Tetrahydrobiopterin (BH_4) (Xia et al. 1998).

11.1.3
Calcium

Prolonged ischemia is associated with severe intracellular Ca^{2+} overload. The depression in Ca^{2+}-regulatory mechanisms by ROS ultimately results in additional intracellular Ca^{2+} overload through increased L-type calcium channel current and increased $[Ca^{2+}]_i$, leading to cell death. Simultaneously, an increase in Ca^{2+} during ischemia induces the conversion of xanthine dehydrogenase to xanthine oxidase and subsequently results in generating superoxide radicals (Garlick et al. 1987). Although initial mitochondrial Ca^{2+} buffering can be cardioprotective (Delcamp et al. 1998), continued mitochondrial buffering may lead to the total collapse of mitochondrial membrane potential and cell death (Halestrap et al. 1998). Since the discussion of the implications of Ca^{2+} overload as the possible cause of ischemia-reperfusion injury is beyond the scope of this chapter, we will not go into further details here.

11.1.4
Apoptosis

During reperfusion, apoptosis may be initiated with the formation of intracellular ROS and/or intracellular calcium overload (Gottlieb et al. 1994; Maulik et al. 1998). After the first step in the cascade that leads to apoptosis, which is the translocation of the pro-apoptotic proteins Bad and Bax from the cytosol to the mitochondrial membrane, heterodimerization of Bad or Bax with the antiapoptotic Bcl-2 or Bcl-xl occurs which can lead to the release of the mitochondrial localized cytochrome c into the cytosol (Kluck et al. 1997; Mentzer et al. 2008). Cytochrome c subsequently forms a complex with apoptosis factor 1 (APAF-1) and caspase-9 in the cytosol, leading to activation of caspase 3 and the cleavage of poly(ADP)-ribosylating protein (PARP) (Mentzer et al. 2008). Activation of PARP is the final event in the process, leading to DNA fragmentation (Yang et al. 1997). The mitochondrial membrane potential collapses by the increased intracellular ROS and/or intracellular calcium overload, leading to mitochondrial permeability transition pore (MPTP) opening, which, if not reversed, can result in the loss of mitochondrial proteins such as cytochrome c (Josephson et al. 1991). However, the physiologic relevance of apoptosis during myocardial ischemia-reperfusion has yet to be determined (Mentzer et al. 2008).

11.1.5
Summary

Ischemia-reperfusion injury (i.e. myocardial stunning, apoptosis, and infarction) appears to be a complex, interconnected process. For instance, apoptosis may proceed to necrosis when mitochondria are no longer able to withstand the intracellular calcium overload and oxidative stress induced by ROS and when oxidative phosphorylation is unable to keep pace with energy demands. Due to the resulting decrease in the myocardial phosphorylation potential, energy-dependent ion pumps cannot maintain normal ion gradients. This results in cell swelling and, ultimately, loss of membrane integrity. Cardioprotection strategies that are designed to reduce cellular and subcellular ROS formation and oxidative stress, are the focus of the remaining chapter.

11.2
Oxygen Radical Scavengers (Antioxidants)

Several attempts have been made to limit the tissue damage caused by oxidative stress after ischemia-reperfusion injury that accompanies cardiopulmonary bypass. One technique used by Tang et al. (2002) was leukocyte depletion by filtering activated leucocytes from the circulation during extracorporal bypass. Although this resulted in less renal injury, not all leukocytes can be removed from the circulation by these methods and therefore end-organ damage by oxidative stress still remains. An alternative strategy for limiting oxidative stress is to scavenge the oxygen radicals by antioxidants or "oxygen radical scavengers". Antioxidants are substances that inhibit or delay the oxidative damage to subcellular proteins, carbohydrates, lipids and DNA. It has been suggested that antioxidants can act through several mechanisms such as (a) direct scavenging of ROS or their precursors, (b) inhibiting the formation of ROS, (c) attenuating the catalysis of ROS generation via binding to metal ions, (d) enhancing endogenous antioxidant generation and (e) reducing apoptotic cell death by up-regulating Bcl-2 (Dhalla et al. 2000; Maulik et al. 1999). Antioxidants can be divided into endogenous antioxidants which are produced by the body itself, and exogenous antioxidants which are produced outside the body. Examples of endogenous antioxidants are catalase, superoxide dismutase, glutathione peroxidase and vitamin E. The mechanisms of action of these endogenous antioxidants were briefly mentioned in section 1b (ROS). Superoxide dismutase is present in the cytoplasm and on the endothelial cell surface (with either copper or zinc) and in the mitochondria (with manganese) (Ohta et al. 1994). It catalyzes the dismutation of superoxide anion (O_2^-) to H_2O_2. Subsequently H_2O_2 is reduced to H_2O and O_2 by peroxidases such as glutathione peroxidase or catalase. Glutathione peroxidase, whose activity in the heart is much higher than catalase (Dhalla et al. 2000) catalyzes the peroxidation of H_2O_2 in the presence of reduced glutathione to form H_2O and oxidized glutathione. Oxidized glutathione is reduced back to glutathione by glutathione reductase, which requires NADPH from the hexose monophosphate shunt (see Fig. 2). Examples of exogenous antioxidants include: thiol-containing compounds like *N*-acetylcysteine, iron chelating agents, allopurinol, vitamins A, C and E, β-adrenergic blockers, angiotensin converting enzyme inhibitors and Ca^{2+} antagonists (Kalaycioglu et al. 1999; Khaper et al. 1997).

11.2.1
N-acetylcysteine

N-acetylcysteine (NAC) is a thiol (sulfhydryl-containing) compound, a precursor of reduced glutathione. NAC has been in clinical use for more than 30 years, primarily as a mucolytic, and is the gold standard for treatment of acetaminophen poisoning (Kelly 1998). It can both enhance intracellular glutathione synthesis and directly scavenge ROS (Kelly 1998), thereby presenting as a powerful antioxidant. In an experimental study by Ceconi et al. (1988) isolated rabbit hearts were pretreated for 60 min with an infusion of NAC (as a sulfydryl donor) before 60 mins low-flow ischemia and 30 min reperfusion. NAC treatment significantly improved post-ischemia function and induced a 38% increase in tissue content of reduced glutathione. They concluded that NAC could contribute in mitigating reperfusion damage incurred during myocardial ischemia. In more recent clinical studies (Arstall et al. 1995; Sochmann et al. 1996), it was shown that when NAC was combined with thrombolytic therapy during evolving acute myocardial infarction, significantly less oxidative stress occurred, together with a better preservation of left ventricular function. In this study, oxidative stress was measured by malondialdehyde as a measure of the extent of lipid peroxidation, by reduced (GSH) and by oxidized (GGSH) glutathione concentrations. Left ventricular function was measured by performing cardiac catheterisation between day 2 and 5 and measuring the cardiac index. The role of NAC administration on the oxidative response of neutrophils in patients subjected to cardiopulmonary bypass (CPB) and cardioplegic arrest was studied by Anderson et al. (1995). NAC was given as a bolus of 100 mg/kg followed by a continuous infusion of 20 mg/kg in the cardiopulmonary bypass circuit from the beginning to the end of bypass. The oxidative burst response of neutrophils in the patients receiving NAC was significantly reduced compared to the control group. In an attempt to identify direct evidence for cardioplegia-induced reperfusion by ROS, Mehlhorn et al. (2003) investigated the effect of cardioplegia-induced ischemia and reperfusion on myocardial distribution and formation of nitrotyrosine as a mediator for peroxynitrite-mediated tissue injury and 8-isoprostane as an indicator for ROS mediated lipid peroxidation. Nitrotyrosine represents the stable end product of cell membrane protein-bound tyrosine nitration by peroxynitrite caused by increased NO (Mihm et al. 2001). 8-isoprostaglandin-$F_2\alpha$ is the stable end product of arachidonic acid oxidation generated by the effect of ROS on membrane phospholipids (Basu et al. 2000; Reilly et al. 1997; Waugh and Murphy 1996). Transmural left ventricle biopsy specimen were collected before and after CPB, from the hearts of ten patients undergoing coronary artery operation. Immunohistochemistry was performed on nitrotyrosine and on 8-isoprostane among other enzymes. Both nitrotyrosine and 8-isoprostane formation increased after CPB in the coronary endothelium, indicating injury mediated by both peroxynitrite and oxygen-derived free radicals. The question of whether NAC could have a therapeutic effect on oxidative stress in the hearts of patients during cardiac surgery involving CPB and cardioplegic arrest was subsequently addressed in a randomized, double-blind, placebo-controlled clinical trial (Tossios et al. 2003). The effects of NAC (100 mg/kg bolus followed by continuous infusion of 20 mg/kg/h during CPB) was compared to placebo on myocardial 8-iso-prostaglandin-$F_2\alpha$ and nitrotyrosine formation as indicators for direct ROS-mediated myocardial alterations in the hearts of patients subjected to coronary artery surgery during CPB. Transmural left ventricle biopsy specimen were collected before and after CPB, and immunostained for 8-iso-prostaglandin-$F_2\alpha$ and nitrotyrosine. They found that NAC prevented formation of 8-iso-prostaglandin-$F_2\alpha$ and nitrotyrosine in left ventricular cardiomyocytes compared to placebo. These results suggest that ROS scavenging with NAC attenuates myocardial oxidative stress in the hearts of patients subjected to CPB and cardioplegic arrest (see Fig. 3).

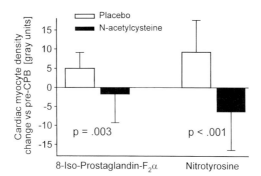

Fig. 3 Change from before CPB to the end of CPB in cardiomyocyte density for 8-iso-prostaglandin-F$_2\alpha$ and nitrotyrosine in both groups. Data are presented as means $\pm$ SD (for 8-isoprostaglandin-F$_2\alpha$, n = 19 in the placebo group and n = 17 in the NAC group; for nitrotyrosine, n = 18 in the placebo group and n = 19 in the NAC group. (Used with kind permission from: The American Association for Thoracic Surgery; (Tossios et al. (2003))

Koramaz (2006) used NAC as an enrichment of cold blood cardioplegia in a study of 30 patients subjected to coronary artery bypass grafting. They added 50 mg/kg of NAC to cold blood cardioplegia and compared this to cold blood cardioplegia alone. Serum samples were collected for measurement of malondialdehyde (MDA), an oxidative product of lipid peroxidation, and Troponin I. In the NAC group, both postoperative troponin I and MDA levels were significantly lower when compared with the control group. These results suggest that NAC-supplementation of cardioplegia minimizes myocardial injury during and after cardiac surgery. Since ROS have also been shown to induce apoptosis in cardiac myocytes subjected to ischemia and reperfusion (Dröge 2002; Von Harsdorf et al. 1999), we (Fisher et al. 2004) proposed that ROS scavenging could potentially prevent myocardial apoptosis. In a randomized study of 40 patients that underwent coronary artery bypass surgery, NAC (100 mg/kg added to CPB prime and 20 mg/kg infusion throughout bypass) was compared to placebo. LV biopsy samples were taken before and at the end of CPB and analyzed for active caspases-3 and -7, the apoptosis signal pathway central effector enzymes. The results showed that, in contrast to the placebo group, cardiac myocytes of the NAC group remained negative for both activated caspases at the end of CPB. It was concluded that NAC prevents cardioplegia-induced apoptosis signal cascade initiation in human LV myocardium.

11.2.2
Allopurinol

Allopurinol is a competitive inhibitor of the superoxide-generating enzyme xanthine oxidase, which catalyses the oxidation of hypoxanthine to xanthine and xanthine to uric acid. During ischemia, hypoxanthine formation from cell metabolism is increased and during reperfusion hypoxanthine is oxidized to uric acid by a process leading simultaneously to the formation of free radicals (Pesonen et al. 1995). Allopurinol reduces the formation of free radicals by inhibiting superoxide formation, hence it acts as an antioxidant but is only a weak radical scavenger (Downey et al. 1988). Because xanthine oxidase is virtually absent from the human heart (Grum et al. 1989), the suppression of xanthine oxidase activity and with it free radicals by allopurinol should take place mainly systemically (Coghlan et al. 1994). In a prospective, randomized, double-blind placebo-controlled study by Coghlan et al. (1994), this question was addressed and the clinical, biochemical and hemodynamic effects of low-dose xanthine oxidase inhibition in patients (n = 25) undergoing coronary artery bypass grafting was analyzed. They found that after the first postoperative hour, cardiac index increased significantly only in the active treatment group (two tablets of 300 mg of allopurinol before operation). In addition, allopurinol treatment significantly reduced the use of inotropic support after the operation and increased the rate of peripheral warming (see Fig. 4). Furthermore, products of lipid peroxidation increased significantly only in the placebo group, both in the systemic circulation and in the coronary sinus. No significant difference was found between the groups with respect to vitamin E release. Systemic radical activity appeared to dominate, because the release of products of lipid peroxidation rose more rapidly in the arterial circulation and no net arteriocoronary sinus difference was found in either group at any time point. However, the use of allopurinol only significantly attenuated the release of products of lipid peroxidation in the coronary sinus blood and not in the systemic circulation.

Allopurinol pretreatment of patients undergoing CPB has previously been reported to reduce postoperative mortality (Jeroudi and Hartley 1994), the use of inotropes (Johnson et al. 1991; Rashid and William-Olsson 1991) and arrhythmias (Rashid and William-Olsson 1991). Tarkka et al. (2000) detected significantly less myocardial production of free radicals, during early reperfusion in allopurinol pre-treated (1 g intravenously immediately prior to CPB and a second portion of 1 g into the CPB line before release of cross-clamping) coronary artery bypass patients (n = 14). In a single-center, randomized, placebo-controlled, blinded trial of 348 infants undergoing heart surgery using deep hypothermic circulatory arrest (DHCA) (Clancy et al. 2001), allopurinol was administered to the study group. Preoperatively three doses were given: the first at 16 h scheduled before surgery (5 mg/kg intravenously (i.v.), the second at 8 h before surgery (5 mg/kg i.v.) and the third dose just before surgery (10 mg/kg i.v.). Perioperatively one dose was given (20 mg/kg), administered in the CPB pump circuitry. Postoperatively nine doses were given (5 mg/kg i.v.) every 8 h. Using clinical endpoints of death, seizures, coma and cardiac events and with a 6 week follow up, it was shown that allopurinol provided significant neurocardiac protection in higher-risk hypoplastic left heart sydrome infants who underwent cardiac surgery using DHCA. Some studies combine allopurinol treatment with other antioxidants. Thus in a study by Sisto et al. (1995), coronary bypass patients (n = 37) who received 600 mg of allopurinol daily for 2 days before the operation in addition to varying doses of vitamin E and C had fewer ischemic electrocardiographic events and required less inotropic support than the placebo groups.

11.2.3
Vitamin E and C

Vitamin E with α-tocopherol as the principal antioxidant constituent is the main lipid-soluble chain-breaking, endogenous antioxidant preventing lipid peroxidation that is found in the

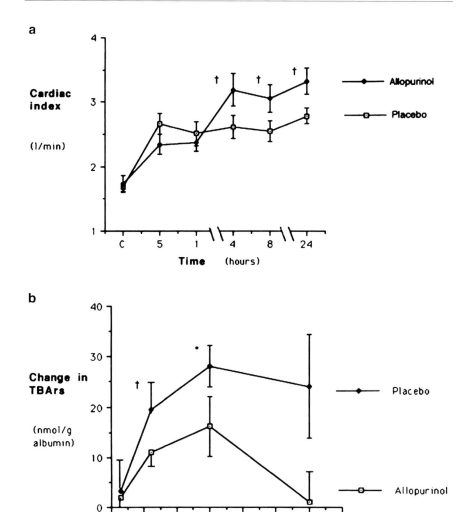

Fig. 4 (**a**) Graph of cardiac index against time during the first postoperative day. Values on *x* axis are hours after bypass. C, Control recordings taken immediately before cannulation for bypass; †, at 4, 8, and 24 h after bypass, the cardiac index in those patients who received allopurinol exceeded the prebypass cardiac index ($p < 0.001$) and the initial postbypass cardiac index after bypass ($p < 0.02$). Used with kind permission from: The American Association for Thoracic Surgery (Coghlan JG, et al. (1994): J Thorac Cardiovasc Surg 107:248–256). (**b**) Increase over control TBArs levels (TBARS means Thiobarbituric acid reactive substances) recorded in the coronary sinus according to treatment group (allopurinol or placebo) at each sampling time after crossclamp removal (mean ± standard error of the mean). Significant increases over baseline were recorded only in the placebo group. †, $p < 0.004$; *, $p < 0.001$. (Used with kind permission from: The American Association for Thoracic Surgery (Coghlan et al. (1994))

lipid membranes of cells. It traps the chain-propagating peroxyl radicals, and thereby reduces the length of the auto-oxidation chains (Cavarochi et al. 1986). Diets deficient in vitamin E result in a greater extent of lipid peroxidation in vitro and in vivo, and supplementation with vitamin E reverses this effect (Cavarochi et al. 1986). Vitamin C is an antioxidant due to its free radical trapping ability and its indirect function via its interaction with vitamin E. Therefore it is the most effective water-soluble antioxidant in the extracellular fluid and the cytoplasm (Frei et al. 1989). However, during CPB, this endogenous antioxidant defense system may be overwhelmed. Attempts have been made to supply exogenously vitamin E and C before and during CPB, with mixed results (Angdin et al. 2003; Cavalca et al. 2008; Cavarochi et al. 1986; Lassnig et al. 2003; Sisto et al. 1995). Studies vary in finding an isolated beneficial clinical effect of exogenously supplied vitamin E and/or C. In conclusion, thus far no clear consistent relevant clinical effects following antioxidant therapy with either vitamin C or E in patients undergoing cardiac surgery with CPB have been established.

11.2.4
Iron Chelators

11.2.4.1
Deferoxamine

Iron chelation with deferoxamine is capable of preventing the generation of hydroxyl radicals from superoxide ions by means of the Fe (II) to Fe (III)-driven Fenton reaction (Menashe et al. 1988). It also acts as a direct scavenger of superoxide radical and thus prevents the secondary generation of hydroxyl radical and hydrogen peroxide (Haber-Weiss cycle) (Dobsak et al. 2002). In two small clinical trails by Menasche et al. (1988, 1990) coronary bypass patients received deferoxamine (given intravenously at 30 mg/kg for 4 h and as an additive to the cardioplegic solution at 250 mg/L. In the first study, right atrial blood samples were taken before, during and after bypass and isolated polymorphonuclear neutrophils were evaluated for their capacity to generate superoxide radicals after they were chemically stimulated. In addition, 6-keto-prostaglandin F1 alpha, the stable derivative of prostacyclin, was used as an index of membrane phospholipid breakdown. They found that polymorphonuclear cells harvested from deferoxamine-treated patients produced significantly fewer superoxide radicals than those of control patients, and that plasma levels of 6-keto-prostaglandin F1 alpha were not significantly different between the two groups. In the second study, plasma lipid peroxidation was assessed. Deferoxamine treated patients showed reduced lipid peroxidation compared to controls. In a further small clinical trial of 14 randomized patients undergoing myocardial revascularisation by Ferreira et al. (1990), deferoxamine (1,000 mg/L) was given as a supplement to the cardioplegic solution. Myocardial biopsy specimens were obtained before ischemia and during reperfusion and were assessed for chemiluminescence (to indirectly determine oxygen-free radical activity) and for electron microscopic studies. Reperfusion samples from the deferoxamine treated group showed a better preservation of myocardial cells with marked reduction of severely damaged mitochondria. In these clinical trials patient outcome was not evaluated. A study by Paraskevaidis et al. (2005) investigated whether deferoxamine infusion during coronary artery bypass grafting reduces reperfusion injury by measuring malondialdehyde (as an index of lipid peroxidation) in plasma, and protects the myocardium against reperfusion injury by evaluating left ventricular ejection fraction (EF) and wall motion score index (WMSI) by transoesophageal echocardiography (TEE). Forty five consecutive male patients scheduled for coronary bypass operation (CABG) were randomly allocated to two groups. Patients either received 4 g of deferoxamine in 250 ml of 5% dextrose solution, continuously infused for 8 h before CPB (study group, n = 25) or 250 ml of 5% dextrose solution for the same period of time and infusion rate, as placebo (n = 20). Determination of malondialdehyde was performed before and during bypass, at the end of the surgical procedure, 8 h after the induction of anaesthesia, and the following day. TEE was performed by two independent experts who were blinded to patients clinical details, immediately and 8 h after the induction of anaesthesia, as well as 12 months after the procedure. Cardiac protective effects conferred by deferoxamine during CABG was additionally evaluated at 12 months after surgery by a complete physical examination and a treadmill exercise test. Interestingly, at 12 months follow up, they discovered a significantly higher left ventricular ejection fraction (LVEF) in treated patients as compared to non-treated patients. This effect was even more pronounced in patients with low LVEF (see Table 1 and Fig. 5). It was concluded, that the resultant improved patient outcome characterized by a better post-ischemic recovery of left ventricular function after CABG using i.v. deferoxamine administration just before CABG can possibly be attributed by the longer period of time of treatment with higher doses of deferoxamine, resulting in a longer protection against reperfusion injury. Overall, the above studies appear to show that iron chelators like deferoxamine can reduce oxygen free radical activity and lipid peroxidation, attenuate apoptotic cell death and preserve myocardial cells and function.

11.2.5
Other Scavengers

Several other oxygen radical scavengers have been investigated experimentally, with varying results; these include β blockers such as propanolol (Khaper et al. 1997) and carvedilol (Cargnoni et al. 2000), cyclosporine (by inhibiting the opening of mitochondrial permeability-transition pores) (Piot et al. 2008), the radical scavenger and antioxidant MCI-186 (Akao et al. 2006; Kotani 2007 and Akao 2006), mannitol (Larsen et al. 2002), selenium (Saito et al. 2003; Venardos et al. 2007), poly(ADP-ribose) polymerase (Yeh et al. 2006), melatonin (Inci et al. 2002), dipyridamole (Kusmic et al. 2000), quercetin (Hayashi et al. 2004), L-arginine (Kronon et al. 1999), and zinc-histidinate/zinc-desferrioxamine/gallium-nitrate/gallium-desferrioxamine (Karck et al. 2001). Taken together, research into the above mentioned wide spectrum of potential antioxidants remains predominantly in the experimental stage. The results have yet to be reproduced and the oxygen radical scavengers need to be tested further in controlled clinical studies.

11.3
Summary

Ischemia-reperfusion injury (i.e. myocardial stunning, apoptosis, and infarction) appears to be a complex, interconnected process. For instance, apoptosis may proceed to necrosis

11 Oxygen Radical Scavengers

Table 1 EF and WMSI after 12 months

	Before CABG	In the ICU	12 months after CABG	P (ANOVA)
Entire study group				
EF%	39.0 ± 8.0	44.6 ± 9.2	48.0 ± 8.6	0.0000[a]
WMSI	2.4 ± 0.2	1.9 ± 0.4	1.8 ± 0.4	0.0000[a]
Control (C) vs. deferoxamine (D) group				
C EF%	38.8 ± 7.9	40.3 ± 10.2	41.7 ± 7.8	
D EF%	39.2 ± 8.2	48 ± 6.6	53.0 ± 5.2	0.000[b]
P	0.841[c]	0.004[c]	0.000[c]	
C WMSI	2.4 ± 0.2	2.2 ± 0.3	2.1 ± 0.3	
D WMSI	2.4 ± 0.2	1.7 ± 0.3	1.5 ± 0.3	0.000[b]
P	0.759[c]	0.000[c]	0.000[c]	
Above (A) vs. below (B) the pre-operative EF median value (38%)				
A EF%	46.8 ± 3.2	50.7 ± 4.8	54.6 ± 3.9	
B EF%	32.2 ± 4	45.5 ± 7.3	51.5 ± 5.9	
A WMSI	2.4 ± 0.2	1.8 ± 0.2	1.7 ± 0.2	
B WMSI	2.5 ± 0.2	1.5 ± 0.3	1.3 ± 0.2	

[a]Greenhouse-Geisser statistic
[b]Wilks lambda statistic
[c]Multiple comparisons with Bonferroni adjustment

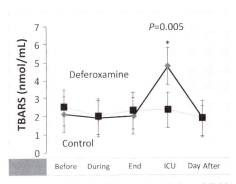

Fig. 5 TBARS (Thiobarbituric acid reactive substances, an index of lipid peroxidation) measurements before and during bypass, at the end of surgical procedure (end), at the intensive care unit (ICU), and the day after. Although at baseline TBARS were similar between the two groups, following CABG they doubled in the control group ($P = 0.01$), but remained unchanged in the deferoxamine group. (Based on: Paraskevaidis et al. (2005))

when mitochondria are no longer able to withstand the intracellular calcium overload and oxidative stress induced by ROS and when oxidative phosphorylation is unable to keep pace with energy demands. Due to the resulting decrease in the myocardial phosphorylation potential, energy-dependent ion pumps cannot maintain normal ion gradients. This results in cell swelling and, ultimately, loss of membrane integrity. ROS are involved in ischemia-reperfusion injury and ROS scavenging attenuates ischemia-reperfusion injury in both the experimental and clinical setting. Taken together, the available clinical data suggest that ROS scavenging may reduce inotropic support and improve myocardial performance. Whether these short-term beneficial effects can be transferred into any durable long-term effects remains to be determined.

References

Akao T, Takeyoshi I, Totsuka O, Arakawa K, Muraoka M, Kobayashi K, Konno K, Matsumoto K, Morishita Y (2006). Effect of the free radical scavenger MCI-186 on pulmonary ischemia-reperfusion injuri in dogs. J Heart Lung Transplant 25:965–971.

Anderson LW, Thiis J, Kharazami A, Rygg I (1995). The role of N-acetylcystein administration on the oxidative response of neutrophils during cardiopulmonary bypass. Perfusion 10:21–26.

Angdin M, Settergren G, Starkopf J, Zilmer M, Zilmer K, Vaage J (2003). Protective efect of antioxidants on pulmonary fuction after cardiopulmonary bypass. J Cardiothorac Vasc Anaesth 17:314–320.

Arstall MA, Yang J, Stafford I, Betts WH, Horowitz JD (1995). N-acetylcysteine in combination with nitroglycerin and streptokinase for the treatment of evolving acute myocardial infarction. Circulation 92:2855–2862.

Basu S, Nozari A, Liu XL, Rubertsson S, Wiklund L (2000). Development of a novel biomarker of free radical damage in reperfusion injury after cardiac arrest. FEBS Lett. 470:1–6.

Bolli R (1990). Mechanism of myocardial stunning. Circulation 82:723–738.

Bolli R, Marban E (1999). Molecular and cellular mechanisms of myocardial stunning. Physiol rev 79:609–634.

Carden DL, Granger DN (2000). Pathophysiology of ischemia-reperfusion injury. J Pathol 190:255–266.

Cargnoni A, Ceconi C, Bernocchi P, Boraso A, Parinello G, Curello S, Ferrari R (2000). Reduction of oxidative stress by carvedilol: role in maintenance of ischemic myocardium viabilità. Cardiovasc Res 47:556–566.

Cavalca V, Colli S, Veglia F, Eligini S, Zingaro L, Squellerio I, Rondello N, Cighetti G, Tremoli E, Sisillo E (2008). Anesthetic propofol enhances plasma (gamma)-tocopherol levels in patients undergoing cardiac surgery. Anaestesiology 108:988–997.

Cavarochi NC, England MD, O Brien JF, Solis E, Russo P, Schaff HV, Orszulak TA, Pluth JR, Kaye MP (1986). Superoxide generation during cardiopulmonary bypass: Is there a role for vitamin E? J Surg Res 40:519–527.

Ceconi C, Curello S, Cargnoni A, Ferrari R, Albertini A, Visioli O (1988). The role of glutathione status in the protection against ischaemic and reperfusion damage: effects of N-acetylcysteine. J Moll Cell Cardiol 20:5–13.

Clancy RR, McGaurn SA, Goin JE, Hirtz DG, Norwood WI, Gaynor W, Jacobs ML, Wernovsky G, Mahle WT, Murphy JD, Nicolson SC, Steven JM, Spray TL (2001). Allopurinol neurocardiac protection trial in infants undergoing heart surgery using deep hypothermic circulatory arrest. Pediatrics 108:61–70.

Coghlan JG, Flitter WD, Clutton SM, Panda R, Daly R, Wright G, Ilsley CD, Slater TF (1994). Allopurinol pre-treatment improves postoperative recovery and reduces lipid peroxidation in patients undergoing coronary artery bypass grafting. J Thorac Cardiovasc Surg 107:248–256.

Delcamp TJ, Dales C, Ralenkotter L (1998). Intramitochondrial [Ca^{2+}] and membrane potential in ventricular myocytes exposed to anoxia-reoxygenation. Am J Physiol 275:H484.

Dhalla NS, Wang X, Beamish RE (1996). Intracellular calcium handling in normal and failing hearts. Exp Clin Cardiol 1:7–20.

Dhalla NS, Elmoselhi AB, Hata T, Makino N (2000). Status of myocardial antioxidants in ischemia-reperfusion injury. Cardiovasc Res 47:446–456.

Dobsak P, Siegelova J, Wolf JE, Rochette L, Eicher JC, Vasku J, Kuchtickova S, Horky M (2002). Prevention of apoptosis by deferoxamine during 4 hours of cold cardioplegia and reperfusion: in vitro study of isolated working rat heart model. Pathophysiology 9:27–32.

Downey MJ, Hearse DJ, Yellon MD (1988). The role of xanthine oxidase during myocardial ischemia in several species including man. J Moll Cell Cardiol 20 (Suppl 2):55–63.

Dröge W (2002). Free radicals in the physiological control of cell function. Physiol Rev 82:47–95.

Ferrari R (1996). The role of mitochondria in ischemic heart disease. J Cardiovasc Pharmacol 28 (suppl 1):S1–S10.

Ferreira R, Burgos M, Milei J, Llesuy S, Molteni L, Hourquebie H, Boveris A (1990). Effect of supplementing cardioplegic solution with deferroxamine on reperfused human myocardium. J Thrac Cardiovasc Surg 100:708–714.

Fisher UM, Tossios UM, Huebner A, Geissler HJ, Bloch W, Mehlhorn U (2004). Myocardial apoptosis prevention by radical scavenging in patients undergoing cardiac surgery. J Thorac Cardiovasc Surg 128:103–108.

Frei B, England L, Ames BN (1989). Ascorbate is an outstanding antioxidant in human blood plasma. Proc Natl Acad Sci 86:6377–6381.

Garlick PB, Davies MJ, Hearse DJ, Slater TF (1987). Direct detection of free radicals in the reperfused rat heart using electron spin resonance spectroscopy. Circ Res 61:757–760.

Goldhaber JL, Weiss JN (1992). Oxygen free radicals and cardiac reperfusion abnormalities. Hypertension 20:118–127.

Gottlieb RA, Burleson KO, Kloner RA (1994). Reperfusion injury induces apoptosis in rabbit cardiomyocytes. J Clin Invest 94:1621.

Gow AJ, Ischiropoulos H (2001). Nitric oxide chemistry and cellular signaling. J Cell Physiol 187:277.

Granger DN (1999). Ischemia-reperfusion:mechanisms of microvascular dysfunction and the influence of risk factors for cardiovascular disease. Microcirculation 6:167–178.

Griendling KK, Alexander RW (1997). Oxidative stress and cardiovascular disease. Circulation 96:3264–3265.

Grum CM, Gallagher KP, Kirsch MM, Shafer M (1989). Absence of detectable xanthine oxidase in human myocardium. J Moll Cell Cardiol 21:263–267.

Halestrap AP, Kerr PM, Javadov S (1998). Elucidating the molecular mechanism of the permeability transition pore and its role in reperfusion injury of the heart. Biochim Biophys Acta 1366:1379.

Hayashi Y, Sawa Y, Nishimura M, Fukuyama N, Ichikawa H, Ohtake S, Nakazawa H, Matsuda H (2004). Peroxynitrite, a product between nitric oxide and superoxide anion, plays a cytotoxic role in the development of post-bypass systemic inflammatory response. Eur J Cardiothorac Surg 26:276–280.

Inci I, Inci D, Dutly A, Boehler A, Weder W (2002). Melatonin attenuates posttransplant lung ischemia-reperfusion injury. Ann Thorac Surg 73:220–225.

Jeroudi MO, Hartley, Bolli R (1994). Myocardial reperfusion injury: role of oxygen radicals and potential therapy with antioxidants. Am J Cardiol 73:2B–7B.

Johnson W, Kayser K, Brenowitz J, Saedi S (1991). A randomised controlled trial of allopurinol in coronary bypass surgery. Am Heart J 121(Pt1):20–24.

Jordan JE, Zhao ZQ, Vinten-Johansen J (1999). The role of neutrophils in myocardial ischemia-reperfusion injury. Cardiovasc Res 43:860–878.

Josephson RA, Silverman HS, Lakatta EG (1991). Study of the mechanisms of hydrogen peroxide and hydroxyl free radical-induced cellular injury and calcium overload in cardiac myocytes. J Biol Chem 266:2354.

Kalaycioglu S, Sinci V, Imren Y, Oz E (1999). Metoprolol prevents ischemia-reperfusion injury by reducing lipid peroxidation. Jpn Circ J 63:718–721

Kaplan P, Lehotsky J, Racay P (1997). Role of sarcoplasmic reticulum in the contractile dysfunction during myocardial ischemia and reperfusion. Physiol Rev 46:333–339.

Karck M, Tanaka S, Berenshtein E, Sturm C, Haverich A, Chevion M (2001). The push-and-pull mechanism to scavenge redox-active transition metals: a novel concept in myocardial protection. J Thorac Cardiovasc Surg 121:1169–1178.

Kawakami M, Okabe E (1998). Superoxide anion radical–triggered Ca^{2+} release from cardiac sarcoplasmic reticulum through ryanodine receptor Ca^{2+} channel. Mol Pharmacol 53:497.

Kelly GS (1998). Clinical applications of N-acetylcysteine. Alt Med Rev 3(2):114–127.

Khaper N, Rigatto C, Seneviratne C, Li T, Singal PK (1997). Chronic treatment with propanolol induces antioxidant changes and protects against ischemia-reperfusion injury. J Moll Cell Cardiol 29:3335–3344.

Kluck RM, Bossy-Wetzel E, Green DR (1997). The release of cytochrome c from mitochondria: A primary site for BCL-2 regulation of apoptosis. Science 275:1132.

Koramaz I, Pulathan Z, Usta S, Karahan SC, Alver A, Yaris E, Kalyoncu NI, Ozcan F (2006). Cardioprotective effect of cold-blood cardioplegia enriched with N-acetylcysteine during coronary artery bypass grafting. Ann Thorac Surg 81:613–618.

Kotani Y, Ishino K, Osaki S, Honjo O, Suezawa T, Kanki K, Yutani C, Sano S (2007). Efficacy of MCI-186, a free-radical scavenger and antioxidant, for resuscitation of nonbeating donor hearts. J Thorac Cardiovasc Surg 133:1626–1632.

Kronon MT, Allen BS, Halldorsson A, Rahman S, Wang T, Albawi M (1999). Dose dependency of L-arginine in neonatal myocardial protection: the nitric oxide paradox. J Thorac Cardiovasc Surg 118:655–664.

Kusmic C, Picano E, Busceti CL, Petersen C, Barsacchi R (2000). The antioxidant drug dipyridamole sparse the vitamin E and thiols in red blood cells after oxidative stress. Cardiovasc Res 47:510–514.

Larsen M, Webb G, Kennington S, Kelleher N, Sheppard J, Kuo J, Unsworth-White J (2002). Mannitol in cardioplegia as an oxygen free radical scavenger measured by malondialdehyde. Perfusion 17:51–55.

Lassnig A, Punz A, Barker R, Keznickl P, Manhart N, Roth E, Hiesmayr M (2003). Influence of intravenous vitamin E supplementation in cardiac surgery on oxidative stress: a double-blinded, randomised, controlled study. Br J Anaesth 91:158.

Lin KT, Xue JY, Sun FF, Wong PY (1997). Reactive oxygen species participate in peroxynitrite-induced apoptosis in HL-60 cells. Biochem Biophys Res Commun 230:115–119.

Ma XL, Lopez BL, Liu GL, Christopher TA, Ischiropoulos H (1997). Peroxynitrite aggravates myocardial reperfusion injury in the isolated perfused rat heart. Cardiovasc Res 36:195–204.

Maulik N, Engelman RM, Rousou JA, Flack III JE, Deaton D, Das DK (1999). Ischemic preconditioning reduces apoptosis by upregulating anti-death gene Bcl-2. Circulation 100:II369–II375.

Maulik N, Yoshida T, Das DK (1998). Oxidative stress developed during the reperfusion of ischemic myocardium induces apoptosis. Free Radic Biol Med 24:869.

Mehlhorn U, Krahwinkel A, Geissler HJ, Larosee K, Fischer UM, Klass O. (2003). Nitrotyrosine and 8-isoprostane formation indicate free radical-mediated injury in hearts of patients subjected to cardioplegia. J Thorac Cardiovasc Surg 125:178–183.

Menashe P, Pasquier C, Belluci S, Lorente P, Jaillon P, Piwnica A (1988). Deferoxamine reduces neutrophil-mediated free radical production during cardiopulmonary bypass in man. J Thorac Cardiovasc Surg 96:582–589.

Menasche P, Antebi H, Alcindor LG, Teiger E, Perez G, Giudicelli Y, Nordmann R, Piwnica A (1990). Iron chelation by deforoxamine inhibits lipid peroxidation during cardiopulmonary bypass in humans. Circulation 82(L5 Suppl):IV 390–396.

Mentzer RM Jr, Jahania MS, Lasley RD (2008). Myocardial protection. In: Cohn L (ed) Cardiac surgery in the adult. New York: McGraw-Hill, 443–464.

Mihm MJ, Coyle CM, Schanbacher BL, Weinstein DM, Bauer JA (2001). Peroxynitrite induced nitration and inactivation of myofibrillar creatine kinase in experimental heart failure. Cardiovasc Res 89:279–286.

Narayan P, Kilpatrick EL, Mentzer RM (2001). Adenosine A1 receptor activation reduces reactive oxygen species and attenuates stunning in ventricular myocytes. J Mol Cell Cardiol 33:121.

Obata T, Hosokawa H, Yamanaka Y (1994). In vivo monitoring of norepinephrine and OH generation on myocardial ischemic injury by dialysis technique. Am J Physiol 266:H903.

Ohta H, Adachi T, Hirano K (1994). Internalization of human extracellular superoxide dismutase by bovine aortic endothelial cells. Free Radic Biol Med 16:501–507.

Palmer RMJ, Rees DD, Ashton DS, Moncada S (1988). L-Arginine is the physiological precursor for the formation of nitric oxide in endothelium dependent relaxation. Biochem Biophys Res Commun 153:1251–1256.

Paraskevaidis IA, Iliodromitis EK, Vlahakos D, Tsiapras DP, Nikolaidis A, Marathias A, Michalis A, Kremastinos DTh (2005). Deferoxamine infusion during coronary bypass grafting ameliorates lipid peroxidation and protects the myocardium against reperfusion injury: immediate and long-term significance. Eur Heart J 26:263–270.

Park JL, Lucchesi BR (1999). Mechanisms of myocardial reperfusion injury. Ann Thorac Surg 68:1905.

Pesonen EJ, Korpela R, Peltola K (1995). Regional generation of free oxygen radicals during cardiopulmonary bypass in children. J Thorac Cardiovasc Surg 110:768–773.

Piot C, Croisille P, Staat P, Thibault H, Rioufol G, Mewton N, Elbelghiti R, Cung TT, Bonnefoy E, Angoulvant D, Macia C, Raczka F, Sportouch C, Gahide G, Finet G, Andre-Fouet X, Revel D, Kirkorian G, Monassier JP, Derumeaux G, Ovize M (2008). Effect of cyclosporine on reperfusion injury in acute myocardial infarction. NEJM 359:473–481.

Pryor WA, Squadrito GL (1995). The chemistry of peroxynitrite: a product from the reaction of nitric oxide with superoxide. Am J Physiol 268: L699–L722.

Rashid MA, William-Olsson G (1991). Influence of allopurinol on cardiac complications in open heart operations. Ann Thorac Surg 52:127–130.

Reilly MP, Delanty N, Roy L, Rokach J, Callaghan PO, Crean P. (1997). Increased formation of the isoprostanes IPF2alpha-I and 8-epi-prostaglandin F2alpha in acute coronary angioplasty: evidence for oxidant stress during coronary perfusion in humans. Circulation 96:3314–3320.

Saito Y, Yoshida Y, Akazawa T, Takahashi K, Niki E. Cell death caused by selenium deficiency and protective effect of antioxidants (2003). J Biol Chem 278:39428–39434.

Sekili S, McCay PB, Li XY (1993). Direct evidence that the hydroxyl radical plays a pathogenetic role in myocardial "stunning" in the conscious dog and demonstration that stunning can be markedly attenuated without subsequent adverse effects. Circ Res 73:705.

Sharikabad MN, Hagelin EM, Hagberg IA (2000). Effect of calcium on reactive oxygen species in isolated rat cardiomyocytes during hypoxia and reoxygenation. J Mol Cell Cardiol 32:441.

Sisto T, Paajanen H, Metsa-Ketela, Harmoinen A, Nordback I, Tarrka M (1995). Pre-treatment with antioxidants and allopurinol diminishes cardiac onset events in coronary artery bypass grafting. Ann Thorac Surg 59:1519–1523.

Sochmann J, Vrbska J, Musilova B, Rocek M (1996). Infarct size limitation: acute N-acetylcysteine defense (ISLAND trial):preliminary analysis and report after the first 30 patients. Clin Cardiol 19(2):94–100.

Staat P, Rioufol G, Piot C, Cottin Y, Cung TT, L'Huillier I, Aupetit JF, Bonnefoy E, Finet G, André-Fouët X, Ovize M (2005). Postconditioning the human heart. Circulation 112:2143–2148.

Stamler JS, Single D, Loscalzo J (1992). Biochemistry of nitric oxide and its redox-activated forms. Science 258:1898–1902.

Steinbeck MJ, Khan AU, Karnovsky MJ (1993). Extracellular production of singlet oxygen by stimulated macrophages quantified using 9,10-diphenylantracene and perylene in a polystyrene film. J Biol Chem 268:15649–15654.

Sulakhe PV, Vo XT, Phan TD (1997). Phosphorylation of inhibitory subunit of troponin and phospholaban in rat cardiomyocytes: Modulation by exposure of cardiomyocytes to hydroxyl radicals and sulfhydryl group reagents. Mol Cell Biochem 175:98.

Sun JZ, Tang XL, Park SW (1996). Evidence for an essential role of reactive oxygen species in the genesis of late preconditioning against myocardial stunning in conscious pigs. J Clin Invest 97:562.

Tanita T, Song C, Kubo H, Hoshikawa Y, Chida M, Suzuki S (1999). Superoxide anion mediates pulmonary vascular permeability caused by neutrophils in cardiopulmonary bypass. Surg Today 29:755–761.

Tang ATM, Alexiou C, Hsu J, Sheppard SV, Haw MP, Ohri SK (2002). Leukodepletion reduces renal injury ion coronary revascularisation: A prospective randomised study. Ann Thorac Surg 74:372–377.

Tarrka MR, Vuolle M, Kaukinen S, Holm P, Eloranta J, Kaukinen U, Sisto T, Kataja J (2000). Effect of allopurinol on myocardial oxygen free radical production in coronary bypass surgery. Scand Cardiovasc J 34:593–596.

Tossios P, Bloch W, Huebner A, Reza Raji M, Dodos F, Klass O, Suedkamp M, Kasper S-M, Hellmich M, Mehlhorn U (2003). N-acetylcystein prevents reactive oxygen species-mediated myocardial stress in patients undergoing cardiac surgery:results of a randomised, double-blind, placebo-controlled clinical trial. J Thorac Cardiovasc Surg 126(5):1513–1520.

Vanden Hoek TL, Shao Z, Li C (1997). Mitochondrial electron transport can become a significant source of oxidative injury in cardiomyocytes. J Mol Cell Cardiol 29:2441.

Vatner DE, Kiuchi K, Manders WT, Vatner SF (1993). Effects of coronary arterial reperfusion on beta-adrenergic receptor-adenylyl cyclase coupling. Am J Physiol 264:H196–H204.

Venardos KM, Perkins A, Headrick J, Kaye DM (2007). Myocardial ischemia-reperfusion injury, antioxidant enzyme systems, and selenium: a review. Curr Med Chem 14: 1539–1549.

Verbunt RJ, Van der Laarse A (1997). Glutathione metabolism in nonischemic and postischemic rat hearts in response to an exogenous prooxidant. Mol Cell Biochem 167:127.

Verma S, Fedak PWM, Weisel RD, Butany J, Rao V, Maitland A, Li R, Dhillon B, Yau TM (2002). Fundamentals of reperfusion injury for the clinical cardiologist. Circulation 105:2332–2336.

Von Harsdorf R, Li P-F, Dietz R (1999). Signaling pathways in reactive oxygen species-induced cardiomyocyte apoptosis. Circulation 99:2934–2941.

Waugh RJ, Murphy RC (1996). Mass spectrometric analysis of four regioisomers of F2 isoprostanes formed by free radical oxidation of arachidonic acid. J Am Soc Mass Spectr 7:490–499.

Xia Y, Tsai AL, Berka V (1998). Superoxide generation from endothelial nitric-oxide synthase: A Ca^{2+}/calmodulin-dependent and tetrahyrobiopterin regulatory process. J Biol Chem 273:25804.

Xu KY, Zweier JL, Becker LC (1997). Hydroxyl radical inhibits sarcoplasmic reticulum $Ca^{(2+)}$-ATPase function by direct attack on the ATP binding site. Circ Res 80:76.

Yang J, Liu X, Bhalla K (1997). Prevention of apoptosis by BCL-2: Release of cytochrome c from mitochondria blocked. Science 275:1129.

Yeh CH, Chen TP, Lee CH, Wu YC, Lin YM, Lin P (2006). Inhibition of poly(adp-ribose) polymerase reduces cardiomyocyte apoptosis after global cardiac arrest under cardiopulmonary bypass. Shock 25:168–175.

Yellon DM, Baxter GF (2000). Protecting the ischemic and reperfused myocardium in acute myocardial infarction:distant dream or near reality? Heart 83:381–387.

New Approaches to Cardioplegia: Alternatives to Hyperkalemia

12

David J. Chambers and Hazem B. Fallouh

12.1 Introduction

The current gold standard for cardioplegic arrest during cardiac surgery is to use a hyperkalemic (elevated potassium) solution (either crystalloid or blood-based). Hyperkalemia induces arrest by shifting the resting membrane potential towards a positive value (i.e. a depolarization) and is, therefore, classified as depolarized arrest. Despite its almost universal usage, depolarized arrest has a number of disadvantages that make hyperkalemia, potentially, a less than optimal means of inducing arrest. Thus, alternative arresting methods and agents, which may be beneficial, have been explored. This chapter describes the disadvantages of depolarized arrest and highlights the alternative agents that could possibly be used in a clinical setting to induce alternative means of arrest, discussing their potential advantages and disadvantages.

12.2 The Induction of Arrest

Elective cardiac arrest forms the cornerstone of myocardial protection for the majority of cardiac procedures (coronary artery bypass surgery and valve surgery) during cardiac operations. This involves the application of a cardioplegic solution to induce rapid myocardial arrest and induce a flaccid diastolic state that allows the surgeon a relaxed non-beating operating field – the induction of "cardioplegia". Cardioplegia can be defined as "an elective, rapid and reversible paralysis of the heart during cardiac surgery". The institution of cardioplegia ensures that myocardial oxygen consumption (MVO_2) is

---

D.J. Chambers (✉) and H.B. Fallouh
Cardiac Surgical Research/Cardiothoracic Surgery, The Rayne Institute (King's College London), Guy's & St. Thomas' NHS Foundation Trust, St. Thomas' Hospital, London, SE1 7EH, UK
e-mail: david.chambers@kcl.ac.uk, david.chambers@gstt.nhs.uk

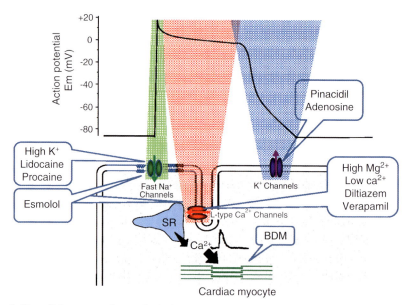

Fig. 1 The cellular targets for cardioplegic arrest and their influence on the action potential with examples of pharmacological agents (Reproduced from Chambers DJ, Fallouh HB. Pharmacol Therap 2010; 127: 41–52, with permission from Elsevier)

significantly reduced (Buckberg et al. 1977), as is the ATP depletion characteristic of severe ischemia. Cardiac arrest can be induced in a number of ways, by targeting specific processes within excitation-contraction coupling (Fig. 1); a brief description of ionic mechanisms associated with the action potential initiation of excitation-contraction coupling is detailed below.

12.2.1
The Physiology of Excitation-Contraction Coupling

The resting membrane potential (E_m) is maintained by selective ionic membrane permeability distribution, predominantly via the potassium gradient, and is therefore close to the potassium equilibrium potential (at around −85 mV). During excitation, either by external stimulation (adjacent cell, external pacing, mechanical excitation) or by spontaneous depolarization via the internal pacemaker cells (Purkinje fibres), the membrane potential rapidly depolarizes triggering the action potential (Fig. 1). This is the net result of a number of ionic currents generated by the activation of various ion channels and pumps in the membrane; these include the fast sodium channel (I_{Na}), the L-type calcium channel ($I_{Ca,L}$), and various potassium channels. These channels are all voltage-gated, and they are of particular interest because they can be pharmacologically targeted to induce myocardial arrest. Stimulation of the cell initiates the action potential via a rapid depolarization of the membrane potential (to around 20 mV) via opening of the sodium channels (Niedergerke and Orkand 1966; Opie 2004). As the membrane potential depolarizes, the L-type calcium channels become activated (at around −40 to −35 mV) allowing calcium to enter the cell; this maintains the membrane potential during the plateau phase of the action potential. The membrane permeability to potassium in an outward direction is also decreased during the plateau phase. The potassium channels are activated generating a small outward potassium current balancing the inward current of the sodium and calcium entry. The rise in intracellular calcium via opening of the L-type calcium channels during the plateau phase leads to activation of the ryanodine receptors (RyR), which are intracellular calcium channels in the sarcoplasmic reticulum (SR). RyR activation leads to a significant release of calcium into the cytosol from the calcium stores in the SR; this process is known as calcium-induced calcium release (CICR). CICR increases the cytosolic calcium concentration (from around 200 nmol/L to around 1,000 nmol/L) and thereby initiates myofilament contraction as a response to the excitation stimulus. This sharp rise in the intracellular calcium concentration by CICR is known as the calcium transient. The L-type calcium channels are inactivated by the depolarized membrane potentials and by the rapid increase in cytosolic calcium concentration. The membrane potential subsequently becomes repolarized by activation of various potassium channels, returning the membrane potential back to its resting value (Opie 2004).

Within the excitation-contraction coupling (ECC) cascade, it is possible to target the ionic mechanisms described above with pharmacological agents that will prevent ECC and thereby induce arrest of the heart. These can be categorized as:

1. Inhibition of fast sodium channels (prevent action potential conduction):
   - Shift resting E_m away from sodium channel activation threshold
     – Induce depolarization (ie. more positive E_m) by extracellular hyperkalemia (eg. St. Thomas' Hospital cardioplegia)
     – Induce hyperpolarization/polarization (ie. close to resting E_m) by potassium channel openers (eg. pinacidil, adenosine)
   - Direct blockade of fast sodium channel activation
     – Induce polarization (ie. close to resting E_m) by sodium channel blockers (eg. tetrodotoxin (TTX), lidocaine, procaine, esmolol).

2. Inhibition of calcium-activated mechanisms (prevent myocyte contraction):
   - Hypocalcemia (eg. zero extracellular calcium in Bretschneider solution (Bretschneider et al. 1975))
   - Direct blockade of sarcolemmal calcium channels (eg. calcium channel blockers – high magnesium, diltiazem, verapamil, esmolol)
   - Direct myofilament inhibition (eg. calcium desensitization – 2,3 butanedione monoxime (BDM))

3. Inhibition of multiple cellular targets (prevent action potential conduction and myocyte contraction)
   - Direct blockade of sodium and calcium channels (eg. esmolol)

12.3
Inhibition of the Fast Sodium Channels

12.3.1
Shift Resting E$_m$ Away from Sodium Activation Threshold

12.3.1.1
Extracellular Hyperkalemia (Depolarized Arrest)

As indicated above, the use of increased extracellular potassium results in a depolarization of the resting membrane potential (normally around −85 mV) to a value that is more positive (ie. less negative) than the resting value and dependent on the extracellular potassium concentration (Fig. 2).

Important threshold values occur (1) when the extracellular potassium concentration is ~10 mmol/L, giving a membrane potential of approximately −65 mV (when the voltage-dependent sodium channel is inactivated, preventing the rapid sodium-induced spike of the action potential) initiating diastolic arrest and (2) at an extracellular potassium level of ~30 mmol/L giving a membrane potential of around −35 mV (activating the calcium channel) leading to calcium uptake into the myocyte (and providing the potential for calcium overload and subsequent ischemia-reperfusion injury) (Opie 2004). Consequently, a relatively narrow protection range exists for the membrane potential (of note, the level of potassium used in the St. Thomas' Hospital cardioplegic solutions (20 or 16 mmol/L in solutions 1 and 2, respectively) fall in the middle of this "window") (Fig. 2).

The activity of the ion channels can be visualized as being controlled by "gates"; these "gates" are either in an activated or inactivated state, depending on the voltage within the

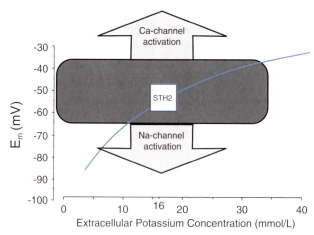

Fig. 2 The relationship between extracellular potassium concentration (mmol/L) and the membrane potential (mV). St. Thomas' Hospital cardioplegia No 2 (STH2) has a potassium concentration (16 mmol/L) that sits midway between the Na-channel inactivation threshold (around −65 mV) and the L-type calcium channel activation threshold (around −35 mV) (Reproduced from Chambers DJ, Fallouh HB. Pharmacol Therap 2010; 127: 41–52, with permission from Elsevier)

action potential. However, the differential activity rates of the "gates" that control the activation and inactivation of channels (Sperelakis et al. 2001) result in non-inactivating currents (termed "window" currents) that remain active at these potentials (Attwell et al. 1979), and allow increases in sodium and calcium (Fig. 3) that will contribute to abnormal myocardial cell ionic gradients. In addition, a "persistent" sodium current that is active at membrane potentials of around −50 mV may also contribute to these abnormal sodium gradients in the myocardial cell (Saint 2006). Attempts to correct these gradients by energy-dependent transmembrane pumps will deplete critical energy compounds (Sternbergh et al. 1989; Hiraoka 2006), and this in turn may contribute to a reduced myocardial recovery.

Consequently, although cardioplegic solutions using moderately elevated potassium concentrations constitute the most popular and widely used procedure for inducing rapid myocardial arrest, it may not be the most optimal means of cardioprotection. This becomes even more important with the changing demographics of cardiac surgery patients who are older, sicker and who have more severe and diffuse disease, and where any improvement in myocardial protection is likely to be of significance. An important characteristic of any effective solution is that it should have a good safety profile, with minimal adverse effects in the systemic circulation during acute (or even chronic) reperfusion. Solutions containing moderate elevations of potassium fulfil these characteristics; they have been shown to be relatively safe, with little post-operative systemic toxic effects and with rapid cardiac reversibility. It is important, therefore, to take into consideration the following criteria when it comes to defining alternative cardioplegic solutions and their constituent agents.

1. *Arrest*: a rapid diastolic arrest is required to keep the myocardium relaxed and to minimize cellular use of high-energy phosphate compounds (ATP and phosphocreatine).
2. *Myocardial protection*: should delay the onset of irreversible injury caused by global ischemia and limit the extent of reperfusion injury.
3. *Reversibility*: arrest should be readily and rapidly reversible on washout for quick resumption of heart function, to enable early weaning off cardiopulmonary bypass.

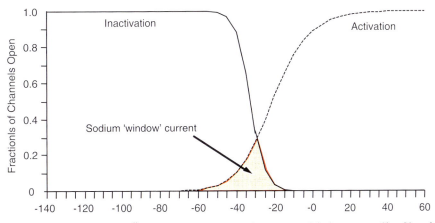

Fig. 3 The sodium "window" current occurs at membrane potentials between −60 mV and −20 mV. The differential activity rates of the channel "gates" at these potentials cause non-inactivating 'window' currents (modified from McAllister et al. (1975)) (Reproduced from Chambers DJ, Fallouh HB. Pharmacol Therap 2010; 127: 41–52, with permission from Elsevier)

4. *Low toxicity*: the cardioplegic agent should have no toxic effects on the heart or other organs after cessation of cardiopulmonary bypass. This is especially important if high concentrations of the pharmacological agent are required to achieve arrest.

Hyperkalemic cardioplegia meets all these criteria, which explains its monopoly of use in cardiac surgery. Any future alternative cardioplegic solution would be expected to offer a similar safety profile for arrest, reversibility and low toxicity, but with improved myocardial protection.

An alternative to inducing depolarized arrest by elevated extracellular potassium concentrations is to induce a hyperpolarized or polarized arrest. This is achieved by using agents that arrest the heart at membrane potentials closer to the "resting" membrane potential than that induced by elevated potassium (depolarization). A number of benefits should ensue, such as reduced ionic imbalance leading to reduced energy utilization, and hence improved protection from a cellular perspective. Hyperpolarized/polarized arrest can be achieved by a number of means using various agents. The different categories of agents, and their mechanism of action, are detailed below.

12.3.1.2
Hyperpolarization/Polarization (Potassium Channel Openers)

The opening of adenosine triphosphate-sensitive potassium channels (K_{ATP}-channels) shifts E_m towards the potassium equilibrium potential (hence a more negative membrane hyperpolarization) and away from the activation threshold of I_{Na}; this should account for the arrest by high concentrations of potassium channel openers. These drugs have been shown to exert protective effects on the myocardium under conditions of ischemia-reperfusion by preventing intracellular calcium overload via a shortening of the action potential duration which can be explained by the metabolism-sensing role of these channels in response to stress (Jahangir and Terzic 2005). K_{ATP}-channel openers are also potent vasodilators, inducing hyperpolarization on vascular smooth muscle cells (Quast et al. 1994), with some evidence that a "hyperpolarizing" cardioplegia protects endothelial function compared to a hyperkalemic "depolarizing" cardioplegia (He and Yang 1997). Studies from Damiano's group have demonstrated the beneficial effect of a variety of K_{ATP}-channel openers (such as aprikalim, pinacidil, nicorandil) to induce a hyperpolarized arrest with either improved or equivalent myocardial protection to hyperkalemic arrest (Maskal et al. 1995; Lawton et al. 1996a, b; Jayawant et al. 1997). However, these studies are not without controversy; we have shown (Walgama et al. 2000a, b) that pinacidil alone is unable to induce arrest per se during aerobic perfusion, even at very high concentrations (1 mmol/L) over extended periods (30 min). In addition, pinacidil alone did not maintain E_m below the threshold of sodium channel activation during ischemia, and required the addition of a sodium channel blocker (procaine, at 1 mmol/L) for complete arrest and improved protection (Walgama et al. 2000a, b). There is also the risk of significant increases in postischemic arrhythmias (Lawton et al. 1996a, b); in addition, the systemic clearance of potassium channel openers is prolonged (Ward et al. 1984) which risks a residual hypotensive effect in patients post-bypass. These limitations make the concept of using a cardioplegia based on K_{ATP}-channel openers as unlikely for future clinical application.

K_{ATP}-channel openers have also been suggested to enhance the cardioprotection of hyperkalemic cardioplegic solutions. Thus, use of these drugs for short pretreatment periods (at least 3 min) before hyperkalemic arrest were shown to improve post-ischemic function (Sugimoto et al. 1994; Dorman et al. 1998; Hebbar et al. 1998), and this may be associated with preconditioning (Menasche et al. 1996). Similar benefits were obtained when potassium-channel openers were used as additives to hyperkalemic cardioplegic solutions (Hosoda et al. 1994; Qiu et al. 1995; Dorman et al. 1997), but these studies remain controversial since others (Galinanes et al. 1992; Ducko et al. 2000) have been unable to show these benefits. Treatment with K_{ATP}-channel openers has also been suggested to prevent the increases in intracellular calcium seen with hyperkalemic solutions (Lopez et al. 1996; Dorman et al. 1997), which may account for the beneficial effects observed. Such benefits may also be associated with the location of the K_{ATP}-channels; improved protection has been observed with mitochondrial-specific K_{ATP}-channel openers such as diazoxide (McCully and Levitsky 2003).

Adenosine, an endogenous purine nucleoside, has been shown to induce complete arrest (at 50 μmol/L) and a hyperpolarization of ~12 mV in the isolated rabbit sino-atrial (SA) node cells via an increased membrane potassium permeability (Belardinelli et al. 1988). It appears to act via an adenosine receptor-activated potassium channel and hence could have similar effects to K_{ATP}-channel openers. This cardioplegic property has been examined in whole hearts, using adenosine either as sole arrest agent (at 10 mmol/L) or as an additive (at 1 mmol/L) to hyperkalemia (Schubert et al. 1989; de Jong et al. 1990; Boehm et al. 1991); adenosine reduced time to arrest and improved post-ischemic recovery of function compared to hyperkalemic cardioplegia. As an additive to hyperkalemic solutions (16 mmol/L potassium), adenosine (1 mmol/L) did not influence the level of depolarization induced by potassium, but did slow the rate of depolarization which reduced the associated intracellular calcium loading (Alekseev et al. 1996). Additionally, it was shown that 1 mmol/L adenosine (but not 0.1 mmol/L) prevented potassium-induced intracellular calcium loading and that this was associated with a PKC-dependent mechanism but not a K_{ATP}-channel dependent mechanism (Jovanovic et al. 1997). Addition of adenosine (at concentrations ranging from 0.1 to 20 mmol/L) to St. Thomas' Hospital cardioplegia was shown to enhance efficacy (Katayama et al. 1997); interestingly, the effects were temperature-dependent, being reduced at hypothermia, and appeared to prevent high-energy phosphate metabolism. Adenosine has also recently been shown to be an effective additive to lidocaine, with improved cardioprotection compared to hyperkalemic cardioplegia (St. Thomas' solution) (Dobson and Jones 2004).

The use of adenosine as an adjunct to hyperkalemic cardioplegic solutions has been examined in a number of clinical studies, but these have had equivocal results. Thus, addition of adenosine (at concentrations ranging from 1 to 250 μmol/L) to warm antegrade blood cardioplegia showed that it was well tolerated up to 25 μmol/L, but higher concentrations induced hypotension (Fremes et al. 1996). Further studies, adding adenosine at 15, 50 or 100 μmol/L to warm antegrade blood cardioplegia showed no benefit to patient outcome in terms of mortality, function or infarction (Cohen et al. 1998). However, a similar study with adenosine added to cold blood cardioplegia (at higher concentrations of 0.5 or 2.0 mmol/L) showed a tendency to reduce adverse events (Mentzer et al. 1999). The clinical studies leave many unanswered questions regarding the efficacy of adenosine as an additive to blood cardioplegia; the short half-life of adenosine (~30 s) may play a role in these effects, and suggest that it may be more effective as a continuous infusion to maintain its effect. Adenosine has been shown to be safe, both experimentally and clinically; its short-acting effect and low potency (requiring relatively high concentrations) is likely to make it more appropriate as an additive to other arresting agents to improve cardioprotection than a cardioplegic agent per se.

12.3.2
Direct Blockade of Sodium Channel Activation (Sodium Channel Blockers)

Direct sodium channel blockade is an effective way to prevent the voltage-activated fast inward sodium-induced depolarization of the action potential (Miller 1998). Tetrodotoxin (TTX) is a potent and rapidly reversible sodium channel blocker, but it is also highly toxic. However, TTX has been shown in experimental studies to act as an effective cardioplegic agent, protecting isolated rat hearts against 60 min of normothermic global ischemia (Tyers et al. 1974). It has been suggested to induce a polarized arrest of the heart, and at a concentration of 25 µmol/L reduced basal metabolic requirements (MVO_2) during ischemic arrest compared to hyperkalemic (depolarized) arrest (Sternbergh et al. 1989). Studies from the authors laboratory, in which TTX (at an optimally defined concentration of 22 µmol/L) was used to induce arrest of isolated working rat hearts subjected to long-term (5–8 h) hypothermic (7.5°C) global ischemic storage, demonstrated significant improvement in protection compared to hyperkalemic (16 mmol/L K^+) arrest (Snabaitis et al. 1997). These studies demonstrated improved post-ischemic function, established that polarized arrest did occur (with a maintained membrane potential during arrest of around −70 mV) and confirmed the reduced metabolic requirements by showing that myocardial content of high-energy phosphate compounds (ATP and phosphocreatine) at the end of ischemia were significantly higher in the TTX-arrested hearts. We were additionally able to establish that polarized arrest resulted in a reduction in the ionic imbalance seen with depolarized (hyperkalemic) arrest (indirectly measured as a reduced efflux of K^+ during ischemia) (Snabaitis et al. 1999). Moreover, the importance of Na^+ and Ca^{2+} overload in the development of myocardial injury was shown (Snabaitis and Chambers 1999) by the sequential addition to the TTX (polarizing) solution of drugs that induced Na/H-exchange inhibition (HOE694), Na/K/2Cl-cotransport inhibition (furosemide) and calcium desensitization (2,3-butanedione monoxime: BDM) to induce additive protective effects on post-ischemic recovery of function when compared to the St. Thomas' Hospital cardioplegic solution. Whilst these studies confirmed the concept that polarized arrest is an effective mechanism to induce arrest and improve myocardial protection, the extreme toxicity of TTX means that it would be unusable clinically as a cardioplegic agent.

Agents with local anesthetic effects (such as procaine and lidocaine) are, however, available clinically and indeed have been widely used either alone or in combination with other agents to induce cardiac arrest (Hearse et al. 1981a, b). Procaine, used at high (~7–11 mmol/L) concentrations as a cardioprotective agent, was used in various early cardioplegic solutions (such as the Bretschneider and Kirsch solutions) (Kirsch et al. 1972; Bretschneider et al. 1975), but later systematic characterisation of both procaine and lidocaine at various concentrations demonstrated significant detrimental effects at these high concentrations (Hearse et al. 1981a, b). The original St. Thomas' Hospital cardioplegic solution No. 1 includes procaine (at 1 mmol/L) as a membrane stabilizer, but it was removed from the No 2 solution to enable its use in the USA (procaine is not authorized by the FDA). Although procaine has been demonstrated to control rhythm disturbances post-operatively (Sellevold et al. 1995), there is also a risk of cardiac arrhythmia and neurological toxicity associated with its use (Brown et al. 1995).

Lidocaine is widely used clinically as a local anesthetic and anti-arrhythmic agent; its mechanism of action is via sodium-channel blockade and, as such, would also appear to be a potentially useful cardioplegic agent. Recently, studies have shown that a combination of lidocaine (500 μmol/L) with adenosine (200 μmol/L) induces a more rapid arrest (suggested to be a "polarized" arrest by estimation of the membrane potential) with improved cardioprotection in rat hearts subjected to prolonged (2 or 4 h) global ischemia compared to a hyperkalemic depolarizing (St. Thomas' Hospital) solution (Dobson and Jones 2004). The calculated membrane potential in these adenosine-lidocaine (AL) arrested hearts was −83 mV, a value similar to that obtained for the resting membrane potential in normal pre-arrest hearts (Kleber 1983). However, our data (Snabaitis et al. 1997), using isolated rat hearts arrested with TTX and in which the membrane potential was measured by sharp electrodes throughout the ischemia (see above), would suggest that these values are unlikely and that some degree of depolarization will be induced during the global ischemia, probably arising from the efflux of potassium from the myocytes. Additional rat heart studies from this group (Sloots et al. 2007) showed no differences in myocardial protection between continuous or intermittent AL solution (at the same concentrations as above) after 40 or 60 min of global tepid (33°C) ischemia; interestingly, intermittent lidocaine alone was less protective than the AL solution, with longer arrest times, increased coronary vascular resistance and reduced recovery of function. This would suggest that adenosine, even at the low concentration of 200 μmol/L, has a significant protective capability. In a more clinically relevant study from the same group (Corvera et al. 2005), it was shown that multidose arrest with a blood-based adenosine-lidocaine (AL-BCP) solution in dogs subjected to cardiopulmonary bypass and global cold (10°C) or warm (37°C) ischemia induced similar protection to that of a corresponding blood-based hyperkalemic (20 mmol/L) solution. Interestingly, this AL-BCP solution was formulated with higher adenosine (400 μmol/L) and lidocaine (750 μmol/L) concentrations to that of the original rat study (Dobson and Jones 2004); despite this, complete arrest was not achieved with cold (10°C) AL-BCP in all hearts, and quiescence was not maintained. This indicates a temperature sensitivity of the solution (possibly due to the lidocaine) and suggested that the solution may be more suitable for tepid or warm ischemic arrest.

Whilst a lidocaine-based solution may appear to be a logical option for improving protection over a hyperkalemic solution, experimental studies have questioned the safety of this drug (despite its clinical use as a local anesthetic and anti-arrhythmic agent, with known side-effects and safety profiles). As a blood-based solution, lidocaine (in combination with magnesium) was shown (Yamaguchi et al. 2007) to effectively arrest dog hearts at a concentration of 1.3 mmol/L; however, this gave systemic concentrations around 20 μg/ml, which is significantly higher than the upper safety margin (~8 μg/ml), and was the first study to examine toxic effects of high sodium channel blocker doses when used as cardioplegic agents (Fallouh and Chambers 2007). Even using lower concentrations of lidocaine may still have potential risks if large doses of cardioplegia were required in prolonged procedures, or in patients with liver impairment or heart failure where the half-life of lidocaine (normally 1.5–2 h) could become significantly longer (Thomson et al. 1973). The risk of lidocaine accumulation in the peripheral circulation could cause problems after weaning off cardiopulmonary bypass.

12.4
Inhibition of Calcium-Activated Mechanisms

As discussed earlier, the intracellular calcium transient increase during each heartbeat is a fundamental part of excitation-contraction coupling. Influencing this increase can have profound effects on the heart; reduction (or abolition) of the calcium transient will prevent mechanical contraction and induce a diastolic arrest. Hence, this should be an effective way to induce cardioplegic arrest; however, caution should be exercised when inhibiting calcium mechanisms as considerable injury can be induced under certain circumstances. The effect of action of agents that influence calcium mechanisms are detailed below.

12.4.1
Hypocalcemia

The complete absence of extracellular calcium from a bathing or perfusion solution of heart muscle effectively prevents calcium influx through the L-type calcium channels and inhibits calcium-induced calcium release from the sarcoplasmic reticulum (SR), so abolishing excitation-contraction coupling of the myofilaments (Rich et al. 1988; Bers 2002) and arresting the heart in diastole (Ringer 1883). Perfusion of hearts with extracellular solutions containing zero calcium risks inducing the "calcium paradox" (Chapman and Tunstall 1987); this reduction of the calcium driving force leads to calcium efflux and sodium loading via the Na/Ca exchanger during the calcium-free period, which is then replaced by calcium loading when subsequently perfused with calcium-containing solutions, leading to a lethal condition of contracture and massive ultrastructural injury. Despite this, a number of cardioplegic solutions have used zero calcium in their composition. The Bretschneider intracellular-type solution (Bretschneider et al. 1975) contained zero calcium but was combined with low-sodium (12 mmol/L) and procaine (7.4 mmol/L); low sodium (and/or high magnesium) will tend to protect against the calcium paradox, as will the conventional hypothermic use of this solution. In reality, there are also often trace contaminants of calcium sufficient to prevent this injury. The low extracellular sodium attenuates the fast sodium current (via the cardiac sodium channel) at the initiation of the action potential; this will tend to maintain membrane potential close to the resting membrane potential, thereby favouring a polarized arrest. Studies comparing the St. Thomas' Hospital solution (normocalcemic and hyperkalemic) to the Bretschneider solution (Jynge et al. 1977; Jynge et al. 1978) demonstrated optimal protection with St. Thomas' solution at all temperatures; in contrast, Bretschneider solution was only protective at hypothermia. The University of

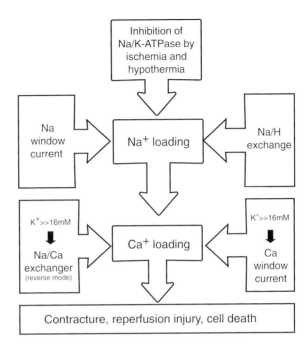

Fig. 4 The mechanisms involved in sodium and calcium loading in cardiac myocytes during depolarized arrest

Wisconsin (UW) intracellular-type organ preservation solution is another zero calcium solution; however, for protection of the heart, it has been shown to be infusion and storage temperature-sensitive with improved protection when calcium and/or magnesium is added (Swanson et al. 1988; Amrani et al. 1992; Fremes et al. 1995).

The stoichiometry between calcium and sodium are inextricably linked to the sodium-calcium exchanger; both these ions need to be reduced to ensure relatively safe myocardial protection, but this relationship is extremely complex (Fig. 4). As a safer alternative, it may be preferable to use drugs that influence calcium movements.

12.4.2
Direct Blockade of Cell Membrane Calcium Channels (Calcium Channel Blockers)

Blockade of the L-type calcium channel decreases calcium influx and inhibits CICR from the SR, which depresses cardiac function. Elevated extracellular concentrations of magnesium can induce myocardial arrest (Shattock et al. 1987), and this is thought to occur by blocking L-type calcium channels via displacement of calcium (Iseri and French 1984). However, these effects are species-dependent; rat myocardium is very sensitive whereas rabbit myocardium is relatively insensitive, possibly reflecting differential sensitivity of the calcium channel to magnesium. Effects on human myocardium are thought to be intermediate to rat and rabbit. Although there have been some examples of magnesium being used as a cardioplegic agent (such as the Kirsch solution, with a magnesium concentration of 160 mmol/L, but in combination with a high (11 mmol/L) concentration of the sodium-channel blocker procaine

(Kirsch et al. 1972)), it has rarely been used in this context. We have recently examined the protective effects of magnesium when used as a cardioplegic agent (Maruyama and Chambers 2008); in combination with a novel perfusion solution (Aqix), it was shown to be effective at an optimal concentration of 25 mmol/L, and to provide improved protection when given as multiple infusions (compared to St. Thomas' Hospital solution). Despite this evidence of efficacy of magnesium alone as a cardioplegic agent, it is more likely to be used for its anti-ischemic effects as an additive to other cardioplegic solutions.

An increase in extracellular magnesium (to levels of 10–20 mmol/L) as an additive to hyperkalemic cardioplegia has been shown to protect against calcium overload during ischemia and reperfusion (Hearse et al. 1978; Brown et al. 1991); improved protection has also been shown in both aged hearts (McCully and Levitsky 1997) and in immature hearts (Kronon et al. 1999). Magnesium is thought to exert its protective effect by influencing the high-energy phosphate content of the myocardium, resulting in improved ATP availability and reduced ATP utilization (Brown et al. 1991; Tsukube et al. 1997). These metabolic effects are associated with reduced intracellular calcium accumulation (Steenbergen et al. 1990) which is linked to the calcium channel antagonistic effects of magnesium (Iseri and French 1984; Shattock et al. 1987). Thus, magnesium appears to be a relatively safe additive for alternative cardioplegic solutions, with considerable protective effects associated with an elevated extracellular concentration (Chakraborti et al. 2002).

In addition to magnesium, there are also drugs that have been specifically developed to act as antagonists of the L-type calcium channel (Fleckenstein and Fleckenstein-Grün 1988). At high concentrations, these calcium antagonists (calcium-channel blockers such as verapamil, diltiazem and nifedipine) can act as cardioplegic agents per se and induce arrest of the heart (Vouhe et al. 1980; Balderman et al. 1992), with comparable protective effects to those of hyperkalemic cardioplegia. However, these agents generally have prolonged negative inotropic effects (such as verapamil with a half-life of >2 h (Popovic et al. 2006)) due to a high affinity of these agents for the L-type calcium channels (Dillon and Nayler 1987). This affinity could result in a slower recovery than that seen with hyperkalemia; this may have both beneficial effects (such as reduced washout by collateral flow and potential for reduced calcium overload during reperfusion) and detrimental effects (prolonged exacerbation of acute stunning leading to low output (Christakis et al. 1986; Breisblatt et al. 1990).

Calcium-channel blockers have also been used as additives to hyperkalemic cardioplegic solutions (de Jong 1986). However, they have been shown to be temperature-sensitive, with no additional protection during hypothermia (Yamamoto et al. 1985), as well as potentially detrimental in patients with severe dysfunction (Christakis et al. 1986). Thus, although calcium-channel blockers are known to be cardioprotective during ischemia, any beneficial effects are likely to be outweighed by the detrimental effects related to dose-dependent, temperature-dependent and time-dependent activity.

12.4.3
Direct Myofilament Inhibition (Calcium Desensitization)

An alternative to influencing effects of calcium at the sarcolemmal level via the calcium channel is to target the intracellular effect of calcium directly on the myofilaments. Direct myofibril desensitization can be induced by 2,3-butanedione monoxime (BDM), which inhibits the force-producing cross-bridge formation between actin and myosin (Gwathmey et al. 1991). BDM was originally developed as an antidote to sarin poisoning, with apparent "chemical phosphatase" activity. Since it is a small and uncharged lipophilic molecule, it can readily exchange with the intracellular milieu, which makes its effects rapidly reversible. As such, it would appear to be a potentially suitable cardioplegic agent; indeed, it has been examined in this role in a number of experimental studies. BDM cardioplegia (using 30 mmol/L BDM) was compared to Bretschneider's HTK solution in porcine and human heart muscle strips (Vahl et al. 1994; Vahl et al. 1995). It was shown that BDM abolished force development despite maintenance of the calcium transient (to a level of around 60% of control), and complete recovery of function was obtained with ischemic periods up to fourfold longer for BDM cardioplegia compared to HTK solution. Studies using isolated rabbit hearts (Jayawant et al. 1999) have also shown that a BDM-based cardioplegia (5 mmol/L BDM) as the arresting agent achieved a similar cardioprotection after 60 min of global ischemia to that of St. Thomas' cardioplegia (hyperkalemia), and despite maintenance of electrical activity for around 34 min.

BDM has also been used as an effective additive to hyperkalemic cardioplegic and long-term preservation solutions. Addition of BDM (at 30 mmol/L) to the University of Wisconsin preservation solution (Stringham et al. 1992) significantly improved the outcome of isolated rabbit hearts stored for 24 h (particularly when calcium was also added) compared to standard UW solution. The addition of BDM prevented contracture formation and reduced high-energy phosphate consumption. Studies from our laboratory have also shown similar synergistic cardioprotective effects with the addition of BDM (at 30 mmol/L) to a "polarized" solution (based on arrest with tetrodotoxin (TTX) used for long-term preservation in isolated working rat hearts (Snabaitis and Chambers 1999) compared to the St. Thomas' Hospital cardioplegic solution; however, in this study we confirmed a calcium-chelating effect of BDM previously seen by others (Garcia-Dorado et al. 1992). When the calcium was titrated back to normal ionic concentrations, the protective effect of BDM was maintained indicating that protection was not associated with this hypocalcemia. Thus, although BDM would appear to have considerable cardioprotective properties, it has not (to our knowledge) been used in any clinical solutions, which raises questions concerning its potential toxic effects (possibly associated with the calcium chelating effect).

12.5
Inhibition of Multiple Cellular Targets

Although induction of arrest can be achieved by inhibition of each of the cellular ionic mechanisms described (Fig. 1), it is possible that inhibition of multiple targets may have synergistic effects to improve protection. Alternatively, it might be that lower concentrations of an arresting agent would be required. This would improve the safety profile of the cardioplegic agents and may also reduce systemic toxicity during reperfusion and improve the rate of reversibility of the agent(s).

12.5.1
Direct Blockade of Both Sodium and Calcium Channels (eg. Esmolol)

Esmolol is an ultra-short-acting cardioselective β_1-blocker that is used clinically for hypertension and tachycardia, and has also been shown to possess myocardial protective effects against ischemia and reperfusion in unstable angina patients (Hohnloser et al. 1991) and during cardiac surgery (Boldt et al. 2004). These properties have been exploited in both experimental (Mehlhorn et al. 1996; Geissler et al. 2000; Booth et al. 2002) and clinical studies (Kuhn-Regnier et al. 1999; Mehlhorn et al. 1999; Kuhn-Regnier et al. 2002) where it has been used during cardiac surgery as a means of inducing "minimal myocardial contraction" (profound bradycardia during maintained continuous normothermic myocardial perfusion, thereby avoiding ischemia) to allow coronary artery bypass surgery on the beating heart. These studies also showed that cardioprotection with esmolol compared favourably to conventional cardioplegic solutions, with an improved protection that may have partly resulted from a reduced myocardial edema formation associated with the continued perfusion and bradycardia.

We (Bessho and Chambers 2001; Bessho and Chambers 2002), and others (Ede et al. 1997), have demonstrated that a high concentration of esmolol (at about 1 mmol/L) induces a diastolic cardiac arrest and thus acts as a cardioplegic agent. Esmolol added to an oxygenated perfusate provided superior cardioprotection (improved recovery of function) to isolated rat hearts when compared to cross-clamp fibrillation (Bessho and Chambers 2001) or St. Thomas' Hospital cardioplegic solution (Bessho and Chambers 2002) after prolonged periods of global ischemia. The β-blocking action of esmolol explains the bradycardia and negative inotropic effect of esmolol, but its arrest invoking action (in an isolated heart with no catecholamine background) requires an alternative explanation for this action, especially as it contrasts other β-blockers (such as atenolol) that do not induce arrest at equipotent doses. Recent studies from our group, and others, have shown that millimolar concentrations of esmolol inhibit the L-type calcium channels (Arlock et al. 2005; Fallouh et al. 2007) and the fast sodium channels (Deng et al. 2006; Fallouh et al. 2008), resulting in a pronounced negative inotropy, a failure of action potential conduction and induction of a diastolic polarized arrest. The short half-life of esmolol (of about 9 min) that results from blood red cell esterase activity (Zaroslinski et al. 1982) gives it independence from renal or hepatic clearance from the systemic circulation, with associated safety profile advantage over some of the other cardioplegic agents described (such as lidocaine, diltiazem, etc). Clinically, the use of relatively high concentrations of esmolol during cardiac surgery (Zaroslinski et al. 1982; Kuhn-Regnier et al. 1999, 2002; Mehlhorn et al. 1999) has demonstrated its safety. However, prolonged infusion periods in excess of 20 min with esmolol concentrations of around 1.5 mmol/L have suggested that the reversibility may be compromised (Pirk et al. 1999); concentrations of ~0.75 mmol/L were optimal for reversibility which casts some doubt on the clinical potential of these higher esmolol concentrations as cardioplegic agents per se.

12.6
Conclusion

During cardiac surgery, the rapid induction of depolarized arrest by a moderately hyperkalemic solution has been the cornerstone of myocardial protection over the past 30 years. Despite this, innumerable studies have been conducted into improving the protection afforded by this technique, without any significant advance over the initial solutions developed in the 1970s. In considering the characteristics of patients who currently receive cardiac surgery in the twentyfirst century compared to those operated in the mid 1970s and 1980s, there is more severe and diffuse disease in a considerably more elderly patient population. Hence, the requirement for improved myocardial protection has never been greater. To achieve this improvement, however, it is likely that new concepts will have to be examined that challenge the traditionally held views concerning the unassailability of hyperkalemic arrest. Using the agents that are potentially available to induce arrest, an important aspect will be providing safety profiles that match those of hyperkalemia. One concept that has gained some momentum regarding potential beneficial advantages to hyperkalemia is that of induction of a polarized arrest, achieved by a variety of agents. These have been described above, and their safety profiles highlighted. Considerably more research will be needed before any of these agents can be accepted clinically and used to determine whether there are clinical benefits that match the potential shown in a number of experimental studies. It is with this in mind that this chapter was written.

References

Alekseev AE, Jovanovic A, Lopez JR, Terzic A (1996). Adenosine slows the rate of K(+)-induced membrane depolarization in ventricular cardiomyocytes: possible implication in hyperkalemic cardioplegia. J Mol Cell Cardiol 28(6): 1193–1202.

Amrani M, Ledingham S, Jayakumar J, Allen NJ, Rothery S, Severs N, Yacoub M (1992) Detrimental effects of temperature on the efficacy of the University of Wisconsin solution when used for cardioplegia at moderate hypothermia. Comparison with the St. Thomas Hospital solution at 4 degrees C and 20 degrees C. Circulation 86(5 Suppl): II280–II288.

Arlock P, Wohlfart B, Sjoberg T, Steen S (2005). The negative inotropic effect of esmolol on isolated cardiac muscle. Scand Cardiovasc J 39(4): 250–254.

Attwell D, Cohen I, Eisner D, Ohba M, Ojeda C (1979). The steady state TTX-sensitive ("window") sodium current in cardiac Purkinje fibres. Pflugers Arch 379(2): 137–142.

Balderman SC, Schwartz K, Aldrich J, Chan AK (1992). Cardioplegic arrest of the myocardium with calcium blocking agents. J Cardiovasc Pharmacol 19(1): 1–9.

Belardinelli L, Giles WR, West A (1988). Ionic mechanisms of adenosine actions in pacemaker cells from rabbit heart. J Physiol 405: 615–633.

Bers DM (2002). Cardiac excitation-contraction coupling. Nature 415(6868): 198–205.

Bessho R, Chambers DJ (2001). Myocardial protection: the efficacy of an ultra-short-acting beta-blocker, esmolol, as a cardioplegic agent. J Thorac Cardiovasc Surg 122(5): 993–1003.

Bessho R, Chambers DJ (2002). Myocardial protection with oxygenated esmolol cardioplegia during prolonged normothermic ischemia in the rat. J Thorac Cardiovasc Surg 124(2): 340–351.

Boehm DH, Human PA, von Oppell U, Owen P, Reichenspurner H, Opie LH, Rose AG, Reichart B (1991). Adenosine cardioplegia: reducing reperfusion injury of the ischaemic myocardium? Eur J Cardiothorac Surg 5(10): 542–545.

Boldt J, Brosch C, Lehmann A, Suttner S, Isgro F (2004). The prophylactic use of the beta-blocker esmolol in combination with phosphodiesterase III inhibitor enoximone in elderly cardiac surgery patients. Anesth Analg 99(4): 1009–1017.

Booth JV, Spahn DR, McRae RL, Chesnut LC, El-Moalem H, Atwell DM, Leone BJ, Schwinn DA (2002). Esmolol improves left ventricular function via enhanced beta-adrenergic receptor signaling in a canine model of coronary revascularization. Anesthesiology 97(1): 162–169.

Breisblatt WM, Stein KL, Wolfe CJ, Follansbee WP, Capozzi J, Armitage JM, Hardesty RL (1990). Acute myocardial dysfunction and recovery: a common occurrence after coronary bypass surgery. J Am Coll Cardiol 15(6): 1261–1269.

Bretschneider HJ, Hubner G, Knoll D, Lohr B, Nordbeck H, Spieckermann PG (1975). Myocardial resistance and tolerance to ischemia: physiological and biochemical basis. J Cardiovasc Surg (Torino) 16(3): 241–260.

Brown DL, Ransom DM, Hall JA, Leicht CH, Schroeder DR, Offord KP (1995). Regional anesthesia and local anesthetic-induced systemic toxicity: seizure frequency and accompanying cardiovascular changes. Anesth Analg 81(2): 321–328.

Brown PS, Jr., Holland FW, Parenteau GL, Clark RE (1991). Magnesium ion is beneficial in hypothermic crystalloid cardioplegia. Ann Thorac Surg 51(3): 359–366; discussion 367.

Buckberg GD, Brazier JR, Nelson RL, Goldstein SM, McConnell DH, Cooper N (1977). Studies of the effects of hypothermia on regional myocardial blood flow and metabolism during cardiopulmonary bypass. I. The adequately perfused beating, fibrillating, and arrested heart. J Thorac Cardiovasc Surg 73(1): 87–94.

Chakraborti S, Chakraborti T, Mandal M, Mandal A, Das S, Ghosh S (2002). Protective role of magnesium in cardiovascular diseases: a review. Mol Cell Biochem 238(1–2): 163–179.

Chapman RA, Tunstall J (1987). The calcium paradox of the heart. Prog Biophys Mol Biol 50(2): 67–96.

Chambers DJ, Fallouh HB (2010). Cardioplegia and cardiac surgery: Pharmacological arrest and cardiac protection during global ischemia and reperfusion. Pharmacol Therap 127(1): 41–52.

Christakis GT, Fremes SE, Weisel RD, Tittley JG, Mickle DA, Ivanov J, Madonik MM, Benak AM, McLaughlin PR, Baird RJ (1986). Diltiazem cardioplegia. A balance of risk and benefit. J Thorac Cardiovasc Surg 91(5): 647–661.

Cohen G, Feder-Elituv R, Iazetta J, Bunting P, Mallidi H, Bozinovski J, Deemar C, Christakis GT, Cohen EA, Wong BI, McLean RD, Myers M, Morgan CD, Mazer CD, Smith TS, Goldman BS, Naylor CD, Fremes SE (1998). Phase 2 studies of adenosine cardioplegia. Circulation 98(19 Suppl): II225–233.

Corvera JS, Kin H, Dobson GP, Kerendi F, Halkos ME, Katzmark S, Payne CS, Zhao ZQ, Guyton RA, Vinten-Johansen J (2005). Polarized arrest with warm or cold adenosine/lidocaine blood cardioplegia is equivalent to hypothermic potassium blood cardioplegia. J Thorac Cardiovasc Surg 129(3): 599–606.

de Jong JW (1986). Cardioplegia and calcium antagonists: a review. Ann Thorac Surg 42(5): 593–598.

de Jong JW, van der Meer P, van Loon H, Owen P, Opie LH (1990). Adenosine as adjunct to potassium cardioplegia: effect on function, energy metabolism, and electrophysiology. J Thorac Cardiovasc Surg 100(3): 445–454.

Deng CY, Lin SG, Zhang WC, Kuang SJ, Qian WM, Wu SL, Shan ZX, Yang M, Yu XY (2006). Esmolol inhibits Na+ current in rat ventricular myocytes. Methods Find Exp Clin Pharmacol 28 (10): 697–702.

Dillon JS, Nayler WG (1987). [3H]-verapamil binding to rat cardiac sarcolemmal membrane fragments; an effect of ischaemia. Br J Pharmacol 90(1): 99–109.

Dobson GP, Jones MW (2004). Adenosine and lidocaine: a new concept in nondepolarizing surgical myocardial arrest, protection, and preservation. J Thorac Cardiovasc Surg 127(3): 794–805.

Dorman BH, Hebbar L, Clair MJ, Hinton RB, Roy RC, Spinale FG (1997). Potassium channel opener-augmented cardioplegia: protection of myocyte contractility with chronic left ventricular dysfunction. Circulation 96(9 Suppl): II253–II259.

Dorman BH, Hebbar L, Zellner JL, New RB, Houck WV, Acsell J, Nettles C, Hendrick JW, Sampson AP, Mukherjee R, Spinale FG (1998). ATP-sensitive potassium channel activation before cardioplegia. Effects on ventricular and myocyte function. Circulation 98(19): II176–II183.

Ducko CT, Stephenson ER, Jr., Jayawant AM, Vigilance DW, Damiano RJ, Jr. (2000). Potassium channel openers: are they effective as pretreatment or additives to cardioplegia? Ann Thorac Surg 69(5): 1363–1368.

Ede M, Ye J, Gregorash L, Summers R, Pargaonkar S, LeHouerou D, Lessana A, Salerno TA, Deslauriers R (1997). Beyond hyperkalemia: beta-blocker-induced cardiac arrest for normothermic cardiac operations. Ann Thorac Surg 63(3): 721–727.

Fallouh HB, Chambers DJ (2007). ICVTS on-line discussion A. The safety of using millimolar doses of lidocaine as cardioplegia. Interact Cardiovasc Thorac Surg 6(2): 176.

Fallouh HB, McLatchie LM, Shattock MJ, Chambers DJ, Kentish JC (2007). Esmolol as a cardioplegic agent: an effect beyond (beta)-blockade. Circulation 116: II323–II324.

Fallouh HB, McLatchie LM, Bardswell SC, Shattock MJ, Chambers DJ, Kentish JC (2008). Myocardial arrest by esmolol: negative inotropy induced by calcium and sodium channel blockade. J Mol Cell Cardiol 44: S49–S50.

Fleckenstein A, Fleckenstein-Grün G (1988) Mechanism of action of calcium antagonists in heart and vascular smooth muscle. Eur Heart J 9(Suppl H): 95–99.

Fremes SE, Levy SL, Christakis GT, Walker SE, Iazetta J, Mallidi HR, Feder-Elituv R, Deemar KA, Cohen EA, Wong BI, Goldman BS (1996) Phase 1 human trial of adenosine-potassium cardioplegia. Circulation 94(9 Suppl II): 370–375.

Fremes SE, Zhang J, Furukawa RD, Mickle DA, Weisel RD (1995). Cardiac storage with University of Wisconsin solution, calcium, and magnesium. J Heart Lung Transplant 14(5): 916–925.

Galinanes M, Shattock MJ, Hearse DJ (1992). Effects of potassium channel modulation during global ischaemia in isolated rat heart with and without cardioplegia. Cardiovasc Res 26(11): 1063–1068.

Garcia-Dorado D, Theroux P, Duran JM, Solares J, Alonso J, Sanz E, Munoz R, Elizaga J, Botas J, Fernandez-Aviles F, Soriano J, Esteban E (1992). Selective inhibition of the contractile apparatus. A new approach to modification of infarct size, infarct composition, and infarct geometry during coronary artery occlusion and reperfusion. Circulation 85(3): 1160–1174.

Geissler HJ, Davis KL, Laine GA, Ostrin EJ, Mehlhorn U, Hekmat K, Warters RD, Allen SJ (2000). Myocardial protection with high-dose beta-blockade in acute myocardial ischemia. Eur J Cardiothorac Surg 17(1): 63–70.

Gwathmey JK, Hajjar RJ, Solaro RJ (1991). Contractile deactivation and uncoupling of crossbridges. Effects of 2,3-butanedione monoxime on mammalian myocardium. Circ Res 69(5): 1280–1292.

He GW, Yang CQ (1997). Superiority of hyperpolarizing to depolarizing cardioplegia in protection of coronary endothelial function. J Thorac Cardiovasc Surg 114(4): 643–650.

Hearse DJ, Braimbridge MV, Jynge P (1981). Protection of the ischemic myocardium: cardioplegia. New York, Raven Press.

Hearse DJ, O'Brien K, Braimbridge MV (1981). Protection of the myocardium during ischemic arrest. Dose-response curves for procaine and lignocaine in cardioplegic solutions. J Thorac Cardiovasc Surg 81(6): 873–879.

Hearse DJ, Stewart DA, Braimbridge MV (1978). Myocardial protection during ischemic cardiac arrest. The importance of magnesium in cardioplegic infusates. J Thorac Cardiovasc Surg 75(6): 877–885.

Hebbar L, Houck WV, Zellner JL, Dorman BH, Spinale FG (1998). Temporal relation of ATP-sensitive potassium-channel activation and contractility before cardioplegia. Ann Thorac Surg 65(4): 1077–1082.

Hiraoka M (2006). Metabolic pathways for ion homeostasis and persistent Na(+) current. J Cardiovasc Electrophysiol 17 Suppl 1: S124–S126.

Hohnloser SH, Meinertz T, Klingenheben T, Sydow B, Just H (1991). Usefulness of esmolol in unstable angina pectoris. European Esmolol Study Group. Am J Cardiol 67(16): 1319–1323.

Hosoda H, Sunamori M, Suzuki A (1994). Effect of pinacidil on rat hearts undergoing hypothermic cardioplegia. Ann Thorac Surg 58(6): 1631–1636.

Iseri LT, French JH (1984). Magnesium: nature's physiologic calcium blocker. Am Heart J 108(1): 188–193.

Jahangir A, Terzic A (2005). K(ATP) channel therapeutics at the bedside. J Mol Cell Cardiol 39(1): 99–112.

Jayawant AM, Lawton JS, Hsia PW, Damiano RJ, Jr. (1997). Hyperpolarized cardioplegic arrest with nicorandil: advantages over other potassium channel openers. Circulation 96(9 Suppl): II240–II246.

Jayawant AM, Stephenson ER, Jr., Damiano RJ, Jr. (1999). 2,3-Butanedione monoxime cardioplegia: advantages over hyperkalemia in blood-perfused isolated hearts. Ann Thorac Surg 67(3): 618–623.

Jovanovic A, Alekseev AE, Lopez JR, Shen WK, Terzic A (1997). Adenosine prevents hyperkalemia-induced calcium loading in cardiac cells: relevance for cardioplegia. Ann Thorac Surg 63(1): 153–161.

Jynge P, Hearse DJ, Braimbridge MV (1977). Myocardial protection during ischemic cardiac arrest. A possible hazard with calcium-free cardioplegic infusates. J Thorac Cardiovasc Surg 73(6): 848–855.

Jynge P, Hearse DJ, Braimbridge MV (1978). Protection of the ischemic myocardium. Volume-duration relationships and the efficacy of myocardial infusates. J Thorac Cardiovasc Surg 76(5): 698–705.

Katayama O, Ledingham SJ, Amrani M, Smolenski RT, Lachno DR, Jayakumar J, Yacoub MH (1997). Functional and metabolic effects of adenosine in cardioplegia: role of temperature and concentration. Ann Thorac Surg 63(2): 449–454; discussion 454–445.

Kirsch U, Rodewald G, Kalmar P (1972). Induced ischemic arrest. Clinical experience with cardioplegia in open-heart surgery. J Thorac Cardiovasc Surg 63(1): 121–130.

Kleber AG (1983). Resting membrane potential, extracellular potassium activity, and intracellular sodium activity during acute global ischemia in isolated perfused guinea pig hearts. Circ Res 52 (4): 442–450.

Kronon MT, Allen BS, Hernan J, Halldorsson AO, Rahman S, Buckberg GD, Wang T, Ilbawi MN (1999). Superiority of magnesium cardioplegia in neonatal myocardial protection. Ann Thorac Surg 68(6): 2285–2291; discussion 2291–2282.

Kuhn-Regnier F, Geissler HJ, Marohl S, Mehlhorn U, De Vivie ER (2002). Beta-blockade in 200 coronary bypass grafting procedures. Thorac Cardiovasc Surg 50(3): 164–167.

Kuhn-Regnier F, Natour E, Dhein S, Dapunt O, Geissler HJ, LaRose K, Gorg C, Mehlhorn U (1999). Beta-blockade versus Buckberg blood-cardioplegia in coronary bypass operation. Eur J Cardiothorac Surg 15(1): 67–74.

Lawton JS, Harrington GC, Allen CT, Hsia PW, Damiano RJ, Jr. (1996). Myocardial protection with pinacidil cardioplegia in the blood-perfused heart. Ann Thorac Surg 61(6): 1680–1688.

Lawton JS, Sepic JD, Allen CT, Hsia PW, Damiano RJ, Jr. (1996). Myocardial protection with potassium-channel openers is as effective as St. Thomas' solution in the rabbit heart. Ann Thorac Surg 62(1): 31–38.

Lopez JR, Jahangir R, Jahangir A, Shen WK, Terzic A (1996). Potassium channel openers prevent potassium-induced calcium loading of cardiac cells: possible implications in cardioplegia. J Thorac Cardiovasc Surg 112(3): 820–831.

Maruyama Y, Chambers DJ (2008). Myocardial protection: efficacy of a novel magnesium-based cardioplegia (RS-C) compared to St. Thomas' Hospital cardioplegic solution. Interact Cardiovasc Thorac Surg 7(5): 745–749.

Maskal SL, Cohen NM, Hsia PW, Wechsler AS, Damiano RJ, Jr. (1995). Hyperpolarized cardiac arrest with a potassium-channel opener, aprikalim. J Thorac Cardiovasc Surg 110(4 Pt 1): 1083–1095.

McAllister RE, Noble D, Tsien RW (1975). Reconstruction of the electrical activity of cardiac Purkinje fibres. J Physiol 251(1): 1–59.

McCully JD, Levitsky S (1997). Mechanisms of in vitro cardioprotective action of magnesium on the aging myocardium. Magnes Res 10(2): 157–168.

McCully JD, Levitsky S (2003). The mitochondrial K(ATP) channel and cardioprotection. Ann Thorac Surg 75(2): S667–S673.

Mehlhorn U, Allen SJ, Adams DL, Davis KL, Gogola GR, Warters RD (1996). Cardiac surgical conditions induced by beta-blockade: effect on myocardial fluid balance. Ann Thorac Surg 62 (1): 143–150.

Mehlhorn U, Sauer H, Kuhn-Regnier F, Sudkamp M, Dhein S, Eberhardt F, Grond S, Horst M, Hekmat K, Geissler HJ, Warters RD, Allen SJ, Rainer de Vivie E (1999). Myocardial beta-blockade as an alternative to cardioplegic arrest during coronary artery surgery. Cardiovasc Surg 7(5): 549–557.

Menasche P, Mouas C, Grousset C (1996). Is potassium channel opening an effective form of preconditioning before cardioplegia? Ann Thorac Surg 61(6): 1764–1768.

Mentzer RM Jr., Birjiniuk V, Khuri S, Lowe JE, Rahko PS, Weisel RD, Wellons HA, Barker ML, Lasley RD (1999). Adenosine myocardial protection: preliminary results of a phase II clinical trial. Ann Surg 229(5): 643–649.

Miller RD (1998). Local anesthetics. In Basic and Clinical Pharmacology. Katzung BG. Stamford, Appleton and Lange: 425–433.

Niedergerke R, Orkand RK (1966). The dependence of the action potential of the frog's heart on the external and intracellular sodium concentration. J Physiol 184(2): 312–334.

Opie LH (2004). Channels, Pumps, and Exchangers. In Heart Physiology From Cell to Circulation. Philadelphia, Lippincott Williams & Wilkins: 73–118.

Pirk J, Kolar F, Ost'adal B, Sedivy J, Stambergova A, Kellovsky P (1999). The effect of the ultrashort beta-blocker esmolol on cardiac function recovery: an experimental study. Eur J Cardiothorac Surg 15(2): 199–203.

Popovic J, Mitic R, Sabo A, Mikov M, Jakovljevic V, Dakovic-Svajcer K (2006). Spline functions in convolutional modeling of verapamil bioavailability and bioequivalence. II: study in healthy volunteers. Eur J Drug Metab Pharmacokinet 31(2): 87–96.

Qiu Y, Galinanes M, Hearse DJ (1995). Protective effect of nicorandil as an additive to the solution for continuous warm cardioplegia. J Thorac Cardiovasc Surg 110(4 Pt 1): 1063–1072.

Quast U, Guillon JM, Cavero I (1994). Cellular pharmacology of potassium channel openers in vascular smooth muscle. Cardiovasc Res 28(6): 805–810.

Rich TL, Langer GA, Klassen MG (1988). Two components of coupling calcium in single ventricular cell of rabbits and rats. Am J Physiol 254(5 Pt 2): H937–H946.

Ringer S (1883). A further Contribution regarding the influence of the different Constituents of the Blood on the Contraction of the Heart. J Physiol 4(1): 29–42.

Saint DA (2006). The role of the persistent Na(+) current during cardiac ischemia and hypoxia. J Cardiovasc Electrophysiol 17(Suppl 1): S96–S103.

Schubert T, Vetter H, Owen P, Reichart B, Opie LH (1989). Adenosine cardioplegia. Adenosine versus potassium cardioplegia: effects on cardiac arrest and postischemic recovery in the isolated rat heart. J Thorac Cardiovasc Surg 98(6): 1057–1065.

Sellevold OF, Berg EM, Levang OW (1995). Procaine is effective for minimizing postischemic ventricular fibrillation in cardiac surgery. Anesth Analg 81(5): 932–938.

Shattock MJ, Hearse DJ, Fry CH (1987). The ionic basis of the anti-ischemic and anti-arrhythmic properties of magnesium in the heart. J Am Coll Nutr 6(1): 27–33.

Sloots KL, Vinten-Johansen J, Dobson GP (2007). Warm nondepolarizing adenosine and lidocaine cardioplegia: continuous versus intermittent delivery. J Thorac Cardiovasc Surg 133(5): 1171–1178.

Snabaitis AK, Chambers DJ (1999). Long-term myocardial preservation: beneficial and additive effects of polarized arrest (Na+-channel blockade), Na+/H+-exchange inhibition, and Na+/K+/2Cl- -cotransport inhibition combined with calcium desensitization. Transplantation 68(10): 1444–1453.

Snabaitis AK, Shattock MJ, Chambers DJ (1997). Comparison of polarized and depolarized arrest in the isolated rat heart for long-term preservation. Circulation 96(9): 3148–3156.

Snabaitis AK, Shattock MJ, Chambers DJ (1999). Long-term myocardial preservation: effects of hyperkalemia, sodium channel, and Na/K/2Cl cotransport inhibition on extracellular potassium accumulation during hypothermic storage. J Thorac Cardiovasc Surg 118(1): 123–134.

Sperelakis N, Sunagawa M, Nakamura M (2001). Electrogenesis of the resting potential. In Heart physiology and pathophysiology. Sperelakis N, Kurachi Y, Terzic A and Cohen MV. San Diego, Academic Press: 175–198.

Steenbergen C, Murphy E, Watts JA, London RE (1990). Correlation between cytosolic free calcium, contracture, ATP, and irreversible ischemic injury in perfused rat heart. Circ Res 66 (1): 135–146.

Sternbergh WC, Brunsting LA, Abd-Elfattah AS, Wechsler AS (1989). Basal metabolic energy requirements of polarized and depolarized arrest in rat heart. Am J Physiol 256(3 Pt 2): H846–851.

Stringham JC, Paulsen KL, Southard JH, Fields BL, Belzer FO (1992). Improved myocardial ischemic tolerance by contractile inhibition with 2,3-butanedione monoxime. Ann Thorac Surg 54(5): 852–859; discussion 859–860.

Sugimoto S, Puddu PE, Monti F, Schiariti M, Campa PP, Marino B (1994). Pretreatment with the adenosine triphosphate-sensitive potassium channel opener nicorandil and improved myocardial protection during high-potassium cardioplegic hypoxia. J Thorac Cardiovasc Surg 108(3): 455–466.

Swanson DK, Pasaoglu I, Berkoff HA, Southard JA, Hegge JO (1988). Improved heart preservation with UW preservation solution. J Heart Transplant 7(6): 456–467.

Thomson PD, Melmon KL, Richardson JA, Cohn K, Steinbrunn W, Cudihee R, Rowland M (1973). Lidocaine pharmacokinetics in advanced heart failure, liver disease, and renal failure in humans. Ann Intern Med 78(4): 499–508.

Tsukube T, McCully JD, Metz KR, Cook CU, Levitsky S (1997). Amelioration of ischemic calcium overload correlates with high-energy phosphates in senescent myocardium. Am J Physiol 273(1 Pt 2): H418–425.

Tyers GF, Todd GJ, Niebauer IM, Manley NJ, Waldhausen JA (1974). Effect of intracoronary tetrodotoxin on recovery of the isolated working rat heart from sixty minutes of ischemia. Circulation 50(2 Suppl II): 175–180.

Vahl CF, Bonz A, Hagl C, Hagl S (1994). Reversible desensitization of the myocardial contractile apparatus for calcium. A new concept for improving tolerance to cold ischemia in human myocardium? Eur J Cardiothorac Surg 8(7): 370–378.

Vahl CF, Bonz A, Hagl C, Timek T, Herold U, Fuchs H, Kochsiek N, Hagl S (1995). "Cardioplegia on the contractile apparatus level": evaluation of a new concept for myocardial preservation in perfused pig hearts. Thorac Cardiovasc Surg 43(4): 185–193.

Vouhe PR, Helias J, Grondin CM (1980). Myocardial protection through cold cardioplegia using diltiazem, a calcium channel blocker. Ann Thorac Surg 30(4): 342–348.

Walgama OV, Shattock MJ, Chambers DJ (2000). Efficacy of a K-ATP channel opener to induce myocardial arrest: species differences. J Mol Cell Cardiol 32: A40.

Walgama OV, Shattock MJ, Chambers DJ (2000). Myocardial arrest and protection: dual effect of a K-channel opener and Na-channel blocker as an alternative to hyperkalemia. J Mol Cell Cardiol 32: A41.

Ward JW, McBurney A, Farrow PR, Sharp P (1984). Pharmacokinetics and hypotensive effect in healthy volunteers of pinacidil, a new potent vasodilator. Eur J Clin Pharmacol 26(5): 603–608.

Yamaguchi S, Watanabe G, Tomita S, Tabata S (2007). Lidocaine-magnesium blood cardioplegia was equivalent to potassium blood cardioplegia in left ventricular function of canine heart. Interact Cardiovasc Thorac Surg 6(2): 172–176.

Yamamoto F, Manning AS, Braimbridge MV, Hearse DJ (1985). Calcium antagonists and myocardial protection during cardioplegic arrest. Adv Myocardiol 6: 545–562.

Zaroslinski J, Borgman RJ, O'Donnell JP, Anderson WG, Erhardt PW, Kam ST, Reynolds RD, Lee RJ, Gorczynski RJ (1982). Ultra-short acting beta-blockers: a proposal for the treatment of the critically ill patient. Life Sci 31(9): 899–907.

Myocardial Protection via the Coronary Venous Route

13

Werner Mohl, Dejan Milasinovic, and Sarah Burki

13.1 Introduction

Perioperative and peri-interventional myocardial protection as well as auxiliary measures to prevent ischemic/reperfusion injury remain an important curative effort in clinical medicine. Whereas global ischemia, myocardial protection and their theoretical pathophysiological interaction are tightly related since the first cardiac operations were performed almost over half a century ago, new innovative "minimally invasive" and peri-interventional procedures require new insight into this technology. There are several important targets that need to be considered:

1. Prevention of iatrogenic myocardial injury mandatory during procedures in a diseased heart.
2. Reversal of disease related changes in myocardial structure, perfusion and metabolism and thus cardiac performance.

To better understand present goals for myocardial protection one has to consider not only new technologies, but also demographic changes and broadened indications spanning from "conservative" cardiac surgery to minimally invasive and also hybrid and interventional procedures. There are new important questions arising as the timing of treatments in relation to myocardial jeopardy and their necessary sequence to potentiate curative efforts. One important problem however remains "the optimal access" to deprived myocardium and its microcirculation.

Long before cardiac surgery was developed the nutrition of the myocardium via the coronary veins has drawn attention and a lot of pathophysiological data have been collected supporting the retrograde approach to the diseased myocardium. An overview on the history of different retrograde arterialization and the advantages and disadvantages of

W. Mohl (✉), D. Milasinovic, and S. Burki
Department of Cardiac Surgery, Medical University of Vienna, Währinger Güertel 18–20, 1090 Vienna, Austria
e-mail: werner.mohl@meduniwien.ac.at

coronary sinus interventions shows the current paradigm shift based on the new understanding and advances in molecular biology (Mohl et al. 2008a, b).

The coronary sinus as a retrograde entrance port to the jeopardized heart has been promoted to achieve myocardial protection in various groups of patients. Its distinct anatomical characteristics open several pathophysiological options and make the coronary sinus route one of the most interesting research spots within the future perspective of cardioprotection, even more than one hundred years after the first description of retroperfusion via coronary sinus by Pratt (1898).

The most prominent application domains of the retrograde myocardial protection via the coronary venous system include:

- Cardioprotection by the means of retrograde cardioplegia during cardiac surgery in combination with anterograde cardioplegia, as the most successful strategy for perioperative myocardial protection in patients with but also more frequently without severe coronary artery disease.
- Peri- and post-interventional protection after acute myocardial ischemia by the means of cell, gene or growth factor delivery via the coronary venous system.

13.2
Perioperative Myocardial Protection Via Coronary Sinus

Myocardial protection has emerged as the most important prerequisite to modern cardiac surgery, contributing immensely to the common goal of long lasting patient benefit. Ventricular dysfunction is known to be one of the detrimental consequences of an ineffective cardioprotection during open-heart surgery. The rapid development of open-heart surgery has increased demand for potent perioperative techniques to facilitate the chemical "arrest" of the heart and forge its protection against intraoperative stress factors, such as ischemia with its imminent and long-term sequelae. Cardioplegic solutions, varying from crystalloid to cold blood solutions, set a firm ground for establishing myocardial protection in cardiac surgery. Myriad recipes have been formulated varying concentrations of electrolytes, vasoactive and cardioprotective drugs. Apart from different recipes and formulas for temperature, timing and amount of delivery, the coronary veins provide the most suitable route because of the dense meshwork of its vasculature allowing optimal protection even in patients with severe coronary artery disease. Furthermore, new data shift the evidence from a mere delivery route towards more complex molecular consequences of myocardial protection via coronary veins that are most probably determined by an exceptional role of venous endothelium as the origin of substance exchange, force detection and cellular defence. These considerations create a completely new environment for our scientific understanding and its application in innovative approaches in order to overcome inherent morphological and physiological burdens on the surgeon's quest for achieving optimal perioperative cardioprotection.

13.2.1
The Coronary Veins and Venous Endothelium

Anatomy of the coronary venous system holds the key for optimal utilization of this pathway in achieving myocardial protection. The great majority of blood flows through epicardial coronary veins that merge together creating the coronary sinus and draining into the right atrium. In 79% of cases the anterior interventricular vein (AIV) runs along the side of the left anterior descending artery (LAD) in the anterior interventricular groove and, turning laterally at the base of the heart, creates the great cardiac vein (GCV), which consequently receives tributaries from the left ventricular surface via the AIV, left marginal and left posterior vein (Jain et al. 2006). Middle cardiac vein (MCV) drains directly into the coronary sinus that ends with a variable Thebesian valve. In contrast, the small cardiac vein (SCV) is responsible for the drainage of the right ventricle and it connects directly the right atrium.

Apart from the described epicardial coronary veins there are also venoluminal interconnections to mention, a special type of Thebesian veins (Vasa cordis minima), which drains venous blood into the ventricles. The Thebesian network further comprises arterioluminal interconnections and communicatory vessels between the capillary bed and the ventricles. Altogether, the Thebesian veins account for 5–10% of the venous return in the heart (Jain et al. 2006).

It may be concluded that these characteristics of the coronary venous system account for many clinical applications, as described later in the chapter. The complex and intricate anatomy of the coronary venous system has played the most appreciated role in the research conducted previously in the field of myocardial protection via the coronary sinus route.

13.2.1.1
Access to the Coronary Sinus

Coronary sinus catheterization is used in cardiac surgery as well as in interventional and electrophysiological approaches. Whereas the technique of coronary sinus catheterization in cardiac surgery is a simple transatrial approach, the access during interventions is more demanding.

For the purpose of intraoperative protection, the positioning of the catheter can be controlled by visual inspection. First, a purse string suture is sutured in the free wall of the right atrium about 5 cm above the pericardial reflection and the entrance of the inferior vena cava. After inserting the catheter into the atrium, the second hand is used to find the entrance of the coronary sinus, which is at the base of the heart and can be felt near the inferior vena cava entrance into the right atrium. The catheter can be advanced easily in most cases. The correct position can be inspected under manual control. As mentioned below the balloon position is normally too far distally, but necessary to assure a stable catheter position. To prevent an air lock this maneuver has to be performed before going on bypass. There are several modifications of the catheter technology, which should facilitate a homogeneous distribution of retrograde flow into all veins especially into the posterior and lateral veins.

In interventional cardiology different approaches can be used. Most commonly the femoral vein for electrophysiology and recently other coronary sinus interventions is used. This access is chosen because of logistic reasons but it is also the most difficult, since one has to rotate the catheter backwards as soon as the tip enters the right atrium. Then the tip should be rotated down to access the coronary sinus orifice and again upwards to advance the catheter into a stable position. This can be successfully performed when a steerable catheter system or a pre-shaped sheet is used. An easier approach is the access from the left subclavian vein or both jugular veins or even the left brachial vein. This approach has become very popular through the growing demand in resynchronization therapy since it uses the curve of the right atrial free wall to guide the catheter near the coronary sinus ostium.

As with all interventions, severe side effects have been experienced with malpositioning of the catheters, and the most dangerous is the blow out defect in the coronary sinus wall, which occurs if a compliant balloon ruptures the wall. This will immediately lead to a pericardial tamponade when used during interventions. Myocardial hemorrhage is another serious adverse effect and can be seen during cardioplegic delivery if the catheter wedges into the vessel wall. We, and others, reported on curative approaches when these traumas occur. Care has to be taken not to occlude the coronary sinus permanently through surgical corrections of these injuries, since this causes severe underperfusion of coronary arteries due to the venous engorgement and impedance to coronary artery inflow and a lack of venous drainage. Aharinejad et al. (1996) and Aigner et al. (2006) have shown that pericardial patch technique poses an effective method to correct coronary sinus rupture, and to successfully circumvent its detrimental complications.

Altogether these complications are very rare and should not prevent the use of retrograde myocardial protection.

13.2.2
Retrograde Cardioplegia

The main delivery pathway for cardioplegia is the anterograde route via the coronary arteries either through direct cannulation of both coronary ostia or via the aortic root. Since the early days of cardiac surgery it has been known that ostial cannulation, used in patients undergoing aortic valve or aortic root surgery, bears some risk of intimal injury and subsequent ostial stenosis with its deleterious consequences. In context of avoiding the aforementioned complications, retroinfusion via the coronary sinus has been evaluated by Menasché et al. (1982) and found to be a safe and effective delivery technique during aortic valve surgery. Despite the fact that new generations of catheters were on the market, and that overall more sophisticated surgical techniques are in use, the occurrence of deleterious complications after anterograde cardioplegia, such as left main coronary artery stenosis, has been confirmed in the 1990s as well (Winkelmann et al. 1993). This was one important reason for incorporating retrograde cardioplegia into the everyday clinical practice in many centres worldwide. Retrograde cardioplegia protects deprived myocardium via the coronary venous microcirculation, totally reversing flow towards the vented or opened aortic root during cross-clamping and is used either alone as an alternative route in patients undergoing aortic valve or aortic root surgery or in combination with anterograde induction to arrest the heart.

More abundant use of retrograde cardioplegia has offered new insights into what is referred to as patchy meshwork of microvessels of heart, a system that has been identified as one of the main targets in modern perioperative myocardial protection. Consequently, retrograde cardioplegia and its impact at the cellular level of cardioprotection have sparked intense research efforts. Retrograde cardioplegia, when administered alone, was shown to inadequately perfuse both the middle portion of the right ventricle and the posteroseptal portion of the left ventricle (Allen et al. 1995), supporting the widely accepted notion that retrograde cardioplegia alone insufficiently protects the right ventricular free wall and the septal portion of the myocardium. These observations are in concordance with the structure of the coronary venous system. In general, there are three venous systems that drain the heart: the coronary sinus, anterior cardiac veins and the venae cordis minimae, also called Thebesian veins (Ruengsakulrach and Buxton 2001). The coronary sinus opens into the right atrium between the ostium of vena cava inferior and the tricuspid orifice. It accounts for 75% of the coronary venous circulation (Mohl 1987), thus leaving some myocardial portions out of its draining range. Coronary sinus anomalies may seriously aggravate the distribution of retrograde cardioplegia and are classified in five categories: (1) absence of the coronary sinus, associated with persistent left superior vena cava, (2) hypoplastic coronary sinus, with a number of cardiac veins directly entering the chambers, (3) atresia or stenosis of the coronary sinus ostium, (4) enlargement of the coronary sinus, with or without left-to-right shunt, (5) "unroofed" coronary sinus, communicating with the left atrium (Ruengsakulrach and Buxton 2001). Additionally, Ludinghausen identified five possible variations of the coronary venous structure. His findings revealed that, in at least 13% of cases, a cardioplegic solution infused retrograde would not reach remote portions of the left ventricle (Ruengsakulrach and Buxton 2001). In addition to morphological variability, the coronary venous system contains Thebesian veins (as indicated above), which are also referred to as venoluminal shunts, thus causing retrograde cardioplegia to escape the myocardium and flow into heart chambers, before reaching the capillary bed. However, this property of the coronary venous system is at the same time advantageous in protecting the myocardium from hemorrhage and edema.

In their comparative study, Louagie and colleagues indicated that continuous retrograde cold blood cardioplegia was more beneficial than intermittent anterograde or retrograde cold blood cardioplegia, as assessed by better left and right ventricular stroke work index during the first 20 min after coronary artery bypass (Louagie et al. 1997). The presented results are especially interesting when considering the fact that most of the right ventricle free wall cannot be reached by retroperfusion of the coronary sinus. Another, prospective and randomized study by the same group (Louagie et al. 2004) confirmed the assumption of more benefit associated with continuous cold blood cardioplegia by comparing it to its intermittent counterpart. Measured estimates of a reduction in myocardial ischemia included lower production of lactate and hypoxanthine in patients treated with continuous cardioplegia, whereas the left ventricular function was characterized by higher left ventricular stroke work index in the continuous cardioplegia group

(Louagie et al. 2004). These results suggested a successful mechanism of self-regulation of the coronary venous system in terms of continuous retrograde infusion of cardioplegia being not detrimental, as one might think based on the varying anatomy, but rather of benefit for preservation of the heart function. Nevertheless, retrograde cardioplegia alone when compared to anterograde cardioplegia was associated with enhanced apoptosis of cardiomyocytes in both right and left ventricle. These results were obtained in an open surgery pig model (Vähäsilta et al. 2005).

Anterograde delivery with simultaneous coronary sinus occlusion seems to be a valuable tool to more uniformly cool the heart in the presence of coronary artery disease (Neumann et al. 1996). This technique of intermittent occlusion of the coronary sinus in a physiologic optimized function (PICSO) can be performed also as a protection against regional ischemia in off pump surgery. It is, however, necessary to mention that during cardioplegic arrest a combination of all three delivery routes has to be performed sequentially to successfully reach all portions of the heart muscle, which are deprived of blood by coronary artery disease or might be left out because of anatomical problems. The upper part of the interventricular septum and parts of the right ventricle are also difficult to protect with the retrograde approach alone because these regions have alternate non-coronary sinus drainage pathways. Another important component is the stability and positioning of catheters in the coronary sinus during retrograde cardioplegic delivery. The posterior interventricular vein branches from the coronary sinus in the near proximity of its orifice and is left out during retrograde delivery. Perfusion in this vessel during retrograde delivery can be seen to be orthograde because of the dense interconnections of veins in the lateral and posterior aspect of the heart. Figs. 1 and 2 depict the anatomy of coronary veins and its important highlights in regard to retrograde cardioplegia.

In summary, the complex anatomy of the coronary venous system and hitherto not fully depicted properties of endothelial cells greatly extended research boundaries in the field of retrograde cardioplegia, thus allowing for simultaneous existence of several schools of thought in the field of perioperative cardioprotection. Especially, anterograde cardioplegia complemented by its retrograde counterpart seem to draw increasing attention from the scientific community in what appears to be a logical step towards an unfolding architecture of perioperative cardioprotection. In this regard, an interesting study from Neumann et al. (1996) investigated a combined cardioplegia regimen consisting of anterograde perfusion and coronary sinus occlusion to mimic effects of retrograde cardioplegia. The study showed no obvious benefit of this regimen as compared to the standard ones. Nevertheless, it pointed out the significance of a sufficient cardioplegic infusion dose for optimal cardioprotection, using either alternative or standard regimens (Neumann et al. 1996).

It can be concluded that a combination of anterograde induction, repetitive doses of retrograde cardioplegia and total reversal of flow during rewarming together with periods of coronary sinus occlusion might be the optimal myocardial protection during cardiac surgery. Demographic changes necessitate prolonging crossclamp times to correct structural heart disease in patients with severe comorbidities and unified research efforts have unveiled the rising potential of the coronary sinus route for sophisticated perioperative myocardial protection complementary to anterograde cardioplegia. Even now after successful research for more than 30 years there is room for further improvements thus warranting continuing research of this "backdoor" alternative.

13   Myocardial Protection via the Coronary Venous Route   227

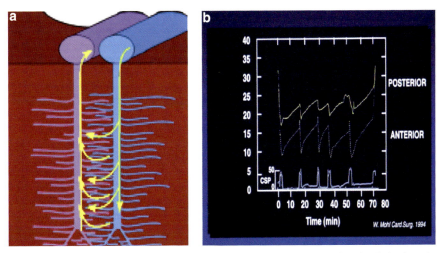

Fig. 1 During aortic cross-clamping cardioplegia flows retrograde via the microcirculation into the coronary arteries as depicted in (**a**) and into the vented aortic root. Under these premises the coronary circulation can be totally reversed and during re-warming at the end of cardioplegic arrest and retrograde perfusion with blood, the heart starts beating spontaneously with the closed cross-clamp in place. (**b**) shows higher temperatures in posterior septum as compared to anterior septum during retrograde infusion. The peaks in coronary sinus pressure (CSP) match with lower temperatures observed

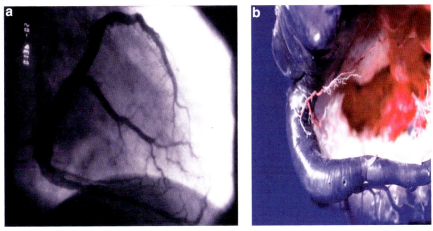

Fig. 2 (**a**) Shows balloon catheter in the coronary sinus during coronary catheterisation. Note that the posterior inferior vein is less perfused and fills via collaterals antegrade from circumflex branches. In surgery because of technical reasons of catheter stability the balloon is even more advanced distally sparing the posterior and lateral portion of the heart from cardioplegic protection. Discrepancies of effects observed in retrograde cardioplegic protection can be explained by the phenomenon of the variability of catheter position. In (**b**) the corrosion cast shows the entrance from the right atrium. This portion is a transition zone overlapping the endocardial/myocardial portion of the coronary sinus with the endothelial/vascular portion. The corrosion cast is rotated to depict the entrance of the coronary sinus ostium from the right atrium. Ideally the balloon should be positioned in the first portion of the vascular part (see *asterix*)

13.3
Peri- and Postinterventional Myocardial Protection: How to Regenerate Ischemic Hearts?

Scientific scope of coronary sinus interventions has now shifted from the surgical perspective towards the potential cure of degenerated chronic failing hearts. In the following we summarise the recent efforts in this field and the interesting connections to the coronary venous system.

13.3.1
Anterograde Intracoronary Cell Transplantation

Latest developments in interventional treatment of coronary artery disease have pointed out the necessity of advanced cardioprotective methods beyond reperfusion techniques, such as percutaneous coronary interventions (PCI) and subsequent stent implantation. Therefore, various adjunctive therapies have been developed in order to supplement the "gold standard" PCI. Common denominator of all adjunctive therapies is the peri- and post-interventional protection of myocardium from detrimental sequelae of ischemia-reperfusion injury and subsequent functional improvement. In analogy to perioperative myocardial protection, research efforts in the field of peri-interventional cardioprotection exhibit main roads and alternative pathways and their combination might provide more insight in the pathophysiological consequences of ischemia-reperfusion phenomenon in the heart. One of the most encouraging therapy regimens involves transplantation of pluripotent stem cells into the ischemia-jeopardized myocardium, aiming at replenishment of cardiomyocytes, neovascularization and better control of inflammatory processes. A series of very important publications demonstrated high potential of stem cells to induce regeneration, but also indicated the need for more in depth analysis of ischemic microenvironment and its susceptibility to allow for engraftment and proliferation of transplanted progenitor cells.

A review by Dimmeler et al. (2008) distinguishes between three different adult stem cell types that have been experimentally indicated to possess the potential for inducing tissue regeneration:

- Bone marrow derived stem cells – hematopoietic stem cells (HSCs), side population cells (SP cells, expressing Abcg2 transporter) and mesenchymal stem cells (MSCs, containing a subset population of multipotential adult progenitor cells).
- Circulating pool of stem and progenitor cells, for one part originating from the bone marrow – endothelial progenitor cells (EPCs).
- Tissue resident stem cells – the cells isolated from adult hearts were marked by the presence of c-kit, sca-1 and cardiac side population (SP) markers.

Several experimental trials compared different cell types in order to detect the most suitable cell line for the transplantation. Bone marrow derived stem cells such as purified mesenchymal stem cells (MSCs) appeared to have the most potential. In line with the notion of identifying the most effective cell type, a recent study (van der Bogt et al. 2008) compared four different types of intracoronary infused cells into the infarct related artery in an acute ischemia mouse model. Mesenchymal stem cells (MSCs), skeletal myoblasts (SkMb), and fibroblasts did not survive longer than 2 weeks after transplantation, whereas bone marrow mononuclear cells (MN) were still present in the myocardium after 6 weeks. Subsequent histological analysis confirmed prolonged existence of mononuclear cells in the myocardium, even though these cells did not undergo transdifferentiation into cardiomyocytes. In spite of this lack of transdifferentiation, left ventricular function was improved in the study arm with mononuclear (MN) cells (van der Bogt et al. 2008).

Experimental trials have been followed by clinical studies in order to further investigate the relevance of this promising therapy regimen in every day clinical setting. Strauer et al. (2002) reported that transplantation of autologous mononuclear bone marrow derived stem cells via intracoronary infusion under clinical conditions was feasible and safe. Subsequent studies explored potential effects of the stem cell therapy proposing myocardial regeneration and neovascularization to be most relevant. Wollert et al. (2004a, b) documented a significant improvement in left ventricular function after intracoronary infusion of autologous bone marrow derived stem cells 6 months after acute myocardial ischemia. Nevertheless, the significant difference in the global function improvement was lost after 18 months. Lunde et al. (2006), on the other hand, found no significant effects of intracoronary infusion of autologous mononuclear bone marrow derived cells (BMC) on global left ventricular function in the same population of patients. Janssens et al. (2006) confirmed the lack of global left ventricular function augmentation, but at the same time advocated possible beneficial effects on infarct remodelling. Finally, Schächinger et al. (2006) proposed intracoronary stem cell infusion to be of great potential to trigger myocardial regeneration and announced future large-scale studies to clarify the true mechanisms behind these observed effects.

Even though different research groups sought uniformity in respect to the protocol, it was hard to maintain the consistency of results. The following parameters seem to have been of decisive influence on the projected outcomes: (1) the time point of transplantation, (2) the number of progenitor cells infused and (3) the type of progenitor cells. Meluzín et al. (2006) showed that intracoronary transplantation of autologous mononuclear BMCs improved regional myocardial function of the infarcted wall in a dose-dependent manner, thus providing one possible explanation for the observed inconsistency. Most of the studies reported set the transplantation time point to be between 3 and 7 days after primary PCI. Bartunek et al. (2005) performed the cell infusion approximately 10 days (11.6 ± 1.4) after infarction using CD 133+ cells derived from bone marrow, as opposed to the great majority of other studies transplanting unfractioned bone marrow mononuclear cells. The protocol was based on previous findings suggesting that selected bone marrow derived cells were of higher engraftment potential than heterogenous mononuclear bone marrow cells (Wollert et al. 2004a, b). Bartunek et al. 2005 documented an improved left ventricular function, whereas a higher rate of cardiac events raised some concerns about the method. Endothelial progenitor cells (EPC) and their substantial role in the process of neovascularization are yet another cell type to be considered for transplantation alongside bone marrow derived stem cells. Initial studies revealed their regenerative potential, in combination with intracoronary application of mesenchymal stem cells (MSCs), expressed through an improvement in left ventricular function and amelioration of reperfusion injury (Katritsis et al. 2005). One of the main problems in the clinical application of EPCs is the fact that there seems to be a rather heterogenous group of blood-circulating cells capable of inducing neovascularization. Initial efforts to characterize the population of endothelial progenitor cells by a combination of markers such as CD133, CD34 and KDR failed to produce consistent results and were challenged by in vitro analyses, which indicated CD34+/CD45− cells to be of greater potential to induce neovascularization (Dimmeler et al. 2008). Furthermore, it has to be taken into account that circulating cells in diseased patients might have only limited vitality to regenerate the heart.

While intracoronary stem cell transplantation started to gain more scientific relevance under clinical conditions, it has become clear that the process of stem cell mobilization and recruitment during ischemic periods is in fact inherent to mammalian hearts. Its importance has become more appreciated due to the lack of sustainable long-term effects of transplanted pluripotent species. Signal pathways of intrinsic mobilization and homing of cells into ischemic portions of the myocardium have inspired a new wave of interest to explore possible options for enhanced attraction and tissue embedment of the transplanted cell species. The Magic trial tested a combined approach using granulocyte colony stimulating factor (G-CSF) to recruit the progenitor cells before harvesting them from the peripheral blood. Even though it showed some improvements, this therapy regimen raised serious concerns due to the fact that the rate of in-stent restenosis was significantly higher in patients treated with the named growth factor (G-CSF) (Kang et al. 2004).

In summary, anterograde intracoronary transplantation of progenitor cells as a means of postinterventional myocardial protection after successful patency restoration of an occluded coronary artery stems from the same general idea of perioperative cardioprotection allowing for myocardium to recover from ischemia. A meta-analysis published in 2007 (Abdel-Latif et al. 2007) supports the notion of transplantation of bone marrow derived stem cells into ischemic myocardium, documenting an improvement in left ventricular ejection fraction, infarct scar size and left ventricular end-systolic volume, as compared to the state of the art therapy. Nevertheless, no significant effects on left ventricular end-diastolic volume were reported, which, as one of the morphological substrates of remodelling, could predict the extent of long-term clinical outcomes (Bolognese et al. 2002).

Of note, the great majority of the presented studies used a balloon catheter to repeatedly occlude an infarct-related vessel while infusing progenitor cells. Thus, the results might have been confounded by an effect of post-conditioning, which has an application mechanism that closely resembles the described intracoronary cell transplantation. More details on the phenomenon of post-conditioning are presented in section 13.3.2.4. All of the listed studies might have underestimated the importance of the endothelial structures necessary for the microenvironmental optimization in the process of tissue regeneration. For instance, the coronary venous endothelium has been indicated to play an important role in the ischemic microenvironment, as in all organs the venous system is responsible for exchange of molecules and interaction between blood-borne molecules and even cells (i.e., tumor cells, bacteria and even viral particles), thus mainly supporting the homeostasis of the organism. Therefore, it may be concluded that despite observed progress in early clinical stem cell research, subsequent clinical studies have exhibited some drawbacks, suggesting that further aspects like adaptation of ischemic microenvironment need to be addressed.

13.3.2
Adjunctive Approaches to Minimize the Reperfusion Injury and Protect Myocardium During Primary PCI: Anterograde Intracoronary Delivery Route

The overarching solution to myocardial ischemia protection involves not only replenishment of lost cardiac myocytes but also restoration of normal oxygen delivery at the microcirculatory level, and halting deleterious processes of the reperfusion injury cascade. The common denominators of research efforts that have been put forth in order to find a way to re-establish complete myocardial perfusion at the microcirculatory level and to block reperfusion injury have been: (1) pharmacological and surgical techniques to minimize the no-reflow phenomenon and (2) pharmacological interference with metabolic processes in oxygen deprived cardiac myocytes. It is common knowledge that ischemic microcirculation cannot be fully reperfused due to clogging of a majority of vessels with cellular debris and activated coagulation and endothelium. Inadequate myocardial perfusion despite TIMI grade 3 flow is termed no-reflow phenomenon and it is most reliably assessed by contrast echocardiography shortly after revascularization. Angiographic no-reflow assessment is a clinically more applicable tool and thus more commonly used in research; its incidence is 5–20% of primary percutaneous interventions (PCI) (Sardella et al. 2008). The no-reflow phenomenon is partially held responsible for left ventricular remodelling, which is the most important prognostic determinant after acute myocardial infarction (AMI) (Bolognese et al. 2002). Reperfusion injury is earmarked by calcium overload and production of superoxide radicals, with both phenomena being potential cardioprotection targets.

Retrograde, pressure-regulated drug administration via the coronary venous system has been an alternative route for delivery of anti-reperfusion-injury substances, and it may be applied adjunctively to established anterograde reperfusion techniques such as PTCA, as will be described in the following sections.

13.3.2.1
Adenosine, Nicorandil

Adenosine has been shown, experimentally, to limit reperfusion injury, reduce infarct size and improve ventricular function. Petronio et al. (2005) documented angiographic improvements after adjunctive intracoronary infusion of adenosine, whereas there was no prevention of left ventricular remodelling. Several other clinical studies confirmed the potential of adenosine to limit no-reflow phenomenon after PCI (Kopecky et al. 2003).

Nicorandil, a hybrid K_{ATP}-channel opener and nicotinamide nitrate, is known to experimentally reduce no-reflow phenomenon and improve cardiac function. It has also been reported that it suppresses radical production after AMI, thus taking an active role in ameliorating reperfusion injury. The findings of an important clinical trial contributed to the search of possible mechanisms of action – improved microvascular function as assessed by myocardial contrast echocardiography (Ito et al. 1999). In addition, Fujiwara et al. (2007) were able to show that nicorandil downsized expression of matrix metalloproteinases (MMPs) that are known for taking an active role in the process of myocardial remodelling.

13.3.2.2
Abciximab, Bivalirudin

Abciximab inhibits platelet aggregation by blocking glycoprotein IIb/IIIa; thus, its adjunctive use could diminish detrimental side effects of PCI such as existence of microemboli. Major studies concentrated on assessing the ability of adjunctive abciximab to ameliorate adverse cardiac events, showing that abciximab was able to reduce their rate (Neumann et al. 2000; Montalescot et al. 2001; Antoniucci et al. 2003). However, reports of the Cadillac trial, which consisted of 1,052 patients in the Abciximab arm, documented no significant difference between long-term effects of PCI alone (PTCA or Stenting) and PCI followed by abciximab (Stone et al. 2002). Bivalirudin, a direct thrombin inhibitor, is proposed to offer the same ischemia protection as heparin plus glycoprotein IIb/IIIa inhibitors, such as abciximab, while reducing the occurrence of bleeding complications. Stone and colleagues (Stone et al. 2008) performed a randomized study using Bivalirudin in patients undergoing primary PCI and thereby documented lower rates of bleeding complications and adverse cardiac events.

13.3.2.3
Distal Microcirculatory Protection Devices

The notion of removing distal remnants of atherosclerotic material after primary PCI, brought about by thrombus dislodgement, offered new possibilities to re-establish microvascular circulation, thus minimizing no-reflow phenomenon and salvaging myocardium. Several smaller studies indicated beneficial effects of such a therapy regimen expressed by reduced infarct size and enhanced event-free survival (Nakamura et al. 2004). Nevertheless, more powerful studies failed to confirm these encouraging effects (Dangas et al. 2008; Gick et al. 2005). From the reported studies it could not be decisively concluded whether distal clearing of dislodged thrombotic material is sufficient to restore microvascular circulation, reduce infarct size and prevent remodelling, thus securing long term left ventricular function recovery.

13.3.2.4
Post-Conditioning

Post-conditioning, much like pre-conditioning, involves transient ischemia periods, which trigger protective cellular cascades delivering strong survival signals to cells deprived of oxygen. It has originally been thought that this phenomenon models the cell to solely fight the reperfusion injury by reducing oxidative stress, minimizing mitochondrial calcium accumulation, improving endothelial function and reducing inflammation (Zhao et al. 2003). Later studies suggested a more active role of post-conditioning as a trigger of transduction signal pathway, which is then responsible for the obtained myocardial protection. This pathway comprises the survival kinase cascade, phosphoinositide 3-kinase (PI3K)-Akt, which is itself one of the mediators of the reperfusion injury salvage pathway, the so called RISK pathway (Hausenloy and Yellon 2007). Thus, the phenomenon of post-conditioning elicited by transient ischemic periods and with the mode of action closely corresponding to ischemic pre-conditioning, is yet another factor to be considered in a sophisticated puzzle of myocardial protection. In addition, recent trials have focussed on techniques that try to remove toxic waste and debris from the reperfused microcirculation using antibodies, with an aim to reduce coagulation in the microcirculatory bed.

13.4 Retrograde Transplantation of Stem Cells and Retroinfusion of Cardioprotective Substances Into Ischemic Myocardium: More than an Alternative Delivery Route

As indicated in previous sections, transplantation of stem and progenitor cells into ischemic hearts has been shown to ameliorate structural damage and to foster left ventricular function recovery. The proposed mode of action is replenishment of damaged cardiac myocytes and neovascularization. What is trying to be accomplished is virtually a functional rebirth of parts of the myocardium, damaged by prolonged periods of ischemia. Myocardial ischemia may be of acute origin, termed acute coronary syndrome (ACS), or it could persist in certain myocardial areas for a longer time span, thus setting ground for a chronic ischemia condition termed ischemic cardiomyopathy. Pathophysiological processes behind the scenes of those two conditions are not completely alike, even though they both stem from the same principle of impaired oxygen delivery at the cellular level. Due to the same origin of acute and chronic myocardial ischemia, therapy regimens for these two conditions ought, in principle, be the same but also account for specificities of both courses of events. In particular, reperfusion injury is of detrimental consequence after restoration of epicardial blood flow in patients experiencing ACS, and requiring distinct modes of action. *Thus, activation of multiple protective pathways is required for the most optimized myocardial protection.* Transplantation of cells capable of replenishing stocks of cardiac myocytes and triggering angiogenesis is, in theory, the most powerful way to protect and revive ischemically modified and functionally impaired myocardium and to prevent remodelling. Although there have been significant breakthroughs in this field of research translating a sound experimental background into steady clinical facts, more research is inevitably in order to adapt this tempting notion to every day clinical situations. In Sect. 13.3.1, various approaches to cell transplantation have been reconsidered. One striking common feature of all listed techniques was the anterograde intracoronary route of application. Among the variety of other factors such as time point of transplantation, number and type of transplanted cells, the only common denominator of all approaches was the route of cell administration via infarct related coronary artery. The logic behind this procedure was to access jeopardized myocardium via the shortest possible route and to avoid intramyocardial administration of cells, which is the most direct but also the most hazardous technique. Intracoronary infusion of cells is being done according to the standard protocol through an over-the-wire balloon catheter, which is repeatedly being inflated for 3 min to impede the backflow of the infused solution. Three minutes of inflation are followed by 3 min of deflation restoring normal coronary flow to avoid extensive ischemic periods. Altogether, three inflation-deflation cycles are conducted for completion of the cell administration. It may be noticed that by transiently occluding a coronary vessel, as it is done during cell infusion, brief ischemia periods are inflicted upon myocardium thus strongly resembling the mechanics of post-conditioning. Therefore, it may be that some of the beneficial effects originally thought to be associated with intracoronary cell transplantation could have been confounded by effects of post-conditioning, which potential for cardioprotection was previously commented on in Sect. 13.3.2.4. Additional delivery techniques include a direct surgical injection of cells into the myocardium. Standard transepicardial surgical approaches do not allow for free access of the septal wall and neglect the importance of microcirculation. Endoventricular systems for delivery of precursor cells are inaccurate due to their instability, expressed by the lack of rotation with the heart (Thompson et al. 2003). On the other hand, an innovative application concept, involving combined intracoronary and percutaneous intramyocardial stem cell injection, has been shown to beneficially affect global left ventricular function when applied as late as 3 weeks after acute myocardial infarction (Gyöngyösi et al. 2009).

Due to a very sophisticated scheme of multiple autologous healing pathways that are convened into existence by the signals of myocardial ischemia, the most efficient cardioprotection ought to include most of them. In order to account for inconsistency and pitfalls of present intracoronary stem cell transplantation procedures, an alternative route of administration via coronary sinus has been taken into consideration. Much like retrograde cardioplegia, the stem cell transplantation via coronary sinus offers more than just an alternative delivery pathway, but rather a distinct research domain of which full utilization is embedded within the framework of modern myocardial protection.

13.4.1 Transvenous Intracoronary Route for Cell Transplantation and Gene/Protein Delivery

To brieØy recapitulate: Hitherto conducted studies on transplantation of progenitor cells provide promising data about its ability to induce myocardial regeneration and thus to protect the heart from an ischemic burden. The arterial route for stem cell transplantation has a potential risk of producing coronary emboli and has a limitation of delivering the cells only to the specific myocardial portions perfused by the chosen artery. Standard intramyocardial delivery of precursor cells may potentially induce an inflammatory response, leading to an impairment of transplanted cell engraftment and myocardial damage (Suzuki et al. 2004a, b). In contrast, the retrograde transplantation of stem cells via coronary sinus is tempting for the following reasons: (1) direct delivery of the cells into the myocardial interstitium, (2) minimal washout of the cells in deprived myocardial zones, (3) controlled time of administration, with prolonged balloon inflation, (4) emigration of inflammatory cells is known to take place in postcapillary venules, rather than at arterioles and capillaries,

(5) finally, coronary sinus cannulation is a well established technique, at present largely in use due to development of cardiac resynchronization therapy (CRT) (Jain et al. 2006).

In addition, any other regimen of interest that incorporated the gained knowledge and experience would need further evaluation: Anterograde infusion of the target coronary artery in combination with pulsatile coronary sinus occlusion in order to potentially facilitate improved engraftment of transplanted cells.

13.4.1.1
Experimental Studies on Transvenous Intracoronary Cell Transplantation

Suzuki and colleagues developed a retrograde infusion technique through the left cardiac vein and conducted initial research in rat hearts, establishing a firm experimental ground in the field of retrograde cell transplantation. The initial research (Suzuki et al. 2004a, b) was conducted in non-ischemic hearts. A skeletal muscle precursor cell line derived from a male heterozygote mouse was infused through the left cardiac vein and its distribution studied. It was then documented that transplanted myoblasts populated layers of the left ventricle free wall 10 min after the transplantation. More interestingly, by day 28, surviving myoblasts had differentiated into multinuclear myotubes (Suzuki et al. 2004a, b). The subsequently observed change in number of myoblasts indicated a potential proliferation of implanted myoblasts to the certain point where the proliferation stopped and differentiation began (Suzuki et al. 2004a, b). When compared to experimental data on anterograde intracoronary cell transplantation the following conclusions emerged, as stated by Suzuki and colleagues:

- Anterograde transplantation resulted in higher entrapment of myoblasts within myocardium. Retrograde infused cells that do not reach interstitial space are prone to be flushed out of the coronary sinus.
- The exact mechanism of cell migration from intravascular into interstitial space has not yet been depicted. Nevertheless, it is known that inflammatory cells migrate rather at venules, a finding that suggested the potential mode of action of the retrograde cell transplantation.
- Retrograde infused cells seemed to exhibit higher survival/proliferation rates.
- Some experimental data on anterograde cell transplantation revealed markedly larger end point grafts compared to retrograde transplantation. Due to inconsistency of cell lines transplanted in these studies, it is difficult to reach a definitive conclusion.

Retrograde transplantation of precursor cells via coronary veins was not associated with increased rate of myocardial hemorrhage, edema or with increased number of inflammatory cells. It has also been concluded that greater numbers of progenitor cells may be transplanted via coronary veins than via coronary arteries, for anterograde cell infusion might lead to an occlusion of microvessels and consequent tissue damage (Suzuki et al. 2004a, b).

Another important experimental study assessed the impact of retrograde cell transplantation on ischemic myocardium in the same rat model (Suzuki et al. 2004a, b). The behaviour of the transplanted cells corresponded to the findings of the study conducted in non-ischemic hearts. Langendorff perfusion was used to assess heart function 28 days after the cell transplantation via coronary veins. It revealed data closely related to echocardiographic results obtained also at day 28: left ventricular ejection fraction was improved, left ventricular end-diastolic dimension was reduced and coronary flow was significantly higher (Suzuki et al. 2004a, b). The observed end-diastolic dimension reduction is of particular importance when compared to anterograde intracoronary cell transplantation that barely had any positive influence on end-diastolic volume. Interestingly the same study found a significant reduction of collagen deposition in the border zones of infarcts (Suzuki et al. 2004a, b), findings that may be put in line with decreased end-diastolic dimensions and thus indicate a potential of retrograde transplanted cell to interfere with the process of remodelling. An interesting observation was also that, at day 28, implanted precursor cells were only detected in border zones of infarction areas, suggesting their inability to survive in the central infarct zones (Suzuki et al. 2004a, b).

Thompson et al. (2003) introduced yet another technique for direct stem cell transplantation utilizing the transvenous entrance port to the myocardium. This group experimentally used the coronary sinus route for intramyocardial delivery of previously harvested bone marrow cells. A catheter equipped with intravascular ultrasound (IVUS) was inserted into the coronary sinus, then further into the great cardiac vein and it finally reached anterior interventricular coronary vein where it was inserted intramyocardially through the vessel wall (Thompson et al. 2003). In this way, the coronary venous system was used as a roadmap to different portions of the heart.

The same group conducted additional experiments in swine hearts to test the ability of the coronary sinus route to bring about an improvement in function of an impaired left ventricle (Thompson et al. 2005). Pigs treated with intramyocardial transplantation of autologous bone performed retrograde marrow cells showed a significant improvement in left ventricular ejection fraction. The route of cell infusion was exactly the same as the one established in non-ischemic hearts and described above. Improvement in contractile function, especially in previously akinetic and hypokinetic regions seemed to have played a major role in enhancing the level of overall heart function. Alongside the improved contractility of the left ventricle, a reduction in infarct size was also documented. Importantly, the described transplantation of bone marrow cells was not associated with higher rate of ventricular tachycardia or fibrillation (Thompson et al. 2005). The main strength of this study is better applicability in the clinical setting than previous experimental protocols conducted in a small-animal model. However, one serious limitation was insufficient histopathological analysis of implanted cells in the course of events following the intervention, so that their embedment into different infarct zones could not reliably be tracked down. The authors pointed out the fact that the cell surface muscular marker desmin was not expressed by transplanted cells, thus suggesting that the overall functional improvement might be attributed to processes other than transdifferentiation. A new hypothesis considered enhancement of dormant host protective pathways to be crucial for the observed results (Thompson et al. 2005; Mohl 2007).

The obtained experimental data on transvenous transplantation of precursor cells unveil two important assets of this delivery route: (1) exposition of larger myocardial areas to the transplanted cells due to specific anatomy of coronary venous system and (2) a possibility for easier migration of cells through postcapillary venules, which are the normal sites of cell migration during inflammatory processes and defence.

13.4.1.2
Clinical Data on Transvenous Intracoronary Cell Transplantation

Despite increasing experimental evidence that the retrograde intracoronary precursor cell transplantation via the coronary venous system allows for successful engraftment of transplanted cells and improves cardiac function, the clinical application of this method is still in its infancy. Siminiak et al. (2005) conducted a phase I clinical trial in order to investigate feasibility and safety of transvenous intracoronary transplantation of skeletal myoblasts. The patient population comprised patients suffering from chronic myocardial ischemia and diagnosed with NYHA II or III. Skeletal myoblasts were injected directly into myocardium through a catheter that was equipped with intravascular ultrasound (IVUS) imaging and that had initially been placed in a particular coronary vein via the coronary sinus. Due to the well- established visibility of adjacent arteries there were no accidental artery punctures recorded or any other sort of adverse events linked to the applied methodology. Out of ten patients, nine received the transplanted skeletal myoblasts via the coronary sinus route, whereas in one patient the coronary sinus cannulation could not be completed. Thus, the authors concluded that the described retrograde injection technique was feasible and safe and that future studies ought to investigate its efficacy (Siminiak et al. 2005). Due to the fact that this study comprises patients with heart failure rather than acute myocardial infarction patients, and uses skeletal myoblasts as opposed to bone derived or circulating progenitor cells, it is difficult to compare it to other clinical regimens for transplantation of progenitor cells, as described in Sect. 13.3.1.

13.4.1.3
Gene and Protein Delivery via Coronary Venous System

Retroinfusion of drugs via coronary sinus in a pressure-regulated manner has been showed to prolong the contact time of a drug with myocardium (Boekstegers et al. 2000). The idea is that a drug would have more time to react on myocardial cells during this longer contact period. Interestingly, there is a significant drug concentration gradient after retroinfusion with highest concentrations found in subendocardial layers and smallest concentrations in epicardial layers of myocardium (Boekstegers and Kupatt 2004). Retroinfusion of cardioprotective substances have demonstrated a significant potential to limit reperfusion injury and to even reduce infarct size. Superoxide dismutase (SOD), glutathione (GTH) and the Na^+/K^+ exchange inhibitor cariporide, have all been shown, in experimental studies, to successfully reach myocardium deploying their beneficial effects by antagonising reperfusion injury (Kupatt et al. 2004). Fukushima et al. (2006) also showed in their rat model that superoxide dismutase was more efficient in attenuating reperfusion injury and consequently improving cardiac function when infused through the coronary venous system, in particular via the left coronary vein, as compared to initially used intravenous application. The retrograde intracoronary route has also been shown to optimally facilitate the delivery of antibodies against intercellular adhesion molecule-1 (ICAM-1) and P-selectin that are known to slow down the inflammatory process and diminish effects of ischemia-reperfusion injury, due to the fact that it allows for transportation of antibodies to the postcapillary venules (Fukushima et al. 2006).

In line with the presented benefits of retrograde infusion of cardioprotective substances, there is historic evidence that retrograde application of thrombolytics results in earlier clot lysis (Meerbaum et al. 1983) and even intermittent pressure elevation in the coronary venous system alone may have resulted in the same beneficial effect of a reduction of clot lysis (Mohl et al. 2008a, b). It therefore can be concluded that clearing of the postischemic microcirculation may be facilitated via the coronary venous route. As it is with progenitor cells, the route of delivery of genes and proteins into damaged myocardium contributes vastly to the overall success of a given therapy regimen. Hoshino compared different injection routes for gelatin hydrogel microspheres, which are proposed to be novel non-viral vectors for gene and protein delivery (Hoshino et al. 2006). Three injection regimens were compared upon infusion of gelatin hydrogel microspheres enriched with basic fibroblast growth factor to induce angiogenesis: anterograde injection via coronary arteries, retrograde injection via coronary veins and intramyocardial injection via the coronary sinus. Anterograde injection had the highest efficiency of delivery and the most homogeneous distribution of the infusate, while retrograde injection produced a scattered, non-homogeneous pattern. The greatest retention rate was documented with the anterograde route (70%), while retrograde and intramyocardial route via coronary sinus had smaller retention rates of 20% and 50%, respectively (Hoshino et al. 2006). Despite the high efficiency of distribution, anterograde injection exhibited important pitfalls, such as focal infarctions due to microembolism produced by occlusion of microarteries by the infusate. It also failed to produce expected outcomes in terms of angiogenesis triggered by the injected basic fibroblast growth factor (Hoshino et al. 2006). Finally, retrograde injection via coronary venous system and intramyocardial injection via the coronary sinus route increased the coronary flow reserve (Hoshino et al. 2006).

Several research groups have tested the ability of percutaneous retrograde transluminal gene delivery (PTRGD) to foster adenoviral gene transfer into myocardium. It was then documented that retroinfusion of adenoviral vectors led to more efficient gene transfer than intramyocardial injection (Raake et al. 2004). At the same time the comparison with anterograde infusion was also in favour of retroinfusion (Boekstegers et al. 2004).

The somewhat surprising results might be explained in part by the aforementioned findings: (1) retrograde infusate has longer contact time with the target microcirculation compared to anterograde infused substances, and (2) retrograde infusion is associated with significantly less damage to myocardium than the intramyocardial injection. The listed favourable outcomes of coronary sinus interventions including retroinfusion of cells, genes and growth factors might be in part explained by pressure characteristics of the coronary venous flow.

13.5
Exceptional Role of Pressure in the Hemodynamics of Coronary Sinus Interventions

The early years of experimental and clinical research in the field of retroinfusion via coronary sinus were marked by a notion of retroinfusion of oxygenated blood into the ischemic myocardium. This idea has been, for the most part, abandoned due to massive expansion of anterograde approach known as percutaneous transluminal coronary angioplasty (PTCA), where the balloon catheter is inserted directly into an occluded vessel. Nevertheless, in some instances, where the anterograde revascularization seems impossible, the coronary sinus retroinfusion still remains an option (Boekstegers and Kupatt 2004). Even though there have been a wide variety of retroinfusion regimens, they all have some kind of pulsatile pressure alteration of the coronary venous flow in common. This common denominator has sparked extensive research to elaborate on potential impact of pulsatile pressure change in the coronary venous flow, pointing out interesting phenomena such as the impact of shear stress and cyclic strain on the venous endothelium.

It has been speculated that delivery pressures of more than 50 mm Hg are detrimental during retrograde cardioplegia, as suggested by findings of Walter (Walter et al. 2002). Nevertheless, it has never been appreciated that the deleterious effects have been obtained during large doses of concomitant simultaneous delivery of cardioplegic solutions both anterograde as well as retrograde. It therefore remains speculative whether this pressure limit withholds scientific scrutiny. However it is important to note that jets of retrograde flow may create lesions and hemorrhage in the coronary sinus vessel wall. Our own experience shows that the retrograde delivery technique may result in severe adverse effects whereupon several methods have been developed by our group to efficiently correct these lesions (Aharinejad et al. 1996; Aigner et al. 2006).

13.5.1
Arterialization of Coronary Veins

Retroinfusion of oxygenated blood seemed to be a logic solution to what sometimes seems to be a problematic anterograde vessel patency restoration. Various techniques such as synchronized coronary venous retroperfusion (SRP) (Boekstegers et al. 1990) and selective synchronized suction and retroinfusion of coronary veins (SSR) (Boekstegers et al. 1994) have shown remarkable potential, but also exhibited serious drawbacks in regard to clinical practicability. Pressure-regulated retroinfusion in high-risk PTCA patients demonstrated better clinical applicability (Boekstegers et al. 1998). This technique utilizes the systolic coronary sinus occlusion pressure in order to avoid over- or underperfusion of ischemic myocardium.

Chronic arterialization of a cardiac vein is preserved as a valuable option for patients who have no other option and are therefore not candidates for standard revascularization procedures. Percutaneous in-situ arterialization of a cardiac vein (PICVA) is a recently developed model which exhibited beneficial effects, but is held back by its limited clinical applicability originating for the most part from the chronic increase in the coronary venous pressure (Oesterle et al. 2001). Another method under on-going developmental study is a ventricle-to-coronary vein bypass; the general idea is to supply retrograde flow during systole and to allow for diastolic draining (Boekstegers and Kupatt 2004). Although the mechanism behind this idea seems controversial, the pressure regulation seems to play an important role in the process of coronary sinus retroinfusion and may be pointed out as a distinct research target.

13.5.2
Pulsatile Cardioplegia

Cardiac muscle is always perfused in a pulsatile manner, with the only exceptions to this rule being elective ventricular fibrillation and cardioplegia delivery during open-heart surgery. It is known that the pulsatility enhances transmural and also regional myocardial flow (Kassab et al. 2006), thus making pulsatile cardioplegia an alluring choice for perioperative myocardial protection.

Heterogeneous cardioplegia distribution in the heart, even in the absence of coronary artery disease (Aldea et al. 1990) has drawn much attention and unified scientific efforts in optimizing anterograde and retrograde cardioplegia. Nevertheless, especially the combined detrimental effects of preoperative regionally ischemic myocardium and seriously aggravated distribution of a cardioplegic solution, found in the subgroup of patients suffering from severe coronary artery disease form an even more challenging population in need of perioperative cardioprotection. The notion of more optimized treatment of ischemic myocardial areas and more evenly distributed cardioplegia during open-heart surgery has sparked in depth research of possible techniques able to supplement the standard regimens. Microcirculatory perfusion has been recognized as one of the strongest fundamentals of myocardial protection, which is neither transparently established nor easily displayed (unlike the patency of epicardial vessels). Thus, scientific attention has been shifted towards avoiding microvasculatory damage and fostering myocyte self-defence potential. Aldea et al. (1990) pointed out the importance of coronary pressure for the proper distribution of a cardioplegic solution. At lower perfusion pressures the heterogeneity of cardioplegia distribution pattern increases nonlinearly, thus suggesting a greater number of myocardial areas being possibly insufficiently perfused. Higher cardioplegia perfusion pressures accounted for less heterogenicity, thus making it more evenly distributed (Aldea et al. 1990). Pulsatile cardioplegia emerged as a tempting research direction after some of the newest publications considered it to be of great potential in protecting the ischemic jeopardized heart at the microvasculature and subsequently cellular level, most probably by the means of improved cardioplegia distribution. It had already been shown to ameliorate detrimental effects of myocardial ischemia on left ventricular function during cardiopulmonary bypass (Mori et al. 1987). An interesting study by Graham et al. (2002) compared standard anterograde cold blood cardioplegia with the same type of cardioplegic solution applied biologically, thus with variable pulsatility. Better perseverance of diastolic cardiac function was documented in patients undergoing cardiopulmonary bypass with biological cardioplegia application (Graham et al. 2002). The authors suggested that beneficial effects of the biologically normal perfusion during cardiac "arrest" are attributed to improved microvasculatory circulation, as a result of fractal delivery of cold blood solution.

Kostelec et al. (2006) conducted a study to compare non-pulsatile with pulsatile cardioplegia in an open failing ventricle model. Pulsatile cardioplegia markedly improved subendocardial perfusion of the open failing ventricle, suggesting better perioperative cardioprotection potential.

The main hypothesis coming from these studies is based on previous works of Goto et al. (1996) who documented vasodilatation to be associated with an increased pulse pressure, and who advocated the notion that precapillary resistance vessels undergo luminal changes when treated with pulsatile flow. Interestingly, the authors proposed this effect to be endothelium independent. Thus, the notion of pulsatile cardioplegia is interesting when put in the context of retrograde cardioplegia delivery. The success of coronary sinus interventions, including retroinfusion of drugs, cells, genes and growth factors and oxygenated blood is closely related to pressure control of the coronary sinus flow, suggesting that pulsatile retrograde cardioplegia could maximize benefit in perioperative cardioprotection.

13.5.3
Controlled Pressure Elevation in the Coronary Sinus: A Common Denominator of Coronary Sinus Interventions

In recent years, strong evidence has been accumulated for a provocative hypothesis suggesting that periodic pressure elevation of the coronary sinus flow, which is known to be associated with a wide variety of coronary sinus interventions, has potential for inducing regeneration by activating venous endothelial cells (Mohl et al. 2008a, b). The backbone of this process is an assumed pluripotency of endothelial cells when exposed to shear stress and cyclic strain. The most crucial observations, which have shaped the hypothesis and still warrant future research to unveil the mode of actions, are presented in the following list:

- Mohl et al. (1984) observed a substantial reduction in infarct size with the technique known as pressure intermittent coronary sinus occlusion (PICSO), where the coronary sinus was occluded intermittently by the means of a balloon catheter being inflated and deflated in a periodic manner. The findings from this study underscored the notion that by solely interacting with coronary sinus pressure without any retroinfusion, beneficial effects on ischemic myocardium may be obtained. More recently a meta-analysis performed by Syeda et al. (2004) revealed a significant reduction in infarct size after periodic coronary sinus elevation.
- Lochner proposed an important role of NO in the process of preconditioning, a finding which was promptly connected to the notion that shear stress-treated endothelial cells are known to release NO (Lochner et al. 2002).
- Zheng et al. (2001) documented up-regulation of vascular endothelial growth factor (VEGF) after exposure of microvascular endothelial cells to shear stress. Vascular endothelial growth factor (VEGF) is known to be one of the inducers of angiogenesis, a process crucial to myocardial regeneration.
- Groenendijk et al. (2004) pointed out a very important role of kinetic blood flow force in the developing heart, postulating its influence on modelling of the development.
- Weigel et al (2007) showed that the use of periodic coronary sinus pressure elevation in ischemic swine hearts was associated with an up-regulation of vascular endothelial growth factor (VEGF) and heme-oxygenase 1 (HO-1). It was also documented that the VEGF up-regulation was positively correlated with an increase in coronary sinus occlusion pressure.
- Recently, Grunewald et al. (2006) suggested that VEGF was capable of inducing perivascular expression of stromal derived factor 1 (SDF1) which is itself thought to

be responsible for homing of progenitor cells. Thus, if pressure elevation in coronary sinus were capable of up-regulating VEGF, positive effects of retrograde transplantation of progenitor cells would also include better recruitment of progenitor cells.

Beneficial clinical outcomes of periodic pressure elevation within the coronary venous system in acute ischemia treatment (Mohl et al. 2008a, b) and the newly established hypothesis of myocardial regeneration induced by pressure activated coronary venous endothelium (Mohl et al. 2008a, b) may inspire future research efforts to fully elucidate the role of coronary venous flow pressure in observed positive effects of an "alternative coronary sinus route".

13.6
Conclusion

Integrating all available results and known effects of myocardial protection as well as the underlying principles of ischemia and reperfusion allow a common proposition. The coronary venous system, in spite of all knowledge gathered in the last decades, is still a black spot in our understanding of its entire role in myocardial protection and myocardial regeneration but we can acknowledge its important role for therapies and the only unlimited access to deprived myocardium.

Many of the effects reported above have one important commonality.

- All efforts to gain access via the coronary venous system induce changes in the pressure and flow relationship in coronary veins.
- Periodic pressure increase in the venous system may activate coronary venous endothelium, a mechanism termed mechanotransduction.
- Permanent pressure increase is detrimental for the nutrition of the heart by inducing a reduction of coronary artery inflow.
- To allow the combination of positive effects and prevention of myocardial underperfusion, a physiologic pressure control is mandatory.
- In global ischemia and retroperfusion of cardioplegia, flow can be reversed totally.
- Pulsatility can induce activation of venous endothelium during global cardiac arrest.
- Activation of venous endothelium might enhance homing or even mobilisation of regenerative cells thus allowing stem cell effects without stem cell transplantation.

Based on the findings that mechanical forces may be transduced into a certain gene expression pattern during angiogenesis and also morphogenesis (Ingber 2002; Patwari and Lee 2008), the activation of venous endothelium by periodic coronary sinus pressure elevation might be recapitulating inborn embryonic pathways in the adult ischemic heart and thus help prevent the sequelae of global and regional ischemia and reperfusion. Even more so it can be speculated that this delivery route will be the core of an improved understanding of myocardial protection and regeneration. Therefore a dream might come true that not only regeneration can be induced during global cardiac arrest but also no option patients with chronic heart failure may be bridged to regeneration.

References

Abdel-Latif A, Bolli R, Tleyjeh IM, Montori VM, Perin EC, Hornung CA, Zuba-Surma EK, Al-Mallah M, Dawn B. (2007) Adult bone marrow-derived cells for cardiac repair: a systematic review and meta-analysis. Arch Intern Med 167:989–997.

Aharinejad S, Baumgartner H, Miksovsky A, Mohl W. (1996) Closure of ruptured coronary sinus by a pericardial patch. Ann Thorac Surg 62(3):889–8891.

Aigner C, Wolner E, Mohl W. (2006) Management of central coronary sinus ruptures using the pericardial patch repair technique. Ann Thorac Surg 81(4):1275–1278.

Aldea GS, Austin RE Jr, Flynn AE, Coggins DL, Husseini W, Hoffman JI. (1990) Heterogeneous delivery of cardioplegic solution in the absence of coronary artery disease. J Thorac Cardiovasc Surg 99(2):345–353.

Allen BS, Winkelmann JW, Hanafy H, Hartz RS, Bolling KS, Ham J, Feinstein S. (1995) Retrograde cardioplegia does not adequately perfuse the right ventricle. J Thorac Cardiovasc Surg 109(6):1116–24; discussion 1124–1126.

Antoniucci D, Rodriguez A, Hempel A, Valenti R, Migliorini A, Vigo F, Parodi G, Fernandez-Pereira C, Moschi G, Bartorelli A, Santoro GM, Bolognese L, Colombo A. (2003) A randomized trial comparing primary infarct artery stenting with or without abciximab in acute myocardial infarction. J Am Coll Cardiol 42(11):1879–1885.

Bartunek J, Vanderheyden M, Vandekerckhove B, Mansour S, De Bruyne B, De Bondt P, Van Haute I, Lootens N, Heyndrickx G, Wijns W. (2005) Intracoronary injection of CD133-positive enriched bone marrow progenitor cells promotes cardiac recovery after recent myocardial infarction: feasibility and safety. Circulation 112(9 Suppl):I178–I183.

Boekstegers P, Diebold J, Weiss C. (1990) Selective ECG synchronised suction and retroinfusion of coronary veins: first results of studies in acute myocardial ischaemia in dogs. Cardiovasc Res 24(6):456–464.

Boekstegers P, Kupatt C (2004) Current concepts and application of coronary venous retroinfusion. Basic Res Cardiol 99(6):373–381.

Boekstegers P, Peter W, von Degenfeld G, Nienaber CA, Abend M, Rehders TC, Habazettl H, Kapsner T, von Lüdinghausen M, Werdan K. (1994) Preservation of regional myocardial function and myocardial oxygen tension during acute ischemia in pigs: comparison of selective synchronized suction and retroinfusion of coronary veins to synchronized coronary venous retroperfusion. J Am Coll Cardiol 23(2):459–469.

Boekstegers P, Giehrl W, von Degenfeld G, Steinbeck G. (1998) Selective suction and pressure-regulated retroinfusion: an effective and safe approach to retrograde protection against myocardial ischemia in patients undergoing normal and high risk percutaneous transluminal coronary angioplasty. J Am Coll Cardiol 31(7):1525–1533.

Boekstegers P, von Degenfeld G, Giehrl W, Heinrich D, Hullin R, Kupatt C, Steinbeck G, Baretton G, Middeler G, Katus H, Franz WM. (2000) Myocardial gene transfer by selective pressure-regulated retroinfusion of coronary veins. Gene Ther 7(3):232–240.

Boekstegers P, Kupatt C. (2004) Current concepts and applications of coronary venous retro-infusion. Basic Res Cardiol. 99(6):373–381.

Bolognese L, Neskovic AN, Parodi G, Cerisano G, Buonamici P, Santoro GM, Antoniucci D. (2002) Left ventricular remodeling after primary coronary angioplasty: patterns of left ventricular dilation and long-term prognostic implications. Circulation 106(18):2351–2357.

Dangas G, Stone GW, Weinberg MD, Webb J, Cox DA, Brodie BR, Krucoff MW, Gibbons RJ, Lansky AJ, Mehran R; EMERALD Investigators. (2008) Contemporary outcomes of rescue percutaneous coronary intervention for acute myocardial infarction: comparison with primary angioplasty and the role of distal protection devices (EMERALD trial). Am Heart J 155(6):1090–1096. Epub 2008 Jan 30.

Dimmeler S, Burchfield J, and Zeiher AM. (2008) Cell-based therapy of myocardial infarction. Arterioscler Thromb Vasc Biol 28:208–216

Fujiwara T, Matsunaga T, Kameda K, Abe N, Ono H, Higuma T, Yokoyama J, Hanada H, Osanai T, Okumura K. (2007) Nicorandil suppresses the increases in plasma level of matrix metalloproteinase activity and attenuates left ventricular remodeling in patients with acute myocardial infarction. Heart Vessels 22(5):303–309. Epub 2007 Sep 20.

Fukushima S, Coppen SR, Varela-Carver A, Brindley G, Yamahara K, Sarathchandra P, Yacoub MH, Suzuki K. (2006) Enhanced efficiency of superoxide dismutase-induced cardioprotection by retrograde Intracoronary administration. Cardiovasc Res 69 459–465

Gick M, Jander N, Bestehorn HP, Kienzle RP, Ferenc M, Werner K, Comberg T, Peitz K, Zohlnhöfer D, Bassignana V, Buettner HJ, Neumann FJ. (2005) Randomized evaluation of the effects of filter-based distal protection on myocardial perfusion and infarct size after primary percutaneous catheter intervention in myocardial infarction with and without ST-segment elevation. Circulation 112(10):1462–1469

Goto M, VanBavel E, Giezeman MJ, Spaan JA. (1996) Vasodilatory effect of pulsatile pressure on coronary resistance vessels. Circ Res 79(5):1039–1045.

Gyöngyösi M, Lang I, Dettke M, Beran G, Graf S, Sochor H, Nyolczas N, Charwat S, Hemetsberger R, Christ G, Edes I, Balogh L, Krause KT, Jaquet K, Kuck KH, Benedek I, Hintea T, Kiss R, Préda I, Kotevski V, Pejkov H, Zamini S, Khorsand A, Sodeck G, Kaider A, Maurer G, Glogar DR. (2009) Combined delivery approach of bone marrow mononuclear stem cells early and late after myocardial infarction: the MYSTAR prospective, randomized study. Nat Clin Pract Cardiovasc Med 6(1):70–81. Epub 2008 Nov 11.

Graham MR, Warrian RK, Girling LG, Doiron L, Lefevre GR, Cheang M, Mutch WA. (2002) Fractal or biologically variable delivery of cardioplegic solution prevents diastolic dysfunction after cardiopulmonary bypass. J Thorac Cardiovasc Surg 123(1):63–71.

Groenendijk BC, Hierck BP, Gittenberger-De Groot AC, Poelmann RE. (2004) Development-related changes in the expression of shear stress responsive genes KLF-2, ET-1, and NOS-3 in the developing cardiovascular system of chicken embryos. Dev Dyn 230(1):57–68.

Grunewald M, Avraham I, Dor Y, Bachar-Lustig E, Itin A, Jung S, Chimenti S, Abramovitch R, Keshet E (2006) VEGF-Induced adult neovascularization: Recruitment, retention and role of accessory cells. Cell 124:175–189

Hausenloy DJ, Yellon DM. (2007) Preconditioning and postconditioning: united at reperfusion. Pharmacol Ther 116(2):173–191. Epub 2007 Jun 30. Review.

Hoshino K, Kimura T, De Grand AM, Yoneyama R, Kawase Y, Houser S, Ly HQ, Kushibiki T, Furukawa Y, Ono K, Tabata Y, Frangioni JV, Kita T, Hajjar RJ, Hayase M. (2006) Three catheter-based strategies for cardiac delivery of therapeutic gelatin microspheres. Gene Ther 13 (18):1320–1327. Epub 2006 May 18.

Ito H, Taniyama Y, Iwakura K, Nishikawa N, Masuyama T, Kuzuya T, Hori M, Higashino Y, Fujii K, Minamino T. (1999) Intravenous nicorandil can preserve microvascular integrity and myocardial viability in patients with reperfused anterior wall myocardial infarction. J Am Coll Cardiol 33(3):654–660.

Ingber DE. (2002) Mechanical signaling and the cellular response to extracellular matrix in angiogenesis and cardiovascular physiology. Circ Res 91(10):877–887.

Jain AK, Smith EJ, Rothman MT. (2006) The coronary venous system: an alternative route of access to the myocardium. J Invasive Cardiol 18(11):563–568.

Janssens S, Dubois C, Bogaert J, Theunissen K, Deroose C, Desmet W, Kalantzi M, Herbots L, Sinnaeve P, Dens J, Maertens J, Rademakers F, Dymarkowski S, Gheysens O, Van Cleemput J, Bormans G, Nuyts J, Belmans A, Mortelmans L, Boogaerts M, Van de Werf F. (2006) Autologous bone marrow-derived stem-cell transfer in patients with ST-segment elevation myocardial infarction: double-blind, randomised controlled trial. Lancet 367(9505):113–121.

Kassab GS, Kostelec M, Buckberg GD, Covell J, Sadeghi A, Hoffman JI. (2006) Myocardial protection in the failing heart: II. Effect of pulsatile cardioplegic perfusion under simulated left ventricular restoration. J Thorac Cardiovasc Surg 132(4):884–890.

Katritsis DG, Sotiropoulou PA, Karvouni E, Karabinos I, Korovesis S, Perez SA, Voridis EM, Papamichail M. (2005) Transcoronary transplantation of autologous mesenchymal stem cells and endothelial progenitors into infarcted human myocardium. Catheter Cardiovasc Interv 65(3):321–329.

Kang HJ, Kim HS, Zhang SY, Park KW, Cho HJ, Koo BK, Kim YJ, Soo Lee D, Sohn DW, Han KS, Oh BH, Lee MM, Park YB. (2004) Effects of intracoronary infusion of peripheral blood stem-cells mobilised with granulocyte-colony stimulating factor on left ventricular systolic function and restenosis after coronary stenting in myocardial infarction: the MAGIC cell randomised clinical trial. Lancet 363(9411):751–756.

Kopecky SL, Aviles RJ, Bell MR, Lobl JK, Tipping D, Frommell G, Ramsey K, Holland AE, Midei M, Jain A, Kellett M, Gibbons RJ. (2003) AmP579 Delivery for Myocardial Infarction REduction study. A randomized, double-blinded, placebo-controlled, dose-ranging study measuring the effect of an adenosine agonist on infarct size reduction in patients undergoing primary percutaneous transluminal coronary angioplasty: the ADMIRE (AmP579 Delivery for Myocardial Infarction REduction) study. Am Heart J 146(1):146–152.

Kostelec M, Covell J, Buckberg GD, Sadeghi A, Hoffman JI, Kassab GS. (2006) Myocardial protection in the failing heart: I. Effect of cardioplegia and the beating state under simulated left ventricular restoration. J Thorac Cardiovasc Surg 132(4):875–883.

Kupatt C, Hinkel R, Horstkotte J, Deiss M, von Brühl ML, Bilzer M, Boekstegers P. (2004) Selective retroinfusion of GSH and cariporide attenuates myocardial ischemia-reperfusion injury in a preclinical pig model. Cardiovasc Res 61(3):530–537.

Lochner A, Marais E, Du Toit E, Moolman J (2002) Nitric oxide triggers classic ischemic preconditioning. Ann NY Acad Sci 962:402–414

Louagie YA, Gonzalez E, Jamart J, Malhomme B, Broka S, Buche M, Eucher PM, Schoevaerdts JC. (1997) Assessment of continuous cold blood cardioplegia in coronary artery bypass grafting. Ann Thorac Surg 63(3):689–696.

Louagie YA, Jamart J, Gonzalez M, Collard E, Broka S, Galanti L, Gruslin A. (2004) Continuous cold blood cardioplegia improves myocardial protection: a prospective randomized study. Ann Thorac Surg 77(2):664–671

Lunde K, Solheim S, Aakhus S, Arnesen H, Abdelnoor M, Egeland T, Endresen K, Ilebekk A, Mangschau A, Fjeld JG, Smith HJ, Taraldsrud E, Grøgaard HK, Bjørnerheim R, Brekke M, Müller C, Hopp E, Ragnarsson A, Brinchmann JE, Forfang K. (2006) Intracoronary injection of mononuclear bone marrow cells in acute myocardial infarction. N Engl J Med 355(12):1199–1209

Meluzín J, Mayer J, Groch L, Janousek S, Hornceck I, Hlinomaz O, Kala P, Panovský R, Prsek J, Kamínek M, Stanícek J, Klabusay M, Korístek Z, Navrtil M, Dusek L, Vinklrkov J. (2006) Autologous transplantation of mononuclear bone marrow cells in patients with acute myocardial infarction: the effect of the dose of transplanted cells on myocardial function. Am Heart J 152(5):975–915.

Menasché P, Kural S, Fauchet M, Lavergne A, Commin P, Bercot M, Touchot B, Georgiopoulos G, Piwnica A. (1982) Retrograde coronary sinus perfusion: a safe alternative for ensuring cardioplegic delivery in aortic valve surgery. Ann Thorac Surg 34(6):647–658.

Meerbaum S, Lang TW, Povzhitkov M, Haendchen RV, Uchiyama T, Broffman J, Corday E. (1983) Retrograde lysis of coronary artery thrombus by coronary venous streptokinase administration. J Am Coll Cardiol 1(5):1262–1267.

Mohl W, Glogar DH, Mayr H, Losert U, Sochor H, Pachinger O, Kaindl F, Wolner E. (1984) Reduction of infarct size induced by pressure-controlled intermittent coronary sinus occlusion. Am J Cardiol 53(7):923–928.

Mohl W (1987) Retrograde cardioplegia via the coronary sinus. Ann Chir Gynaecol 76(1):61–67.
Mohl W (2007) Embryonic recall: myocardial regeneration beyond stem cell transplantation. Wien Klin Wochenschr. 119(11–12):333–336.
Mohl W, Komamura K, Kasahara H, Heinze G, Glogar D, Hirayama A, Kodama K. (2008) Myocardial protection via the coronary sinus. Circ J 72(4):526–533.
Mohl W, Mina S, Milasinovic D, Kasahara H, Wei S, Maurer G. (2008) Is activation of coronary venous cells the key to cardiac regeneration? Nat Clin Pract Cardiovasc Med 5(9):528–530.
Montalescot G, Barragan P, Wittenberg O, Ecollan P, Elhadad S, Villain P, Boulenc JM, Morice MC, Maillard L, Pansiéri M, Choussat R, Pinton P; ADMIRAL Investigators. (2001) Abciximab before direct angioplasty and stenting in myocardial infarction regarding acute and long-term follow-up. Platelet Glycoprotein IIb/IIIa inhibition with coronary stenting for acute myocardial infarction. N Engl J Med 344(25):1895–1903.
Mori F, Ivey TD, Itoh T, Thomas R, Breazeale DG, Misbach G. (1987) Effects of pulsatile reperfusion on postischemic recovery of myocardial function after global hypothermic cardiac arrest. J Thorac Cardiovasc Surg 93(5):719–727.
Nakamura T, Kubo N, Seki Y, Ikeda N, Ishida T, Funayama H, Hashimoto S, Yasu T, Fujii M, Kawakami M, Saito M. (2004) Effects of a distal protection device during primary stenting in patients with acute anterior myocardial infarction. Circ J 68(8):763–768
Neumann FJ, Kastrati A, Schmitt C, Blasini R, Hadamitzky M, Mehilli J, Gawaz M, Schleef M, Seyfarth M, Dirschinger J, Schömig A. (2000) Effect of glycoprotein IIb/IIIa receptor blockade with abciximab on clinical and angiographic restenosis rate after the placement of coronary stents following acute myocardial infarction. J Am Coll Cardiol 35(4):915–921.
Neumann F, Mohl W, Griesmacher A, Simon P, Zweytick B, Kupilik N, Stix G, Moidl R, Wolner E. (1996) Perioperative myocardial injury with different modes of Anterograde and retrograde cardioplegic delivery. Eur J Cardiothorac Surg 10(3):185–193.
Oesterle SN, Reifart N, Hauptmann E, Hayase M, Yeung AC. (2001) Percutaneous in situ coronary venous arterialization: report of the first human catheter-based coronary artery bypass. Circulation 103(21):2539–2543
Patwari P, Lee RT. (2008) Mechanical control of tissue morphogenesis. Circ Res;103(3):234–243. Review
Petronio AS, De Carlo M, Ciabatti N, Amoroso G, Limbruno U, Palagi C, Di Bello V, Romano MF, Mariani M. (2005) Left ventricular remodeling after primary coronary angioplasty in patients treated with abciximab or intracoronary adenosine. Am Heart J 150(5):1015.
Pratt FH. (1898) Nutrition of the heart through vessels of the thebesian and coronary veins. Am J Physiol 1:86–103
Raake P, von Degenfeld G, Hinkel R, Vachenauer R, Sandner T, Beller S, Andrees M, Kupatt C, Schuler G, Boekstegers P. (2004) Myocardial gene transfer by selective pressure-regulated retroinfusion of coronary veins: comparison with surgical and percutaneous intramyocardial gene delivery. J Am Coll Cardiol 44(5):1124–1129.
Ruengsakulrach P, Buxton BF. (2001) Anatomic and hemodynamic considerations influencing the efficiency of retrograde cardioplegia. Ann Thorac Surg 71(4):1389–1395. Review.
Sardella G, Mancone M, Nguyen BL, De Luca L, Di Roma A, Colantonio R, Petrolini A, Conti G, Fedele F. (2008) The effect of thrombectomy on myocardial blush in primary angioplasty: the Randomized Evaluation of Thrombus Aspiration by two thrombectomy devices in acute Myocardial Infarction (RETAMI) trial. Catheter Cardiovasc Interv 71(1):84–91.
Schächinger V, Erbs S, Elsässer A, Haberbosch W, Hambrecht R, Hölschermann H, Yu J, Corti R, Mathey DG, Hamm CW, Süselbeck T, Assmus B, Tonn T, Dimmeler S, Zeiher AM; REPAIR-AMI Investigators. (2006) Intracoronary bone marrow-derived progenitor cells in acute myocardial infarction. N Engl J Med 355(12):1210–1221.
Siminiak T, Fiszer D, Jerzykowska O, Grygielska B, Rozwadowska N, Kamucki P, Kurpisz M. (2005) Percutaneous trans-coronary-venous transplantation of autologous skeletal myoblasts in

the treatment of post-infarction myocardial contractility impairment: the POZNAN trial. Eur Heart J 26(12):1188–1195. Epub 2005 Mar 10.

Stone GW, Grines CL, Cox DA, Garcia E, Tcheng JE, Griffin JJ, Guagliumi G, Stuckey T, Turco M, Carroll JD, Rutherford BD, Lansky AJ; Controlled Abciximab and Device Investigation to Lower Late Angioplasty Complications (CADILLAC) Investigators. (2002) Comparison of angioplasty with stenting, with or without abciximab, in acute myocardial infarction. N Engl J Med 346(13):957–966.

Stone GW, Witzenbichler B, Guagliumi G, Peruga JZ, Brodie BR, Dudek D, Kornowski R, Hartmann F, Gersh BJ, Pocock SJ, Dangas G, Wong SC, Kirtane AJ, Parise H, Mehran R, HORIZONS-AMI Trial Investigators. (2008) Bivalirudin during primary PCI in acute myocardial infarction. N Engl J Med 358(21):2218–2230.

Strauer BE, Brehm M, Zeus T, Köstering M, Hernandez A, Sorg RV, Kögler G, Wernet P. (2002) Repair of infarcted myocardium by autologous intracoronary mononuclear bone marrow cell transplantation in humans. Circulation 106(15):1913–1918.

Suzuki K, Murtuza B, Smolenski RT, Yacoub MH. (2004) Selective cell dissemination into the heart by retrograde intracoronary infusion in the rat. Transplantation 77(5):757–759.

Suzuki K, Murtuza B, Fukushima S, Smolenski RT, Varela-Carver A, Coppen SR, Yacoub MH. (2004) Targeted cell delivery into infarcted rat hearts by retrograde intracoronary infusion: distribution, dynamics, and influence on cardiac function. Circulation 110(11 Suppl 1):II225–II230.

Syeda B, Schukro C, Heinze G, Modaressi K, Glogar D, Maurer G, Mohl W. (2004) The salvage potential of coronary sinus interventions: meta-analysis and pathophysiologic consequences. J Thorac Cardiovasc Surg 127(6):1703–1712.

Thompson CA, Nasseri BA, Makower J, Houser S, McGarry M, Lamson T, Pomerantseva I, Chang JY, Gold HK, Vacanti JP, Oesterle SN (2003) Percutaneous transvenous cellular cardiomyoplasty. A novel nonsurgical approach for myocardial cell transplantation. J Am Coll Cardiol 41(11):1964–1971.

Thompson CA, Reddy VK, Srinivasan A, Houser S, Hayase M, Davila A, Pomerantsev E, Vacanti JP, Gold HK. (2005) Left ventricular functional recovery with percutaneous, transvascular direct myocardial delivery of bone marrow-derived cells. J Heart Lung Transplant;24(9):1385–1392.

Vähäsilta T, Saraste A, Kytö V, Malmberg M, Kiss J, Kentala E, Kallajoki M, Savunen T. (2005) Cardiomyocyte apoptosis after Anterograde and retrograde cardioplegia. Ann Thorac Surg 80(6):2229–2234.

van der Bogt KE, Sheikh AY, Schrepfer S, Hoyt G, Cao F, Ransohoff KJ, Swijnenburg RJ, Pearl J, Lee A, Fischbein M, Contag CH, Robbins RC, Wu JC. (2008) Comparison of different adult stem cell types for treatment of myocardial ischemia. Circulation 118(14 Suppl):S121–S129.

Walter PJ, Kindl F, Podzuweit T, Schaper J. (2002) Metabolic and ultrastructural changes in the ischemic human myocardium due to additional perfusion of the coronary sinus with "Bretschneider cardioplegic solution". In: International Working group of Coronary sinus interventions. Vol. 5, http://www.coronarysinus.com.

Weigel G, Kajgana I, Bergmeister H, Riedl G, Glogar HD, Gyöngyösi M, Blasnig S, Heinze G, Mohl W (2007) Beck and back: a paradigm change in coronary sinusinterventions–pulsatile stretch on intact coronary venous endothelium. J Thorac Cardiovasc Surg 133:1581–1587.

Winkelmann BR, Ihnken K, Beyersdorf F, Eckel L, Skupin M, März W, Herrmann G, Spies H, Schräder R, Sievert H. (1993) Left main coronary artery stenosis after aortic valve replacement: genetic disposition for accelerated arteriosclerosis after injury of the intact human coronary artery? Coron Artery Dis 4(7):659–667.

Wollert KC, Meyer GP, Lotz J, Ringes-Lichtenberg S, Lippolt P, Breidenbach C, Fichtner S, Korte T, Hornig B, Messinger D, Arseniev L, Hertenstein B, Ganser A, Drexler H. (2004) Intracoronary autologous bone-marrow cell transfer after myocardial infarction: the BOOST randomised controlled clinical trial. Lancet 364(9429):141–148.

Wollert KC, Meyer GP, Lotz J, Ringes-Lichtenberg S, Lippolt P, Breidenbach C, Fichtner S, Korte T, Hornig B, Messinger D, Arseniev L, Hertenstein B, Ganser A, Drexler H. (2004) Monitoring of bone marrow cell homing to the infarcted human myocardium. Circulation 110 (suppl III): III–436. Abstract.

Zhao ZQ, Corvera JS, Halkos ME, Kerendi F, Wang NP, Guyton RA, Vinten-Johansen J. (2003) Inhibition of myocardial injury by ischemic postconditioning during reperfusion: comparison with ischemic preconditioning. Am J Physiol Heart Circ Physiol 285(2):H579–H588. Erratum in: Am J Physiol Heart Circ Physiol. 2004 Jan 286(1):H477.

Zheng W, Seftor EA, Meininger CJ, Hendrix MJ, Tomanek RJ (2001) Mechanisms of coronary angiogenesis in response to stretch: role of VEGF and TGF-beta. Am J Physiol Heart Circ Physiol 280:H909–H917

Donor Heart Preservation by Continuous Perfusion

Andreas Zuckerman, Arezu Aliabadi, and Gernot Seebacher

14.1 Introduction

Cardiac transplantation is the best option for end-stage heart failure (Taylor et al. 2008). Transplantation techniques, immunosuppressive protocols and a better understanding of short and long-term complications have increased survival significantly over the last 40 years; however, graft preservation has changed little during that period. Hearts are still preserved by flushing them with cold potassium-based crystalloid solution, with subsequent storage in a sterile container filled with preservation solution containing ice to maintain organ hypothermia. This technique limits a safe preservation time to 4–6 h.

Due to the good results after transplantation, more patients have been put on transplant waiting lists, which increased the waiting times for a donor heart and the mortality on the waiting list. To counterbalance this development, transplant centers have accepted more marginal donor hearts and have tolerated longer ischemic times (Marasco et al. 2007; Wittwer and Wahlers 2008; Morgan et al. 2003; Kirklin et al. 2003; Russo et al. 2007; Banner et al. 2008; Goldsmith et al. 2009). However working in such a setting increases the risk of primary graft dysfunction, leading to higher morbidity and mortality (Russo et al. 2007; Banner et al. 2008; Goldsmith et al. 2009). Moreover, primary graft dysfunction increases time on intensive care units and prolongs in-hospital stay, which is associated with higher costs of transplant procedures (Marasco et al. 2007). Therefore new preservation technologies are necessary to overcome these problems and to increase transplant numbers and improve outcome after cardiac transplantation.

A. Zuckerman (✉), A. Aliabadi, and G. Seebacher
Department of Cardiac Surgery, Medical University of Vienna, Währinger Gürtel 18–20, 1090 Vienna, Austria
e-mail: andreas.zuckermann@meduniwien.ac.at

14.2
Current Concept of Preservation

Cold static storage is a simple, relatively inexpensive and reliable method for preserving donor hearts during a short time period (4–6 h). As a result of generally good outcomes, it is the current standard of care. However, cold storage cannot completely block metabolism within the graft. A low-level but persistent anaerobic metabolism persists within the heart at even low temperatures (Buckberg et al. 1977; Parolari et al. 2002). As a consequence, myocytes and endothelial cells within the graft are damaged by hypoxia, adenosine triphosphate (ATP) depletion, increased acidosis, up-regulation of cytokines and adhesion molecules and depletion of anti-oxidants. This injury is mainly responsible for early graft dysfunction, evidenced by the need for significant inotropic or mechanical support after transplantation (Segovia et al. 1998). Early graft dysfunction appears in 10–25% of cardiac transplants. Patients requiring post-operative mechanical support have significantly increased mortality (Segovia et al. 1998; Lima et al. 2006); in fact, early graft failure is accountable for 40% of early deaths after heart transplantation (International Society for Heart and Lung Transplant. Overall heart and adult heart transplant statistics). This makes the need for better preservation techniques even more imperative when considering the use of hearts from marginal donors that are likely to be at higher risk for developing primary graft dysfunction.

14.3
Rationale of Continuous Machine Perfusion

It may seem logical that a system that provides continuous circulation of oxygenated blood or preservation solution to the explanted donor heart may reduce damage during transport and storage.

The oxygenated blood or solution should allow ongoing aerobic metabolism in the heart, and lead to better preservation of cellular ATP stores and potentially better preservation of membrane conditions. In addition, the continuous perfusion will wash out metabolites that accumulate during the ischemic process such as lactate or adenosine. Lactate accumulation in the heart has been associated with impaired ventricular performance after ischemia in several models and adenosine, resulting from breakdown of ATP, may have deleterious effects upon reperfusion by serving as a substrate for free radical generation through the xanthine oxidase pathway (Rosenbaum et al. 2008a, b; Neely and Grotyohann 1984; Rao et al. 2001a, b; Abd-Elfattah et al. 1998a, b). Finally, machine perfusion systems can precisely control the temperature of the circulating solution and the myocardium, avoiding myocyte damage arising from very low temperatures that are frequently seen with static (ice chest) storage (Hendry et al. 1989). As a result, providing an ongoing supply of oxygenated substrate to the myocardium will diminish the ischemic burden to the heart, reduce reperfusion injury, and avoid thermal damage.

There is also some suggestion that grafts that sustain less early ischemic damage (including endothelial injury) have other long-term benefits and may be subjected to a lower incidence of chronic rejection or cardiac allograft vasculopathy (Valentine 2003). Although encouraging, this possibility remains to be established.

14.4
History

It is interesting to note that the procurement of the donor heart for the first successful human heart transplant was done using a system that enabled the graft to remain perfused with donor blood for most of the storage interval, despite the fact that donor and recipient were located in adjacent operating rooms (Barnard 1967). This donor heart was not removed until cardiac activity had ceased (i.e. a non-heart beating donor), a factor that may have played a role in the choice of the preservation method.

14.5
History of Normothermic Oxygenated Blood Perfusion

The first description of ex vivo autoperfusion for heart-lung preservation occurred as early as 1969 from Robiscek's group (Robiscek et al. 1969; Tam et al. 1969). In these experiments preservation times of 2–6 h were examined and showed no evidence of myocardial ischemia. Hemodynamic and histological observations suggested that myocardial perfusion with blood by this technique was satisfactory even without exogenous substrates or medications. Cooper and colleagues used the same technology to test myocardial viability of resuscitated hearts after 30 min of anoxic arrest (Cooper 1975a, b; Cooper 1977). In 1985, Morimoto and coworkers used a modified version of the Robiscek model to extend preservation to 8 h in lungs and 12 h in hearts (Morimoto et al. 1984; Stewart et al. 1985). The first clinical use of autoperfusion was by the Pittsburgh group of Griffith and Hardesty (Hardesty and Griffith 1987). In 1987, they reported on 14 donor heart-lung blocks that were successfully preserved by autoperfusion (Hardesty and Griffith 1987). Ten patients survived the peri-operative period and had adequate graft function. Further studies, however, showed problems of hemolysis, substrate depletion and contamination in long-term support (Ladowski et al. 1985; Kontos et al. 1987, 1988a, b; Adachi et al. 1987; Ueda et al. 1987; Miyamoto et al. 1988; Muskett et al. 1988; Naka et al. 1989). Moreover, portability problems and the complexity of autoperfusion systems have prevented more broad uptake and use. Prieto and coworkers (Prieto et al. 1988a, b) tested ex vivo multiple organ preservation using normothermic autoperfusion with whole blood. Initially, problems with edema and organ damage occurred; however, improved surgical technique, pharmacologic management, and chamber development resulted in improved results (Prieto et al. 1988a, b). Riveron (Riveron et al. 1988) showed that substrate infusion (15% dextrose, 4.25% amino acids, 8 mEq magnesium sulfate, 30 IU/dl insulin, and 10% lipids) could improve results in the autoperfusion setting. Chien et al. developed a multiorgan autoperfusion system that could preserve organs for 48 h without damage. This group also reported successful lung transplantation in canines after 24 h of autoperfusion (Chien et al. 1988, 1989, 1991a, b, 1997). Hassanein et al. (1998) were the first to report of a portable perfusion apparatus that could preserve donor hearts in a beating state with warm oxygenated blood. They showed less acidosis and myocardial edema, together with better metabolic, contractile and vasomotor function in the blood perfused group compared to a group preserved with University of Wisconsin (UW) solution in a cold static environment (Hassanein et al. 1998 47). Based on these studies, the device was further improved and has become the first commercially available perfusion system for donor heart preservation. The Organ Care System (OCS) by Transmedics has been designed to minimize time dependent ischemia and reperfusion injury by perfusing the heart with warm oxygenated donor blood supplemented with a solution that replenishes nutrients and other blood components necessary for heart function (Transmedics 2009).

14.6
History of Hypothermic Oxygenated Blood Perfusion

Two years before the first successful cardiac transplantation, Levy et al. (1965) were the first to describe an ex vivo continuous technique for cardiac preservation by using an oxygenator, with hearts being perfused for 11 hours (Levy et al. 1965). In 1966, Manax et al. were able to prolong preservation up to 72 h by using hyperbaric oxygenation, hypothermia and substrate substitution (Manax et al. 1966). However, the technical settings were extreme complex and it was controversial to use high pressures in a hypothermic setting. Two years later, Proctor and Parker (1968) reported an outstanding study with hypothermic continuous perfusion, where a mechanical pump was used to perfuse the aortic root. Although the group considered using blood or plasma, they decided to work with Krebs-Henseleit solution (good buffering capacity) because the potential risk of viscosity of blood at low temperatures outweighed its value as nutritional and gas exchange media. The perfusate was mixed with sub-physiologic calcium concentrations, dextran (to increase oncotic pressure), insulin and hydrocortisone. The entire circuit was stored for 72 h in a refrigerator at a constant temperature of 5°C. Afterwards the hearts were flushed with modified Krebs solution at 20°C and 35°C. These hearts were then tested for their mechanical performance and electrical activity after transplantation in the heterotopic position. The mechanical performance and histologic appearance of perfusion preserved hearts were virtually identical to fresh control hearts. This landmark investigation by Proctor and Parker laid the blueprint for future cardiac preservation perfusion circuits. These results also demonstrated the power of perfusion techniques for the long-term preservation of cardiac allografts.

Further investigation into perfusion preservation technique, however, was largely absent for a decade until, in 1981 and 1982, Wicomb et al. (1982a, b, 1984) reported ex vivo functional evaluation of pig or baboon hearts after 24 h of continuous hypothermic perfusion preservation Subsequently, in 1984, they reported on heterotopic heart transplantation in four human patients after continuous hypothermic perfusion preservation of the donor hearts in a portable perfusion system for ex vivo periods ranging from 7 to 16 h (Wicomb et al. 1984). Three of the four patients survived for at least 3 months, although long-term survival was not reported. In two patients, initially poor donor heart function was followed by donor heart recovery within 1 day. A third patient experienced irreversible rejection of the heart after 5 days. However, the fourth patient experienced immediate and excellent donor heart function; on publication, this patient's heart had been functioning well for 15 months (Wicomb et al. 1984).

Following these reports, research groups started to compare perfusion preservation to cold static perfusion. All could demonstrate better protection with continuous perfusion in terms of function, metabolism and vascular integrity (measured by water content) (Wicomb et al. 1982a, b; Spray et al. 1960; Kioka et al. 1986; Ohtaki et al. 1996; Calhoon et al. 1996; Nickless et al. 1998a, b); moreover, there was less histologic damage (Spray et al. 1960).

14.7
Machine Perfusion Systems

A number of new and promising studies using machine heart perfusion have emerged over the past decade, and some attempts are currently being made to translate this technology to patients. In the following sections, the two main philosophies of machine perfusion – hypothermic and normothermic perfusion – will be discussed. In hypothermic perfusion, a non-beating heart is perfused with cold substrate-enriched oxygenated perfusion solution whereas, in normothermic perfusion, a beating heart is perfused with warm, substrate-enriched oxygenated blood.

The following sections describe the working concept, perfusate composition, mechanisms of protection, potential advantages and disadvantages of these two technologies. Furthermore, clinical data in cardiac, as well as other solid organ transplantation, will be reviewed.

14.8
Hypothermic Oxygenated Blood Perfusion

14.8.1
Cold Perfusion Concept and Mechanism of Protection

Donor hearts undergo cardioplegic arrest and are connected to the perfusion machine. Flow- and pressure-controlled cold oxygenated preservation solution is pumped into the coronaries. During perfusion, the heart remains in diastolic arrest.

The mechanism of benefit for hypothermic continuous perfusion preservation is thought to be "reduction of myocardial energy requirements, the supply of oxygen and substrate to meet basal aerobic metabolic demands, and the washout of metabolic products" (Cobert et al. 2008).

14.8.2
Perfusion Route

All experimental setups have used a connector to the ascending aorta of the graft. Via this connector the aorta is perfused retrogradely, providing continuous antegrade coronary perfusion. After perfusion of the heart, the perfusate drains (via the coronary sinus) into the organ storage chamber. Over the last decade experimental settings were refined and perfusion machines have been redesigned and reduced in size. Two companies have produced small portable devices that will be clinically tested in cardiac transplantation in the near future (Organ Transport Systems 2009; Organ Recovery Systems 2009).

14.8.3
Perfusion Pressure and Flow

Toledo-Pereyra and associates (Toledo-Pereyra et al. 1979) reported that canine hearts perfused at a systolic pressure of 25 mm Hg had both better perfusion and transplantation results than hearts perfused at 50 or 80 mmHg and did better than simple hypothermically stored hearts or fresh allografts. Other studies have used aortic pressures of 5 mm Hg to 15 or 20 mm Hg (Gohra et al. 1989; Ohtaki et al. 1996). Overall, perfusion pressures of 15–30 mm Hg are probably best; lower perfusion pressure leads to a decreased oxygen supply to the myocardium, whereas pressures that are too high cause damage to the capillary beds and lead to edema. (Kioka et al. 1986).

Currently, however, most systems use flow measurement that allows a coronary flow of between 30 and 50 ml/h (or 10 ml/100 g/min). Peltz et al. (2008) demonstrated increasing tissue perfusion with flows up to 15 ml/100 g/min. Perfusion at lower flow rates resulted in decreased capillary flow and greater non-nutrient flow, whereas increased tissue perfusion correlated with lower myocardial lactate accumulation but greater edema (Peltz et al. 2008). Ozeki et al. (2007) demonstrated excellent results with a modification of perfusion. Machine perfusion was performed with continuous 15 mm Hg aortic pressure, which could induce coronary flow of 80 ml/h at 4–6°C, and with a transient increase in temperature of the perfusate to 25°C for 30 min at the initiation of perfusion followed by return to 4–6°C for the remaining interval (Ozeki et al. 2007). Earlier studies (Tveita et al. 1999) have shown midrange temperatures reduce the tendency for vasospasm and allow for endothelial dependent vasodilatation in perfused hearts.

14.8.4
Perfusate Oxygenation

Although the ideal partial pressure of oxygen for optimal support of aerobic metabolism has not been established, it is generally understood that an adequate oxygen supply is one of the major factors contributing to improved preservation of the donor heart (Smulowitz et al. 2000). Oxygen pressure varies from 250 mm Hg to between 500 and 700 mm Hg during perfusion preservation (Gohra et al. 1989; Ohtaki et al. 1996). However, experimental evidence shows that functional, biochemical, and structural alterations that follow reoxygenation are similar to changes that follow reperfusion after ischemia (Buckberg 1995). Only a few studies have examined the effect of supraphysiologic oxygenation on perfused organs (Steinberg et al. 1991; Ledingham et al. 1988).

Modern devices (LifeCradle [Organ Transport Systems, Inc, Frisco, TX, USA] and Heart Transporter [OrganRecovery Systems; Des Plaines IL, USA]) are equipped with bubble oxygenators with pO_2 levels aimed between 200 and 400 mmHg (Organ Transport Systems 2009; Organ Recovery Systems 2009).

14.8.5
Perfusate Composition

The earliest perfusion preservation experiments used simple crystalloid solutions as perfusate, such as Krebs-Henseleit buffer solution containing half the physiologic calcium concentration (Proctor and Parker 1968). Although experimental evidence suggests the superiority of perfusion preservation with simple crystalloid solutions over a standard immersion technique, considerable effort has been spent to modify existing solutions or find alternatives to crystalloid solutions that might offer the potential for better cardiac preservation. Smulovitz reviewed different potential perfusate compositions that might have a positive impact on machine perfusion (Smulowitz et al. 2000). Most recent studies have described the use of extracellular solutions (e.g. Celsior, Genzyme, Cambridge, MA, USA) for machine preservation (Koike et al. 2003; Poston et al. 2004; Peltz et al. 2005, 2008; Nameki et al. 2006; Rosenbaum et al. 2007, 2008a, b; Collins et al. 2008), with only one study examining the intracellular UW solution (Oshima et al. 2005). The high potassium levels (125 mmol/l) of UW solution might be associated with vasoconstriction during coronary perfusion and endothelial dysfunction (Koike et al. 2003; Tsutsumi et al. 2001; He 1997) leading to inhomogeneous tissue perfusion (Ozeki et al. 2007; Rosenbaum et al. 2007; Garcia-Poblete et al. 1998; Koike et al. 2007; Tveita et al. 1999).

14.8.6
Effects of Hypothermic Oxygenated Perfusion Tested in Transplant Models

The historical development of hypothermic perfusion has been described above. Most recent work in this area has come from two centres – one in Japan and the other in USA. In Japan, a group lead by Matsumoto and Morishita have reported on early graft function and histologic examination in hearts from non-heart beating canine donors (Koike et al. 2003; Nameki et al. 2006; Oshima et al. 2005). They compared cold organ storage for 4 h against 1 h of coronary perfusion with Celsior, followed by 3 h of cold preservation. Recovery of cardiac output was significantly faster and higher in the perfusion group, with the cold storage group having higher tissue water content and more histopathological damage after transplantation (Koike et al. 2003). Subsequent studies (Oshima et al. 2005) showed an improvement in early graft function if an anti-inflammatory agent (FR167653) was used during the 12-hour perfusion period with UW solution. Hemodynamic recovery was significantly higher in the treatment group and TNF-α levels from coronary sinus were significantly lower after reperfusion; however, both treated and untreated groups showed well-protected myofilaments in ultrastructural measurements (Oshima et al. 2005). Recently, they demonstrated that a short-term perfusion following cold static preservation may provide satisfactory results, compared to continuous perfusion in long-term heart preservation (Nameki et al. 2006).

In the USA, Jessen and colleagues (Rosenbaum et al. 2007, 2008a, b) used the Life-Cradle device to examine canine and pig transplant models for analysis of early graft function after 4 h of machine perfusion compared to cold static preservation. Donor hearts sustained less functional impairmen and, lower tissue lactate accumulation without increasing myocardial edema after storage with continuous perfusion (Rosenbaum et al. 2007, 2008a, b).

14.8.7
Advantages of Hypothermic Oxygenated Perfusion

The strengths of the cold oxygenated machine perfusion approach is the potential to increase transportation time for cardiac transplantation. Improved hemodynamics and endothelial function, reduced myocardial acidosis, energy utilisation, apoptosis and oxidative/ischemia-reperfusion injury might result from even long term machine perfusion. Finally, machine perfusion systems can precisely control the temperature of the circulating solution and the myocardium and may avoid myocyte damage arising from very low temperatures that are frequently seen with static (ice chest) systems (Hendry et al. 1989).

14.8.8
Disadvantages of Hypothermic Oxygenated Perfusion

One potential disadvantage is the risk of edema development during the perfusion interval. Some experimental studies report an increase in heart weight or water content with machine perfusion (Poston et al. 2004; Fitton et al. 2004; Nickless et al. 1998a, b; Ferrera et al. 1993). Water content can increase by up to 40% over a 12-h period of hypothermic perfusion in a preservation device (Ferrera et al. 1994). Multiple factors are likely involved, including perfusate composition, perfusion pressure, and flow rates. Perfusion at higher flow rates through the myocardium appears to increase the risk of myocardial edema development (Peltz et al. 2005). Therefore, device manufacturers look for the ideal flow rate and find a balance between sufficient oxygen and substrate supply and a minimized risk of developing myocardial edema. In addition, the composition of the preservation solution is likely to have a substantial impact on myocardial edema development and vasoconstriction. Lastly, this technology is more expensive than cold static preservation, especially if additional procurement team members are needed.

14.8.9
Clinical Data

In cardiac transplantation, there are currently no clinical studies in human hearts using mechanical cardiac perfusion. However, a recent clinical trial in renal transplantation has proven less delayed graft function and better one-year survival in the machine perfusion group (Moers et al. 2009). Based on these encouraging results, clinical trials with hypothermic perfusion might soon be started in cardiac transplantation.

14.9
Normothermic Oxygenated Blood Perfusion

14.9.1
Working Concept and Mechanisms of Protection

Donor hearts undergo cardioplegic arrest and are then connected to the perfusion machine. Flow-, pressure- and temperature-controlled oxygenated preservation solution (mostly blood) is pumped into the coronaries. The mechanism of protection of normothermic continuous perfusion is thought to be homogenous distribution of substrate and oxygen with minimization of edema through better oncotic pressure, which should maintain the heart in a more physiological state.

14.9.2
Perfusion Route

Historically, heart-lung blocs were used for perfusion. Lungs were ventilated and blood was pumped from the aorta to a bag, where it was collected and re-infused into the upper vena cava. Currently, one such system has been used successfully in clinical application (Organ Care System, Transmedics, Andover, MA, USA) (Transmedics 2009). Hearts are connected to the machine via the aorta, and another cannula is placed into the pulmonary artery. Both venae cavae are closed and blood is pumped retrogradely into the aorta and flows antegrade into the coronaries (resting mode), similar to the Langendorff perfusion mode. The blood is then drained via the coronary sinus to the right atrium and then circulated via the pulmonary artery to an oxygenator and a blood reservoir. From there, a pulsatile pump moves the blood through a blood warmer back to the aorta. The machine can also be used to perfuse the heart in the working mode (similar to the ejecting isolated heart, described by Neely) (Neely et al. 1967). In this mode, the blood flows into the left atrium and is pumped by the heart into the aorta. The blood flows through the aortic connector into the machine and is collected in the blood reservoir. A variable clamp mimics afterload, the coronary arteries are drained as described above.

In experimental settings, different designs have been published over the last years. Hassanein and colleagues used a working heart model, as described above

(Hassanein et al. 1998). Rao used tepid blood perfusion in an arrested heart, with a configuration similar to cold perfusion (Rao et al. 1997, 2001a, b), whereas Hirota and coworkers used cardiolpulmonary bypass in a mixed resting/working mode setting for non-heart beating donation (Hirota et al. 2006). Other groups have used tepid or normal temperatures in a resting mode model (Hirota et al. 2006; Jones et al. 2001, 2003; Aupperle et al. 2007a, b; Garbade et al. 2008; Osaki et al. 2006).

14.9.3
Perfusion Pressure and Flow

Hassanein showed that pig hearts developed excellent cardiac function with warm oxygenated blood. He used the working mode in an experimental setting (Hassanein et al. 1998). Left ventricular pressure was 77 ± 29 mm Hg and coronary perfusion pressure was 52 ± 6 mm Hg during the perfusion period of 12 h. Other groups used pressures between 20 and 90 mm Hg without finding a perfect pressure that fits all systems (Rao et al. 2001a, b; Jones et al. 2003; Aupperle et al. 2007a, b; Osaki et al. 2006).

In the clinical setting with the Organ Care System (OCS), the target pressures in resting mode are between 40 and 60 mm Hg. The pump flow is 0.7 L/min. Pressure and flow can be used to detect problems associated with heart pathology. In working mode the pump flow is increase to 2–4 L/min depending on volume of the blood in the system.

14.9.4
Perfusate Oxygenation

As described earlier, there is no clear evidence for the ideal oxygen pressure for optimal aerobic metabolism; however, all groups target oxygen pressure between 200 and 600 mm Hg (Hassanein et al. 1998; Jones et al. 2001, 2003). Only warm perfusion after non-heart beating donation use lower oxygenation pressures (80 mm Hg) according to earlier studies that report a better myocardial protection in this setting (Cope et al. 1996). The OCS uses a membrane oxygenator and targeted pO_2 levels of 200–600 mm Hg (up to 20 h).

14.9.5
Perfusate Composition

Almost all studies with normothermic perfusion have used donor blood or a combination of donor blood, crystalloid solutions and substrates. Hypometabolic polyethylene glyconated bovine hemoglobin perfusate (PEG-Hb) has been reported (Jones et al. 2001, 2003), using moderate hypothermia (20°C) and a heart rate of 40 beats per minute. PEG-Hb solution affords a mechanism for oxygen delivery, and preferentially remains in the vascular space secondary to its size, structure and oncotic nature (Conover et al. 1998; Tsai and Intaglietta 2002 Mar). PEG-Hb was favoured due to its acelluar nature, making it interesting for prolonged periods of perfusion.

The main problems of long-term perfusion with normothermic perfusion are: hemolysis, inflammation, substrate depletion and contamination. Different pump types and cannulas have been evaluated to reduce the risk of hemolysis (Hassanein et al. 1998; Rao et al. 1997; Hirota et al. 2006; Jones et al. 2001, 2003; Aupperle et al. 2007a, b; Garbade et al. 2008; Osaki et al. 2006). There have been reports of adverse interactions between blood and the synthetic surface of extracorporeal circuits (Menasché 1995), therefore all studies use anti-inflammatory drugs, mostly steroids, during perfusion. Similarly, contamination has been shown to be a problem in the early experience of autoperfusion (Ladowski et al. 1985; Kontos et al. 1987, 1988a, b; Adachi et al. 1987; Ueda et al. 1987; Miyamoto et al. 1988; Muskett et al. 1988; Naka et al. 1989), and hence all studies use antibiotic prophylaxis in their perfusion systems.

Although it is thought that blood has the best ability to protect the heart during perfusion, long-term support is associated with substrate depletion, which has a negative impact on preservation (Ladowski et al. 1985; Kontos et al. 1987, 1988a, b; Adachi et al. 1987; Ueda et al. 1987; Miyamoto et al. 1988; Muskett et al. 1988; Naka et al. 1989). Today, most experimental long-term perfusion settings have a number of different substrates added to the perfusion (electrolytes, glucose, buffer systems, substances that influence oncotic perfusion pressure). Hassanein used 1,500–2,000 ml of fresh homologous blood after 6 h of perfusion (Hassanein et al. 1998). The OCS uses 1,000–1,500 ml of donor blood that is collected through the aorta just before cardioplegic arrest of the heart in the donor. The blood is heparinized and infused into the OCS via a leucocyte-depleting filter. The OCS is primed with a crystalloid solution that contains steroids, substrates, electrolytes and buffers. After starting the preservation perfusion, another solution (that includes insulin, low dose epinephrine and adenosine) is slowly infused into the system. Based on the blood gases examined during the machine perfusion, different drugs or electrolytes can be added to the system.

14.9.6
Effects of Normothermic Oxygenated Perfusion Tested in Transplant Models

Rao and associates (Rao et al. 2001a, b) using their mild hypothermic system, demonstrated that pig-hearts that were perfused with donor blood and insulin had a better recovery after transplantation than hearts perfused only with blood. However, the studies were conducted in a non-heart beating condition and hearts were put on ice during perfusion.

In a non-heart beating donor condition (30 min warm ischemia), Osaki et al. (2006) showed that pig-hearts recovered significantly better if they were perfused with luke-warm blood cardioplegic solution at 40 mm Hg for 20 min. Hearts were implanted while being perfused and beating (Osaki et al. 2006).

14.9.7
Advantages of Normothermic Oxygenated Perfusion

The main advantage of normothermic perfusion with a beating heart is significant reduction of ischemic time. By perfusing the donor heart with warm oxygenated donor blood throughout transport and assessment, the OCS system demonstrated (for the first time) the ability to limit ischemia time to <90 min regardless of the transport distance or time to transplant. In the PROTECT-I trial, it was demonstrated that cold ischemic times were reduced to 76 min with an average total extracorporeal time of 4.9 ± 0.8 h.

Other beneficial factors are a better distribution of the substrate, minimization of edema and an almost normal physiological condition of the heart during perfusion (Hassanein et al. 1998). One of the most important benefits is that organ function can be evaluated ex-vivo. In two cases during the trials, previously undiagnosed, hidden pathologies were uncovered using the OCS. These pathologies would have resulted in potentially fatal consequences using cold ischemic preservation. Lastly, therapeutic interventions to optimize donor heart function ex-vivo are possible during perfusion if blood analysis or hemodynamic data show pathologic results.

14.9.8
Disadvantages of Normothermic Oxygenated Perfusion

The OCS is the first machine perfusion system that is commercially available, therefore it is very expensive. Hospital authorities might be reluctant to invest in a new technology without extensive testing in trials and economic analysis. Another disadvantage is the requirement of donor blood. Treatment of donors is not uniformly performed in donor hospitals. High vasopressor- or inotropic-drug support, low hematocrit or potential contamination by abdominal perfusion are risks for perfusion of the heart on the OCS. Lastly, the difference in metabolism of a heart that is hypothermic and arrested versus warm and beating significantly influences the engineering demands of machine perfusion with a more complex device design increasing the risk of malfunction.

14.9.9
Clinical Data

The OCS (Transmedics, Andover, MA, USA) has been tested in two trials, one in Europe (PROTECT-1) and one in the USA (PROCEED), and was proven to be well designed, effective and not prone to malfunction.

The PROTECT-I trial in Europe evaluated the safety and performance of the OCS^{TM} for the maintenance of hearts for use in transplantation (Tenderich et al. 2008). The trial was a prospective, multi-center study, and the primary endpoint of the trial was 7-day patient survival, which was 100%. In addition, 30-day patient survival, 7-day organ, or graft, survival and 30-day graft survival were all also 100%. Twenty patients from four centers were included in the trial. Two other procedures were excluded by trial design. Nineteen patients could be weaned off bypass at the first attempt. One patient was weaned at the second attempt. No Patient developed primary graft dysfunction. Median time on ventilator and stay in intensive care unit were 10.7 h and 24 h, respectively. Six serious events were recorded during the trial; none was associated with the use of the OCS^{TM}.

The PROCEED trial included 15 patients from four US-centers (McCurry et al. 2008). The primary endpoint was again 7-day survival. The secondary endpoints of the clinical feasibility phase of the trial were 30-day patient survival, 30-day graft survival, physiologic functioning state of the heart during transport in the OCS™ as evaluated by heart rate, coronary flow, aortic root pressure and lactate levels, and incidence of all serious adverse events through 30 days after transplantation or, if later, hospital discharge. In addition to these endpoints, the sponsor collected data regarding post-transplant care and related costs. Of the 15 patients enrolled in the pilot trial, five patients experienced a serious adverse event, one of which consisted of poor heart function resulting in patient death. The other patients who experienced a serious adverse event, in some cases with additional medical therapy, recovered without any ongoing medical complications resulting from the serious adverse events. Thirty-day survival for the 15 patients involved in the pilot study was 93%.

As of December 31, 2008, the overall experience worldwide consists of 84 hearts were maintained and assessed on the OCS (68 in Europe and 16 in the US), 75 patients were transplanted using hearts maintained on the OCS (60 in Europe and 15 in the US). In addition, nine hearts were turned down for heart transplantation after assessment on the OCS revealed significant pathologies that were not detected in the donor. Had these donor hearts been transplanted, the post-transplant clinical outcomes of the recipients would have been compromised. An analysis of the clinical outcomes of these patients demonstrates the following key clinical benefits of the OCS:

1. Excellent clinical outcomes after heart transplantation
2. Significantly reduced cold ischemic time, the major known risk factor impacting short- and long-term outcomes after heart transplantation
3. For the first time, ex-vivo assessment of donor hearts was enabled, potentially eliminating the risk of transplanting diseased hearts that result in poor outcomes
4. The ability to transplant hearts that normally go unutilized when cold ischemic preservation is used, resulting in better utilization of donor organs and the potential to expand the number of successful transplants.

14.10
Conclusion

Cold storage causes damage to the donor heart regardless of preservation strategy, only the degree of injury varies. Good quality grafts tolerate preservation periods of 4–6 h, while marginal grafts probably should be implanted much earlier. Unfortunately, the number of good quality donors has decreased over the last decade. Old age, hypertrophic myocardium, cerebral vascular accident and high inotropic support before procurement are all factors that increase the risk for primary graft dysfunction after transplantation, especially with longer ischemic times. Machine perfusion might be beneficial in such cases. Moreover, with warm oxygenated beating heart perfusion, pathologies undetected before procurement might be discovered and detrimental outcome prevented. With more knowledge on machine perfusion interventional therapies to treat pathologies might be applied (coronary artery disease) to reduce the risk for patients. Better early protection might attenuate the development of graft vasculopathy (Schmauss and Weis 2008).

Machine perfusion may permit longer preservation intervals allowing greater mobility of the heart between centers. Moreover, organ utilization may be improved as more available organs may now be within range of more seriously ill recipients. The coordination of the transplant operation may be simplified if a safe, longer storage interval can be assured, as organs could be harvested even when the preoperative recipient preparation is not completed. Organs that arrive in the operating room when there is still a need for surgical dissection or setup may be at a reduced risk of ischemic damage.

Finally, another potential benefit of machine perfusion may be the ability to expand the donor pool to non-heart beating donors. Early reports have been encouraging in carefully selected patients (Whiting et al. 2006; Boucek et al. 2008). Although non-heart beating donation has not achieved significant use in cardiac transplantation, machine perfusion would appear to offer the best opportunity to allow attempts at "resuscitation" of ischemically injured hearts including those from non-heart beating donation donors. Early experimental results in animal models have provided encouraging data that this may become a reality (Koike et al. 2003; Osaki et al. 2006). This may then allow more patients with end-stage heart disease to receive the life-saving therapy of cardiac transplanation.

References

Abd-Elfattah AS, Jessen ME, Lekven J, et al (1998) Myocardial reperfusion injury. Role of myocardial hypoxanthine and xanthine in free radical-mediated reperfusion injury. Circulation 5(Pt 2):III224–III235.

Abd-Elfattah AS, Jessen ME, Lekven J, Wechsler AS (1998) Differential cardioprotection with selective inhibitors of adenosine metabolism and transport: role of purine release in ischemic and reperfusion injury. Mol Cell Biochem 180:179–189.

Adachi H, Fraser CD, Kontos GJ, Borkon AM, Hutchins GM, Galloway E, Brawn J, Reitz BA, Baumgartner WA (1987) Autoperfused working heart-lung preparation versus hypothermic cardiopulmonary preservation for transplantation. J Heart Transplant 6(5):253–260.

Aupperle H, Garbade J, Ullmann C, Krautz C, Barten MJ, Dhein S, Schoon HA, Gummert FJ. (2007) Ultrastructural findings in porcine hearts after extracorporeal long-term preservation with a modified Langendorff perfusion system. J Vet Med A Physiol Pathol Clin Med 54(5):230–237.

Aupperle H, Garbade J, Ullmann C, Schneider K, Krautz C, Dhein S, Gummert JF, Schoon HA. (2007) Comparing the ultrastructural effects of two different cardiac preparation- and perfusion-techniques in a porcine model of extracorporal long-term preservation. Eur J Cardiothorac Surg 31(2):214–221.

Banner NR, Thomas HL, Curnow E, Hussey JC, Rogers CA, Bonser RS (2008) Steering Group of the United Kingdom Cardiothoracic Transplant Audit. The importance of cold and warm cardiac ischemia for survival after heart transplantation. Transplantation 86(4):542–547.

Barnard CN (1967) The operation: a human cardiac transplant. S Afr Med J 41:1271–1274.

Buckberg GD, Brazier JR, Nelson RL, Goldstein SM, McConnell DH, Cooper N (1977) Studies of the effects of hypothermia on regional myocardial blood flow and metabolism during cardiopulmonary bypass. I. The adequately perfused beating, fibrillating, and arrested heart. J Thorac Cardiovasc Surg 73:87–94

Boucek MM, Mashburn C, Dunn SM, Frizell R, Edwards L, Pietra B, Campbell D (2008) Denver Children's Pediatric Heart Transplant Team. Pediatric heart transplantation after declaration of cardiocirculatory death. N Engl J Med 359(7):709–714.

Buckberg GD (1995): Studies of hypoxemic/reoxygenation injury: Linkage between cardiac function and oxidant damage. J Thorac Cardiovasc Surg 110: 1164–1170

Calhoon JH, Bunegin L, Gelineau JF, et al (1996): Twelve-hour canine heart preservation with a simple, portable, hypothermic organ perfusion device. Ann Thorac Surg 62: 91–93.

Chien S, Diana JN, Oeltgen PR, Todd EP, O'Connor WN, Chitwood WR Jr. (1989) Eighteen to 37 hours' preservation of major organs using a new autoperfusion multiorgan preparation. Ann Thorac Surg 47(6):860–867.

Chien S, Diana JN, Todd EP, O'Connor WN, Marion T, Smith K (1988) New autoperfusion preparation for long-term organ preservation. Circulation 78(5 Pt 2):III58–II165.

Chien S, Maley R, Oeltgen PR, O'Connor W, Wu G, Zhang F, Salley RK. (1997) Canine lung transplantation after more than twenty-four hours of normothermic preservation. J Heart Lung Transplant 16(3):340–351.

Chien S, Oeltgen PR, Diana JN, Shi X, Nilekani SP, Salley R. (1991) Two-day preservation of major organs with autoperfusion multiorgan preparation and hibernation induction trigger. A preliminary report. J Thorac Cardiovasc Surg 102(2):224–234.

Chien SF, Diana JN, Oeltgen PR, Salley R. (1991) Functional studies of the heart during a 24-hour preservation using a new autoperfusion preparation. J Heart Lung Transplant. 10(3):401–8.

Cobert ML, West LM, Jessen ME (2008) Machine perfusion for cardiac allograft preservation. Curr Opin Organ Transplant 13(5):526–530

Collins MJ, Moainie SL, Griffith BP, Poston RS. (2008) Preserving and evaluating hearts with ex vivo machine perfusion: an avenue to improve early graft performance and expand the donor pool. Eur J Cardiothorac Surg 34(2):318–325.

Conover C, Linberg R, Lejeune L, Gilbert C, Shum K, Shorr RG. (1998) Evaluation of the oxygen delivery ability of PEG-hemoglobin in Sprague Dawley rats during hemodilution. Artif Cells Blood Subst Immobil Biotechnol 26(2):199–212.

Cooper DK (1975) Donor heart resuscitation and storage. Surg Gynecol Obstet 140(4):621–31.

Cooper DK (1975) Haemodynamic studies during short-term preservation of the autoperfusing heart-lung preparation. Cardiovasc Res 9(6):753–763.

Cooper DK (1977) The Haematoxylin-basic Fuchsin-picric acid staining reaction as a test of myocardial viability in resuscitated and preserved hearts. Histochem J 9(3):285–291.

Cope JT, Mauney MC, Banks D, Binns OA, De Lima NF, Buchanan SA, Shockey KS, Wilson SW, Kron IL, Tribble CG. (1996) Controlled reperfusion of cardiac grafts from non-heart-beating donors. Ann Thorac Surg 62(5):1418–1423.

Ferrera R, Larese A, Marcsek P, et al. (1994) Comparison of different techniques of hypothermic pig heart preservation. Ann Thorac Surg 57:1233–1239.

Ferrera R, Marcsek P, Larese A, et al. (1993) Comparison of continuous microperfusion and cold storage for pig heart preservation. J Heart Lung Transplant 12:463–469.

Fitton TP, Lin R, Bethea BT, et al. (2004) Impact of 24 h continuous hypothermic perfusion on heart preservation by assessment of oxidative stress. Clin Transplant 18:22–27.

Garbade J, Krautz C, Aupperle H, Ullmann C, Lehmann S, Kempfert J, Borger MA, Dhein S, Gummert JF, Mohr FW. (2008) Functional, metabolic, and morphological aspects of continuous, normothermic heart preservation: effects of different preparation and perfusion techniques. Tissue Eng Part A. Dec 30.

Garcia-Poblete E, Alvarez L, Fernandez H, Escudero C, Torralba A. (1998) Cape Town solution in prolonged myocardial preservation: structural and ultrastructural study. Histol Histopathol 13:21–27.

Gohra H, Mori F, Esato K: (1989) The effect of fluorocarbon emulsion on 24-hour canine heart preservation by coronary perfusion. Ann Thorac Surg 48 96–103.

Goldsmith KA, Demiris N, Gooi JH, Sharples LD, Jenkins DP, Dhital KK, Tsui SS (2009) Life-years gained by reducing donor heart ischemic times. Transplantation 87(2):243–248.

Hardesty RL, Griffith BP (1987) Autoperfusion of the heart and lungs for preservation during distant procurement. J Thorac Cardiovasc Surg 93(1):11–18.

Hassanein WH, Zellos L, Tyrrell TA, Healey NA, Crittenden MD, Birjiniuk V, Khuri SF. (1998) Continuous perfusion of donor hearts in the beating state extends preservation time and improves recovery of function. J Thorac Cardiovasc Surg 116(5):821–830.

He GW. (1997) Hyperkalemia exposure impairs EDHF-mediated endothelial function in the human coronary artery. Ann Thorac Surg 63:84–87.

Hendry PJ, Walley VM, Koshal A, et al. (1989) Are temperatures attained by donor hearts during transport too cold? J Thorac Cardiovasc Surg 98:517–522.

Hirota M, Ishino K, Fukumasu I, Yoshida K, Mohri S, Shimizu J, Kajiya F, Sano S. (2006) Prediction of functional recovery of 60-minute warm ischemic hearts from asphyxiated canine non-heart-beating donors. J Heart Lung Transplant 25(3):339–344.

International Society for Heart and Lung Transplant. Overall heart and adult heart transplant statistics [slide 56]. [Updated 2008]. Available from www.ishlt.org/registries/slides.asp?slides=HeartLungRegistry.

Jones BU, Serna DL, Beckham G, West J, Smulowitz P, Farber A, Kahwaji C, Connolly P, Steward E, Purdy RE, Milliken JC. (2001) Recovery of cardiac function after standard hypothermic storage versus preservation with Peg-hemoglobin. ASAIO J 47(3):197–201.

Jones BU, Serna DL, Smulowitz P, Connolly P, Farber A, Beckham G, Shrivastava V, Kahwaji C, Steward E, Purdy RE, Parker WL, Ages B, Milliken JC. (2003) Extended ex vivo myocardial preservation in the beating state using a novel polyethylene glycolated bovine hemoglobin perfusate based solution. ASAIO J 49(4):388–394.

Kioka Y, Tago M, Bando K, et al (1986) Twenty-four hour isolated heart preservation by perfused method with oxygenated solution containing perfluorochemicals and albumin. J Heart Transplant 5: 437–443.

Kirklin JK, Naftel DC, Bourge RC, McGiffin DC, Hill JA, Rodeheffer RJ, Jaski BE, Hauptman PJ, Weston M, White-Williams C (2003) Evolving trends in risk profiles and causes of death after heart transplantation: a ten-year multi-institutional study. J Thorac Cardiovasc Surg 125(4):881–890.

Koike N, Takeyoshi I, Ohki S, Tsutsumi H, Matsumoto K, Morishita Vohringer M, Mahrholdt H, Yilmaz A, Sechtem U. (2007) Significance of late gadolinium enhancement in cardiovascular magnetic resonance imaging (CMR). Herz 32:129–137.

Koike N, Takeyoshi I, Ohki S, Tsutsumi H, Matsumoto K, Morishita Y. (2003) The effect of short-term coronary perfusion using a perfusion apparatus on canine heart transplantation from non-heart- beating donors. J Heart Lung Transplant 22(7):810–817.

Kontos GJ Jr, Adachi H, Borkon AM, Cameron DE, Baumgartner WA, Hall TS, Hutchins G, Brawn J, Reitz BA (1987) Successful four-hour heart-lung preservation with core-cooling on cardiopulmonary bypass: a simplified model that assesses preservation. J Heart Transplant 6(2):106–111.

Kontos GJ Jr, Borkon AM, Baumgartner WA, Hutchins GM, Peeler M, Brawn J, Reitz BA. (1988) Neurohumoral modulation of the pulmonary vasoconstrictor response in the autoperfused working heart-lung preparation during cardiopulmonary preservation. Transplantation 45(2):275–279.

Kontos GJ Jr, Borkon AM, Baumgartner WA, Fonger JD, Hutchins GM, Adachi H, Galloway E, Reitz BA (1988) Improved myocardial and pulmonary preservation by metabolic substrate enhancement in the autoperfused working heart-lung preparation. J Heart Transplant 7(2):140–144.

Ladowski JS, Kapelanski DP, Teodori MF, Stevenson WC, Hardesty RL, Griffith BP (1985) Use of autoperfusion for distant procurement of heart-lung allografts. J Heart Transplant 4(3):330–333.

Ledingham SJ, Braimbridge MV, Hearse DJ (1988) Improved myocardial protection by oxygenation of St. thomas' Hospital cardioplegic solutions. Studies in the rat. J Thorac Cardiovasc Surg 95:103–111

Levy JF, Bernard HR, Monafo WF (1965) Isolation and storage of artificially oxygenated mammalian hearts. JAMA 191: 1006.

Lima B, Rajagopal K, Petersen RP, Shah AS, Soule B, Felker GM, Rogers JG, Lodge AJ, Milano CA (2006) Marginal cardiac allografts do not have increased primary graft dysfunction in alternate list transplantation. Circulation 114:I27–132.

Manax WG, Largiader F, Lillehei RC (1966) Whole canine organ preservation: Prolongation in vitro by hypothermia and hyperbaria. JAMA 196: 1121–1124.

Marasco SF, Esmore DS, Richardson M, Bailey M, Negri J, Rowland M, Kaye D, Bergin PJ (2007) Prolonged cardiac allograft ischemic time–no impact on long-term survival but at what cost? Clin Transplant 21(3):321–329.

McCurry K, Jeevanandam V, Mihaljevic T, et al. (2008) Prospective multi-center safety and effectiveness evaluation of the Organ Care System device for cardiac use (PROCEED). J Heart Lung Transplant 27: 166.

Menasché P. (1995) The inflammatory response to cardiopulmonary bypass and its impact on postoperative myocardial function. Curr Opin Cardiol 10(6):597–604

Miyamoto Y, Lajos TZ, Bhayana JN, Bergsland J, Celik CF (1988) Beneficial effects of prostaglandin E1 on autoperfused heart-lung preservation. J Heart Transplant 7(2):135–139.

Moers C, Smits JM, Maathuis MH, Treckmann J, van Gelder F, Napieralski BP, van Kasterop-Kutz M, van der Heide JJ, Squifflet JP, van Heurn E, Kirste GR, Rahmel A, Leuvenink HG, Paul A, Pirenne J, Ploeg RJ. (2009) Machine perfusion or cold storage in deceased-donor kidney transplantation. N Engl J Med 360(1):7–19.

Morgan JA, John R, Weinberg AD, Kherani AR, Colletti NJ, Vigilance DW, Cheema FH, Bisleri G, Cosola T, Mancini DM, Oz MC, Edwards NM (2003) Prolonged donor ischemic time does not adversely affect long-term survival in adult patients undergoing cardiac transplantation. J Thorac Cardiovasc Surg 126(5):1624–1633.

Morimoto T, Golding LR, Stewart RW, Harasaki H, Matsushita S, Shimomitsu T, Kasick J, Olsen E, Loop FD, Nose Y (1984) A simple method for extended heart-lung preservation by autoperfusion. Trans Am Soc Artif Intern Organs 30:320–324.

Muskett A, Burton NA, Grossman M, Gay WA Jr (1988) The rabbit autoperfusing heart-lung preparation. J Surg Res 44(2):104–108.

Naka Y, Hirose H, Matsuda H, Shirakura R, Miyagawa S, Fukushima N, Kawashima Y. (1989) Prevention of pulmonary edema developing in autoperfusing heart-lung preparation by leukocyte depletion. Eur J Cardiothorac Surg 3(4):355–358.

Nameki T, Takeyoshi I, Oshima K, Kobayashi K, Sato H, Matsumoto K, Morishita Y. (2006) A comparative study of long-term heart preservation using 12-h continuous coronary perfusion versus 1-h coronary perfusion following 11-h simple immersion. J Surg Res 135(1):107–112.

Neely JR, Libermeister H, Battersby EJ, Morgan HE (1967) Effect of pressure development on oxygen consumption by isolated heart. Am J Physiol Heart Cic Physiol 291: 255–256

Neely JR, Grotyohann LW. (1984) Role of glycolytic products in damage to ischemic myocardium. Circ Res 55:816–824.

Nickless DK, Rabinov M, Richards SM, Conyers RAJ, Rosenfeldt FL (1998) Continuous perfusion improves preservation of donor rat hearts: Importance of the implantation phase. Ann Thorac Surg 65: 1255–1272.

Nickless DK, Rabinov M, Richards SM, et al. (1998) Continous perfusion improves preservation of donor rat hearts: Importance of the implantation phase. Ann Thorac Surg 65:1265–1272.

Ohtaki A, Ogiwara H, Kazuhiro S, Takahashi T, Morishita Y: (1996) Long-term heart preservation by the combined method of simple immersion and coronary perfusion. J Heart Lung Transplant 15: 269–274,

Organ Recovery Systems. Trials. Des Plaines, IL: Organ Recovery Systems. [Updated 2009] Available from http://www.organ-recovery.com/home.php

Organ Tranport Systems. Research. Frisco, TX: Organ Transport Systems, Inc. [Updated 2009] Available from http://allezoe.com/default.aspx

Osaki S, Ishino K, Kotani Y, Honjo O, Suezawa T, Kanki K, Sano S. (2006) Resuscitation of non-beating donor hearts using continuous myocardial perfusion: the importance of controlled initial reperfusion. Ann Thorac Surg 81(6):2167–2171.

Oshima K, Takeyoshi I, Mohara J, Tsutsumi H, Ishikawa S, Matsumoto K, Morishita Y. (2005) Long-term preservation using a new apparatus combined with suppression of pro-inflammatory cytokines improves donor heart function after transplantation in a canine model. J Heart Lung Transplant 24(5):602–608.

Ozeki T, Kwon MH, Gu J, Collins MJ, Brassil JM, Miller Jr MB, Gullapalli RP, Zhuo J, Pierson 3rd RN, Griffith BP, Poston RS. (2007) Heart preservation using continuous ex vivo perfusion improves viability and functional recovery. Circ J 71:153–159.

Parolari A, Rubini P, Cannata A, Bonati L, Alamanni F, Tremoli E, Biglioli P (2002) Endothelial damage during myocardial preservation and storage. Ann Thorac Surg 73(2):682–690.

Peltz M, Cobert ML, Rosenbaum DH, West LM, Jessen ME. (2008) Myocardial perfusion characteristics during machine perfusion for heart transplantation. Surgery 144(2):225–232.

Peltz M, He TT, Adams GA IV, Koshy S, Burgess SC, Chao RY, Meyer DM, Jessen ME. (2005) Perfusion preservation maintains myocardial ATP levels and reduces apoptosis in an ex vivo rat heart transplantation model. Surgery 138(4):795–805.

Poston RS, Gu J, Prastein D, Gage F, Hoffman JW, Kwon M, Azimzadeh A, Pierson RN 3rd, Griffith BP. (2004) Optimizing donor heart outcome after prolonged storage with endothelial function analysis and continuous perfusion. Ann Thorac Surg 78(4):1362–1370

Prieto M, Androne PA, Baron P, Gomez-Fleitas M, Runge WA, Jamieson SW, Kaye MP. (1988) Multiple organ retrieval and preservation with normothermic autoperfusion. Transplant Proc 20(5):827–828.

Prieto M, Baron P, Andreone PA, Runge WJ, Edwards B, Jamieson SW, Kaye MP. (1988) Multiple ex vivo organ preservation with warm whole blood. J Heart Transplant 7(3):227–237.

Proctor E, Parker R (1968) Preservation of isolated heart for 72 hours. Br Med J 4 296–298.

Rao V, Feindel CM, Cohen G, Borger MA, Ross HJ, Weisel RD. (2001) Effects of metabolic stimulation on cardiac allograft recovery. Ann Thorac Surg 71(1):219–225.

Rao V, Feindel CM, Weisel RD, Boylen P, Cohen G. (1997) Donor blood perfusion improves myocardial recovery after heart transplantation. J Heart Lung Transplant 16(6):667–673.

Rao V, Ivanov J, Weisel RD, et al (2001) Lactate release during reperfusion predicts low cardiac output syndrome after coronary bypass surgery. Ann Thorac Surg 71:1925–1930.

Riveron FA, Ross JH, Schwartz KA, Casey G, Sanders O, Eisiminger R, Magilligan DJ Jr. (1988) Energy expenditure of autoperfusing heart-lung preparation. Circulation 78(5 Pt 2): III103–III109.

Robicsek F, Tam W, Daugherty HK, Robiscok LK (1969) The stabilized autoperfusing heart-lung preparation as a vehicle for extracorporeal preservation. Transplant Proc 1(3):834–839.

Rosenbaum DH, Peltz M, DiMaio JM, et al (2008) Perfusion preservation vs. static preservation for cardiac transplantation: effects on myocardial function and metabolism. J Heart Lung Transplant 27:93–99.

Rosenbaum DH, Peltz M, DiMaio JM, Meyer DM, Wait MA, Merritt ME, Ring WS, Jessen ME. (2008) Perfusion preservation versus static preservation for cardiac transplantation: effects on myocardial function and metabolism. J Heart Lung Transplant 27(1):93–99.

Rosenbaum DH, Peltz M, Merritt ME, Thatcher JE, Sasaki H, Jessen ME. (2007) Benefits of perfusion preservation in canine hearts stored for short intervals. J Surg Res 140 (2):243–249.

Russo MJ, Chen JM, Sorabella RA, Martens TP, Garrido M, Davies RR, George I, Cheema FH, Mosca RS, Mital S, Ascheim DD, Argenziano M, Stewart AS, Oz MC, NakaY (2007) The effect of ischemic time on survival after heart transplantation varies by donor age: an analysis of the United Network for Organ Sharing database. J Thorac Cardiovasc Surg 133(2):554–559.

Schmauss D, Weis M. (2008) Cardiac allograft vasculopathy: recent developments. Circulation 117 (16):2131–2141

Segovia J, Pulpon LA, Sanmartin M, Tejero C, Serrano S, Burgos R, Castedo E, Ugarte J (1998) Primary graft failure in heart transplantation: a multivariate analysis. Transplant Proc 30:1932.

Smulowitz PB, Serna DL, Beckham GE, Milliken JC. (2000) Ex vivo cardiac allograft preservation by continuous perfusion techniques. ASAIO J 46(4):389–396.

Spray TL, Watson DC, Roberts WC: (1960) Morphology of canine hearts after 24 hours' preservation and orthotopic transplantation. J Thorac Cardiovasc Surg 73: 880–886.

Steinberg JB, Doherty NE, Munfakh NA, Geffin GA, Titus JS, Hoaglin DC, Denenberg AG, Daggett WM (1991) Oxygenated cardioplegia: the metabolic and functional effects of glucose and insulin Ann Thorac Surg. 51(4): 620–629

Stewart R, Morimoto T, Golding L, Harasaki H, Olsen E, Nose Y (1985) Canine heart-lung autoperfusion. Trans Am Soc Artif Intern Organs 31:206–210.

Tam W, Robicsek F, Daugherty HK (1969) The autoperfusing heart-lung preparation: a vehicle for the preservation of the resuscitated cadaver heart. J Thorac Cardiovasc Surg 58(6):879–885

Taylor DO, Edwards LB, Aurora P, Christie JD, Dobbels F, Kirk R, Rahmel AO, Kucheryavaya AY, Hertz MI (2008) Registry of the International Society for Heart and Lung Transplantation: twenty-fifth official adult heart transplant report–2008. J Heart Lung Transplant 27(9):943–956.

Tenderich G, Tsui S, El-Banayosy A, et al. (2008) The 1-year follow-up results of the PROTECT patient population using the Organ Care System. J Heart Lung Transplant 27: 166.

Toledo-Pereyra LH, Chee M, Lillehei RC: (1979) Effects of pulsatile perfusion pressure and storage on hearts preserved for 24 hours under hypothermia, for transplantation (Abstract). Ann Thorac Surg 27: 24–31.

Transmedics. Heart transplantation. Andover, MA: Transmedics, Inc. [Updated 2009] Available from http:\\www.transmedics.com.

Tsai AG, Intaglietta M. (2002) The unusual properties of effective blood substitutes. Keio J Med 51 (1):17–20.

Tsutsumi H, Oshima K, Mohara J, Takeyoshi I, Aizaki M, Tokumine M, Matsumoto K, Morishita Y. (2001) Cardiac transplantation following a 24-h preservation using a perfusion apparatus. J Surg Res 96:260–267.

Tveita T, Hevroy O, Refsum H, Ytrehus K. (1999) Coronary endothelium-derived vasodilation during cooling and rewarming of the in situ heart. Can J Physiol Pharmacol 77:56–63.

Ueda K, Hatanaka M, Kyo S, Takamoto S, Yokote Y, Arima T, Yamashina M, Omoto R (1987) Effect of prostacyclin analog on pulmonary edema in isolated heart-lung autoperfusion model. J Heart Transplant 6(3):155–161.

Valentine H. (2003) Cardiac allograft vasculopathy: central role of endothelial injury leading to transplant 'atheroma'. Transplantation 76:891–899

Whiting JF, Delmonico F, Morrissey P, et al. (2006) Clinical results of an organ procurement organization effort to increase utilization of donors after cardiac death. Transplantation 81:1368–1371.

Wicomb W, Boyd ST, Cooper DK, Rose AG, Barnard CN: (1981) Ex vivo functional evaluation of pig hearts subjected to 24 hours' preservation by hypothermic perfusion. S Afr Med J 60 245–248.

Wicomb W, Cooper DK, Hassoulas J, Rose AG, Barnard CN: (1982) Orthotopic transplantation of the baboon heart after 20 to 24 hours' preservation by continuous hypothermic perfusion with an oxygenated hyperosmolar solution. J Thorac Cardiovasc Surg 82:133–140.

Wicomb WN, Cooper DK, Barnard CN: (1982) Twenty-four hour preservation of the pig heart by a portable perfusion system. Transplantation 34: 246–250.

Wicomb WN, Cooper DK, Novitsky D, Barnard CN: (1984) Cardiac transplantation following storage of the donor heart by a portable hypothermic perfusion system. Ann Thorac Surg 37: 243–248.

Wittwer T, Wahlers T. (2008) Marginal donor grafts in heart transplantation: lessons learned from 25 years of experience. Transpl Int 21(2):113–125.

Visualization of Cardioplegia Delivery

Lawrence S. Lee, Vakhtang Tchantchaleishvili, and Frederick Y. Chen

15.1
Introduction

Homogeneous delivery of cardioplegia to the heart is essential for myocardial protection during the ischemic cross clamp period. Inadequate cardioplegia is a known and recognized cause of delayed postoperative ventricular recovery. In current clinical practice, however, cardioplegia delivery is performed in an essentially blind manner by surgeons. The surgeon knows neither the anatomic distribution nor the adequacy of the cardioplegia administered. Experimentally and in rare clinical practices, cardioplegia efficacy has been assessed by indirect methods such as myocardial temperature and pH measurement, electrocardiographic monitoring, and coronary venous blood sampling. These methods, however, have significant limitations and shortcomings that have prevented their widespread adoption in clinical practice – they are either too invasive, not consistently reliable, or not feasible in real-time. In addition, these methods rely on sampling only several points within the myocardium. These samples may or may not be representative of the remaining myocardium. As such, surgeons today do not have a truly objective means to assess either the distribution or the efficacy of the cardioplegia they administer and are forced to rely on experience and judgment.

Thus, a substantial clinical need exists for more accurate and efficient cardioplegia delivery. Though several methods of cardioplegia monitoring have been developed and are gaining increasing attention, the most promising method currently under investigation utilizes the actual *visualization* of cardioplegia itself to achieve these aims. The fundamental principle underlying these techniques is the use of a contrast agent admixed with the cardioplegia solution and then visualizing the contrast agent. We describe two such techniques in this chapter.

L.S. Lee, V. Tchantchaleishvili, and F.Y. Chen
Division of Cardiac Surgery, Brigham and Women's Hospital, Harvard Medical School, 75 Francis Street, Boston, MA 02115, USA
e-mail: fchen@partners.org

15.2
Myocardial Contrast Echocardiography (MCE)

15.2.1
Background

Myocardial contrast echocardiography (MCE) is a rapidly evolving technique that is currently used in a number of clinical applications and settings to assess myocardial blood flow. One area of investigation is the intraoperative use of MCE to evaluate the adequacy of cardioplegia delivery. The underlying premise of MCE is the use of an ultrasonic contrast agent in conjunction with simultaneous two-dimensional echocardiographic imaging. The ultrasonic contrast agent, typically composed of gas microbubbles, causes an acoustic mismatch at the air-liquid interface in the myocardial circulation. This, in turn, increases the echocardiographic intensity of myocardium receiving perfusion. The direct visualization of such areas is therefore possible.

Direct imaging of myocardial perfusion using contrast echocardiography was first reported in 1980, when myocardial opacification was seen after injection of contrast agent into the coronary circulation (DeMaria et al. 1980). MCE was used intraoperatively in humans for the first time in 1984 during a coronary artery bypass graft surgery to estimate areas of hypoperfused myocardium and thereby direct the sequence of bypass grafting (Goldman and Mindich 1984). Improvements to MCE techniques and technology since then have allowed MCE to evolve into an effective method to assess intraoperative myocardial perfusion.

15.2.2
Characteristics of Ultrasound Contrast Agents

All forms of MCE rely on the fact that gas microbubbles in the blood are strong reflectors of ultrasonic signals. Reflectivity of a microbubble is substantially greater than that of tissue, and therefore, it creates a highly reflective target that can be detected by ultrasound. This applies to the simplest contrast agent, agitated saline, as well as to other modern, commercially available perfluorocarbon-based agents.

The earliest contrast agents for MCE included saline, diatrizoate meglumine, hydrogen peroxide mixtures, and manufactured gelatin microspheres. These compounds resulted in contrast bubbles that were relatively large (up to 100 µm in diameter) and did not traverse the capillary bed, thereby making it difficult to assess perfusion of the myocardial tissue itself (Kaul et al. 1987). The introduction in 1983 of a technique known as sonication allowed the production of much smaller contrast microbubbles (4–5 µm in diameter) that were capable of capillary transit (Feinstein et al. 1984). This technique provided the basis that ultimately led to the development of modern contrast agents.

Sonication is the exposure of a liquid media (most commonly, phospholipid, albumin, or synthetic polymer solution) to high-energy sound waves that transform the gas present in the solution (air, SF_6, C_3F_8, or other perfluorocarbons) into microbubbles and embeds them within the medium (Feinstein et al. 1984). The size and quantity of these microbubbles can be adjusted during the sonication process by altering the type of liquid media, the ultrasound energy level, and the duration of exposure to the sound waves. High-molecular weight gases such as perfluorocarbons are advantageous because of their low solubility in water and their resultant low diffusion rates, which increase contrast stability and duration of echogenicity. The newer contrast agents are constructed with a thin deformable shell made of various components (albumin, phospholipids, sugars, biopolymers). The presence of a shell stabilizes the microbubbles against dissolution and increases bubble elasticity, resulting in varying acoustic resonance frequencies. The half-life of these agents varies significantly and is influenced by several factors, including the composition of the microbubbles, the surrounding liquid media, and the ultrasound imaging method applied (Villarraga et al. 1996).

While the large size of the earliest microbubbles precluded their use as effective myocardial contrast agents, modern microbubbles are no larger than erythrocytes. As a result, these microbubbles are able to travel through capillaries and exhibit kinetic properties that are similar to red blood cells in the microcirculation. These agents also generally do not interact with or adhere to the vascular lining under normal physiologic conditions (Keller et al. 1989; Jayaweera et al. 1994). However, there have been reports of albumin microbubbles exhibiting altered behavior when used with cold hyperkalemic crystalline cardioplegia perfusion (Keller et al. 1990; Villanueva et al. 1992; Keller et al. 1991). With this cardioplegia solution these albumin microbubbles appear to interact with damaged microvascular endothelial glycocalyx, leading to a dramatic prolongation of microbubble transit time and myocardial opacification effect (Lindner et al. 1998a, b). This effect is not seen when the contrast agent is administered in a normal blood-perfused heart. Such findings suggest that certain contrast agent–endothelial interactions may influence the data obtained from MCE and that the surgeon should be aware of such potential variations should this method be used for cardioplegia visualization.

The acoustic behavior of microbubbles varies depending on the type of ultrasonic energy applied. Low magnitude ultrasound waves will induce microbubbles to oscillate and emit frequencies that are linearly related to the applied energy, while high amplitude ultrasound waves cause the microbubbles to react in a non-linear manner (de Jong et al. 2002). Depending on the specific composition of the microbubble, the frequencies emitted can range from the fundamental frequency to higher resonance frequencies such as harmonics. Newer methods for echocardiographic imaging can capitalize on such variable acoustic properties and permit the acquisition of particular types of data. Thus, understanding the behavior of microbubbles exposed to various ultrasound beams plays a key role in selecting the appropriate contrast-specific techniques required for a particular application.

15.2.3
Data Acquisition and Analysis

MCE is performed by administering the selected contrast agent simultaneously with cardioplegia solution via any of the routes by which cardioplegia is delivered. Both antegrade and retrograde approaches can be utilized with contrast agents at the discretion of the surgeon. Like conventional echocardiography, cross sectional images are then obtained using either transesophageal echocardiography or direct epicardial echocardiography. Visual inspection of the images gives rapid, qualitative information about the degree of tissue perfusion (Fig. 1). More specific regional assessment can be performed by dividing the heart into segments depending on the major coronary supply (or the distribution of the vessel where contrast agent was injected) and imaging each segment separately. This facilitates surgeon determination of the optimal route for cardioplegia delivery as well as help to evaluate the adequacy of myocardial protection after the heart is arrested. Some previous studies have shown that the use of MCE to ascertain homogeneous cardioplegia administration is associated with improved immediate postoperative cardiac function and ventricular recovery (Zaroff et al. 1994).

Assessment of cardioplegia distribution using MCE is generally a qualitative technique that is performed by visually inspecting the ultrasound images at the time of contrast agent injection. Three aspects of myocardial contrast opacification are considered: signal intensity, pattern of filling, and rate of filling. Because this is a qualitative process, the interpretation is mostly operator dependent and subjective. In the simplest analysis, the absence of contrast in the ventricular myocardium implies the absence of significant capillary level flow, and therefore inadequate cardioplegia distribution. Conversely, rapid, uniform opacification of the myocardium implies normal capillary flow and sufficient cardioplegia distribution. Intermediate levels of contrast appearance indicate varying levels of

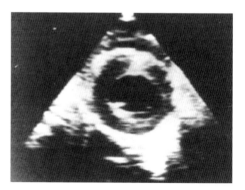

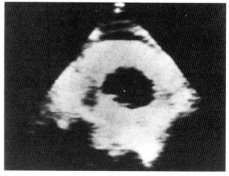

Fig. 1 Two-dimensional echocardiographic short-axis view of the left ventricle before (*top*) and after (*bottom*) intracoronary injection of a contrast agent (Sheil et al. 1996)

cardioplegia distribution, and the decision to re-administer cardioplegia solution is dependent on the interpreting surgeon.

Given the highly variable degree of cardioplegia administration associated with qualitative analysis, efforts have been made to develop quantitative methods of interpreting MCE data. Quantitative assessment of regional cardioplegia distribution would permit more accurate and normalized techniques of cardioplegia administration. In a beating heart, a bolus injection of microbubbles into a coronary artery results in a myocardial contrast effect that peaks and then gradually disappears over time. In an arrested heart, the peak intensity is less and the contrast effect is more prolonged. Based on this signal intensity, myocardial blood flow may be quantitated. One technique is to acquire sequential echocardiographic images, digitize them, and then utilize videodensitometry to calculate time intensity curves. Using these curves, computer algorithms can derive various parameters of curve width, height, and contrast washout to quantify myocardial blood flow (Lindner et al. 1998a, b; DeMaria et al. 1984; Jayaweera et al. 1990; Jayaweera and Kaul 1993; Aaronson et al. 1991; Hirata et al. 1994; Sheil et al. 1996; Porter et al. 1993; Keller et al. 1988). However, in order to apply such analysis to the arrested heart, the aortic root volume, aortic flow, cardioplegia flow, and the rate of contrast injection must remain constant so as to standardize the results. These quantitative techniques can be performed intraoperatively but require more time to complete than the qualitative approach and as such, most surgeons appear to favor the latter.

Recent advances in ultrasound image acquisition technology and instrumentation have enabled more sensitive intramyocardial detection of injected microbubbles (Porter and Xie 1995). Contrast-specific echocardiographic modes have been developed that can exploit the variable acoustic properties of microbubbles. Harmonic and pulse inversion imaging algorithms, for instance, can detect the nonlinear emission of harmonics by resonant microbubbles, which allows for significantly improved separation of true contrast echo signals from background scatter. This results in enhanced and more sensitive images for real-time visualization of myocardial perfusion (Burns 1996; Ophir and Parker 1990; Neppiras et al. 1983; Burns et al. 1992; Simpson et al. 2001).

15.2.4
Limitations

One limitation of MCE is the ephemeral stability of contrast agent microbubbles. These bubbles are sensitive to both hydrostatic and acoustic pressure, and interaction with an ultrasound beam of significant amplitude results in disruption of microbubble integrity with subsequent loss of its reflectivity. These damaged microbubbles initially emanate intense ultrasound signals followed immediately afterwards by a complete loss of signal. While certain imaging techniques intentionally induce bubble disruption in order to capture the transient echo signal, the best method to combat bubble destruction is to understand the acoustic properties of the contrast agent used and to utilize a contrast-specific imaging algorithm appropriate for the required study (Burns 2002).

Perhaps more significant, another limitation of MCE is that this technique, like other methods of echocardiography, is highly operator dependent. A substantial amount of technical skill and expertise as well as specialized imaging equipment is required for its appropriate utilization. Experience is the most effective solution to this particular issue, but not all centers may have the resources necessary to successfully apply MCE in the operating room.

15.2.5
Future Directions

As techniques of microbubbles synthesis become increasingly sophisticated and precise, attention has been focused on molecularly targeted imaging by engineering microbubbles that can localize exclusively to tissues with defined pathologic characteristics. For instance, ischemically stressed endothelial cells overexpress the vascular endothelial growth factor (VEGF) receptor, while acute myocardial ischemia-reperfusion injury is associated with upregulation of leukocyte adhesion molecules on the endothelial cell surface (Demos et al. 1999; Krieglstein and Granger 2001; Kurose et al. 1994). Specifically, the adhesion molecule P-selectin is rapidly mobilized to the endothelial surface from preformed cytoplasmic granules, followed by delayed, transcription-dependent endothelial overexpression of E-selectin, ICAM-1, and VCAM (Krieglstein and Granger 2001; Kurose et al. 1994). Investigators have hypothesized that binding of contrast agents to such adhesion molecules displayed by activated endothelial cells could be used to echocardiographically detect regions of early ischemia in the myocardium. Animal studies using microbubbles synthesized with ligands targeted to such endothelial cell surface receptors show that the identification, localization, and spatial quantification of ischemic regions is possible (Villanueva et al. 2007; Villanueva et al. 2002). Such molecularly directed targeting can allow for highly accurate detection of ischemia and help the surgeon in deciding adequacy of cardioplegia administration. Clearly, however, this approach is in its infancy and requires further investigation to become clinically viable.

15.3
Near-Infrared Fluorescence Imaging

Near-infrared (NIR) fluorescence imaging is a new optical imaging technique that has gained significant attention over the past several years as a novel method of *in vivo* visualization for different clinical scenarios, including cardiac surgery and cardioplegia administration. While MCE and NIR fluorescence imaging are similar in that both employ the injection of an exogenous contrast agent to permit visualization of the region of interest, their fundamental difference is the type of energy utilized for visualization: MCE is based on sound waves, while NIR fluorescence involves application of a specific spectrum of light.

15.3.1
Background

NIR light, electromagnetic radiation with wavelengths between 700 and 900 nm, is the spectrum of light with wavelengths too long to be detected by the human eye and yet shorter than standard infrared light. Living tissue has minimal absorbance and autofluorescence in the NIR wavelength range. This fact makes this spectrum of light particularly well suited for *in vivo* visualization. Moreover, NIR light penetrates tissue and blood with minimal alteration of tissue properties.

When NIR light encounters a fluorescent molecule, that molecule then emits a signal with spectral characteristics that can be detected with an emission filter and captured with a charge-coupled device camera. In living tissue, there are several such endogenous molecules, including hemoglobin, cytochromes, flavins, and porphyrins. However, most of these endogenous molecules generate little NIR fluorescence contrast, and exogenous contrast agents are required to perform in vivo studies for imaging, including cardioplegia and myocardial perfusion monitoring.

15.3.2
Fluorescent Dyes and Their Characteristics

The exogenous contrast agents used for NIR imaging are composed of fluorophores, molecules which absorb energy of a specific wavelength and re-emit energy at a different wavelength thereby causing the agent to become fluorescent. Fluorophores can be divided into organic and inorganic types. The amount and wavelength of the absorbed and emitted energy depend on the particular fluorophore and its surrounding environment. The most widely used organic fluorophores are the heptamethine indocyanines, which belong to the polymethines group. Peak excitation of this class is at 760–800 nm, and peak emission at 790–830 nm. Indocyanine green (ICG) is the most well studied and well known of the organic agents and has been used for more than 40 years in the clinical setting for ophthalmologic angiography, liver function testing, and cardiac output measurement (Fox et al. 1957; Flower and Hochheimer 1973). ICG is an FDA approved, partially water soluble molecule that is hepatically metabolized and has a half life of approximately 2 minutes. It is nontoxic and has an excellent safety record with minimal adverse reactions (Benya et al. 1989). Several other heptamethine fluorophores have been developed with various alterations in properties such as improved solubility and quantum yield, a measure of the efficiency with which the fluorophore emits energy (Flanagan et al. 1997; Lin et al. 2002). Some of these newer agents can be constructed with surface ligands so they can target specific molecular structures. Organic fluorophores in general have several limitations, however, including low quantum yields, difficulty controlling exact excitation and emission wavelengths, and photochemical destruction.

To counter the limitations inherent in organic fluorophores, inorganic fluorophores have been developed. Inorganic fluorophores, also called quantum dots, are semiconductor nanocrystals that are comprised of an inorganic core and shell. The properties of the core and shell affect the overall behavior of the fluorophore, most notably the emission wavelength. An outer layer of an aqueous compatible organic coating must be added in order to perform *in vivo* studies with inorganic fluorophores. Depending on the composition of the inorganic core and shell, the fluorescence emission of the fluorophore can be altered to virtually any discrete wavelength. Quantum dots absorb all wavelengths below their emission one, which allows multiple fluorophores with different fluorescent emissions to be excited by a single wavelength (Lim et al. 2003). Solubility depends on the organic outer layer covering the inorganic shell, and several different types of coatings have been described (Dubertret et al. 2003; Chan and Nie 1998; Bruchez et al. 1998; We et al. 2003). Inorganic fluorophores are remarkably resistant to photochemical destruction, and the metal shell and organic outer coating permit the conjugation of specific targeting molecules to the surface of each fluorophore. Because of the multi-layer composition, however, inorganic fluorophores are relatively large molecules, making them difficult to clear from the circulation (Frangioni 2003). This is one of the most significant current limitations precluding their widespread use in humans as a clinical tool. Inorganic fluorophores were used for vascular imaging for the first time in 2003 in an animal model (Lim et al. 2003). Although still in its infancy, NIR imaging using inorganic fluorophores is an exciting technology that holds significant promise for application in cardiac surgery.

15.3.3
Data Acquisition and Analysis

Fluorescent cardioplegia solution is produced by incorporation of a fluorescent contrast agent, either organic or inorganic, into normal cardioplegia solution. This fluorescent cardioplegia solution may then be administered via any of the routes by which cardioplegia is delivered. When the tissue is illuminated by NIR light at the excitation wavelength of the particular contrast agent present in the solution, the contrast molecules absorb the NIR light and emit fluorescence. This signal is then detected by an NIR fluorescence camera and displayed on a video monitor. Surgeons are then able to visualize the distribution of cardioplegia within the myocardium.

NIR imaging requires several electronic components for a full imaging system. Of particular importance is the selection of appropriate filters, lenses, cameras, and optical cables to ensure the adequate acquisition of images. While commercial NIR imaging systems are available, most research involving NIR imaging has utilized proprietary imaging systems assembled for particular investigational models (De Grand and Frangioni 2003; Soltesz et al. 2007; Frangioni 2003; Rangaraj et al. 2008). Fig. 2 is a schematic of one such NIR imaging system.

Since NIR light is invisible to the human eye, it is possible to irradiate a surgical field simultaneously with visible light as well as NIR light. This allows for the simultaneous acquisition of normal color video and NIR fluorescent images. The visible white light source illuminating the surgical field must be devoid of all NIR and IR light; otherwise, unwanted stimulation of the fluorophores would occur. Normal color video and the NIR images are acquired simultaneously by separate cameras specific to those wavelengths; i.e., a color camera for the visible color video and an NIR fluorescence camera for the NIR images. The images are then processed separately, and the resultant output are real-time

15 Visualization of Cardioplegia Delivery 277

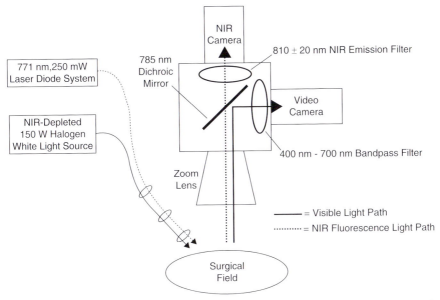

Fig. 2 Schematic of a simultaneous color video/NIR fluorescence imaging system (Nakayama et al. 2002)

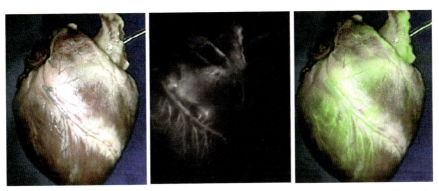

Fig. 3 Retrograde near-infrared fluorescence imaging in a sheep heart. Image corresponding to the surgical field illuminated by visible light (*left*), fluorescent signals captured by the NIR camera (*middle*), and a merged picture of the visible light and NIR images (*right*)

color and NIR images on a monitor in the operating room. These images can be viewed separately or can be merged into one image by overlaying the NIR images on the color ones (Fig. 3).

Because this process allows for real-time visualization, the images can be qualitatively assessed in the operating room to determine adequacy of cardioplegia delivery and the need to re-administer cardioplegia throughout the cross clamp period. By detecting areas of suboptimal cardioplegia distribution the surgeon can also locate regions that may be particularly prone to ischemic injury – for example, animal studies have demonstrated that NIR imaging can identify defects in distal distribution of antegrade cardioplegia due to critical coronary lesions which could be successfully addressed by administering retrograde cardioplegia (Rangaraj et al. 2008). For more precise determination of cardioplegia delivery, quantitative videodensitometric analysis can be performed. Signals from the regions of interest are transferred to a densitometer, where the optical density of the dye is measured and quantified using various software algorithms. Preliminary animal studies have shown the feasibility of such intraoperative quantification of cardioplegia delivery (Soltesz et al. 2007).

15.3.4
Limitations

The field of NIR imaging applied to cardiac surgery is advancing rapidly but is still in its early stages. The major limitations at present involve the depth of penetration of NIR light into tissue, contrast agent behavior, and the difficulty in constructing a fully operational imaging system.

The simple reflectance type of NIR imaging systems that are currently utilized have a limited depth penetration in living tissue. Because of intensity decay and scatter, any target deeper than approximately 0.5 cm may not be adequately imaged (Frangioni 2003). When applied to cardioplegia distribution, this means that NIR is able to reliably image the epicardium and the outermost myocardium but not necessarily the deeper endocardial layers. Because the endocardium is often the most vulnerable and most difficult to protect region of the heart, this is potentially a significant limitation of NIR imaging in cardioplegia. However, recent advances in optical tomographic imaging technology may allow depth penetration of up to 4 cm in the future, which would allow visualization through to the endocardium (Ntziachristos et al. 2003).

The principal limitations of current contrast agents, both organic and inorganic, have been described above. Organic fluorescent agents, while generally nontoxic, are prone to photochemical destruction and may pose difficulty with controlling excitation and emission wavelengths. The newer inorganic fluorescent agents, on the other hand, are more resistant to destruction and are easier to manipulate in terms of fluorescence emission, but are difficult to excrete from the body and have been quite toxic in animal studies. Improvement in contrast dye construction may overcome these limitations, particularly with inorganic agents, thus allowing more precise, non-toxic imaging.

Lastly, most of the NIR imaging systems have been constructed for use as investigational tools rather than for clinical use. At present, there is one commercially available, self-contained NIR imaging system that can be used intraoperatively in humans. While the first use of this product was for oncologic operations to image and highlight malignant tissue, this system has also been approved for use in visualization of coronary vasculature during coronary artery bypass surgery. Additional devices and imaging systems dedicated to cardiac surgery applications will likely follow as advances are made in this field.

15.4
The Future

Seeing is believing. Though in its infancy, imaging techniques of cardioplegia will ultimately change the way cardioplegia is delivered and administered. One can easily imagine a scenario whereby not only cardioplegia distribution is visualized, but also *myocardial ischemia*. If markers of reversible myocardial ischemia (such as lactate level) were tied into NIR, for example, then one could envision a system where the surgeon would administer cardioplegia during the clamp period, ascertain uniform and proper distribution over the entire myocardium, and then simply watch for a color changes indicating the beginning of ischemia. Once the presence of ischemia is detected, the surgeon would then administer another dose of cardioplegia. What is now performed blindly and empirically would be performed precisely and systematically.

15.5
Summary

Cardioplegia delivery is one aspect of cardiac surgery that is currently widely performed in an empiric manner. There is thus an immediate and significant need for objective methods by which adequate cardioplegia administration can be achieved. The most promising techniques involve the visualization of cardioplegia delivery via the use of contrast agents and imaging modalities. While each method discussed has inherent advantages and limitations, there has been substantial progress in recent years toward accomplishing efficacious and accurate cardioplegia administration. With technological advances incorporating molecular biological markers into contrast agents, the ultimate goal of truly precise and safe cardioplegia delivery may be possible in the near future.

References

Aaronson S, Lee BK, Weincek JG, Feinstein SB, Roizen MF, Karp RB, Ellis JE (1991) Assessment of myocardial perfusion during coronary artery bypass surgery with two dimensional transesophageal contrast echocardiography. Anesthesiology 75:433–440
Benya R, Quintana J, Brundage B (1989) Adverse reactions to indocyanine green: a case report and a review of the literature. Cathe Cardiovasc Diagn 17:231
Bruchez M Jr, Moronne M, Gin P, Weiss S, Alivisatos AP (1998) Semiconductor nanocrystals as fluorescent biological labels. Science 281:2013–2016
Burns PN (1996) Harmonic imaging with ultrasound contrast agents. Clin Radiol 51(Suppl 1):50–55
Burns PN (2002) Instrumentation for contrast echocardiography. Echocardiography 19:241–258
Burns PN, Powers JE, Fritzsch T (1992) Harmonic imaging: a new imaging and doppler method for contrast-enhanced ultrasound. (abstract) Radiology 185:142
Chan WCW, Nie SM (1998) Quantum dot bioconjugates for ultrasensitive nonisotopic detection. Science 281:2016–2018

De Grand AM, Frangioni JV (2003) An operational neari-infrared fluorescence imaging system protoype for large animal surgery. Technol Cancer Res Treat 6:553–562

De Jong N, Bouakaz A, Frinking P (2002) Basic acoustic properties of microbubbles. Echocardiography 19:229–240

DeMaria AN, Bommer WJ, Rigga K, Dejee A, Keown M, Ling Kwan O, Mason DT (1980) Echocardiographic visualization of myocardial perfusion by left heart and intracoronary injection of echo contrast agent (abstract). Circulation 60(Suppl II):II-143

DeMaria AN, Bommer WJ, Kwan OL, Riggs K, Smith M, Waters J (1984) In vivo correlation of thermodilution cardiac output and videodensitometric indicator-dilution curves obtained from contrast 2-dimensional echocardiograms. J Am Coll Cardiol 3:999–1004

Demos SM, Alkan-Onyuksel H, Kane BJ (1999) In vivo targeting of acoustically reflective liposomes for intravascular and transvascular ultrasonic enhancement. J Am Coll Cardiol 33:867–875

Dubertret B, Skourides P, Norris DJ, Noireaux V, Brivanlou AH, Libchaber A (2003) *In vivo* imaging of quantum dots encapsulated in phospholoipid micelles. Science 298:1759–1762

Feinstein SB, Ten Cate F, Zwehl W, Ong K, Maurer G, Tei C, Shah PM, Meerbaum S, Corday E (1984) Two-dimensional contrast echocardiography, I: *in vitro* development and quantitative analysis of echo contrast agents. J Am Coll Cardiol 3:14–20

Flanagan JH Jr, Khan SH, Menchen S, Soper SA, Hammer RP (1997) Functionalized tricarbocyanine dyes as near-infrared fluorescent probes for biomolecules. Bioconju Chem 8:751–756

Flower RW, Hochheimer BF (1973). A clinical technique and apparatus for simultaneous angiography of the separate retinal and choroidal circulations. Invest Ophthalmol 12:248–261

Fox IJ, Brooker LG, Heseltime DW, Essex HE, Wood EH (1957) A tricarbocyanine dye for continuous recording of dilution curves in whole blood independent of variations in blood oxygen saturation. Proc Staff Meet Mayo Clin 32:478–484

Frangioni J (2003) In vivo near-infrared fluorescence imaging. Curr Opin Chem Biol 7:626–634

Goldman ME, Mindich BP (1984) Intraoperative cardioplegic contrast echocardiography for assessing myocardial perfusion during open heart surgery. J Am Coll Cardiol 4:1029

Hirata N, Shimazaki Y, Nakano S, Sakai K, Sakaki S, Matsuda H (1994) Evaluation of regional myocardial perfusion in areas of old myocardial infarction after revascularization by means of intraoperative myocardial contrast echocardiography. J Thorac Cardiovasc Surg 108:1119–1124

Jayaweera AR, Edwards N, Glasheen WP, Villanueva FS, Abbott RD, Kaul S (1994) *In vivo* myocardial kinetics of air-filled albumin microbubbles during myocardial contrast echocardiography: comparison with radiolo-labeled red blood cells. Circ Res 74:1157–1165

Jayaweera AR, Kaul S (1993) Quantifying myocardial blood flow with contrast echocardiography. Am J Cardiac Imag 7:317–335

Jayaweera AR, Matthew TL, Sklenar J, Spotnitz WD, Watson DD, Kaul S (1990) Method for the quantitation of myocardial perfusion during myocardial contrast two dimensional echocardiography. J Am Soc Echo 3:91–98

Kaul S, Pandian NG, Guerrero JL, Gillam LD, Okada RD, Weyman AE (1987) Effects of selectively altering the collateral driving pressure on regional perfusion and function in the occluded coronary bed in the dog. Circ Res 61:77–85

Keller MW, Geddes L, Spotnitz W, Kaul S, Duling BR (1991) Microcirculatory dysfunction following perfusion with hyperkalemic, hypothermic, cardioplegic solutions and blood reperfusion. Circulation 84:2485–2494

Keller MW, Glasheen W, Smucker ML, Burwell LR, Watson DD, Kaul S (1988) Myocardial contrast echocardiography in humans. II. Assessment of coronary blood flow reserve. J Am Coll Cardiol 12:925–934

Keller MW, Segal SS, Kaul S, Duling B (1989) The behavior of sonicated albumin microbubbles within the microcirculation: a basis for their use during myocardial contrast echocardiography. Circ Res 65:458–467

Keller MW, Spotnitz WD, Matthew TL, Glasheen WP, Watson DD, Kaul S (1990) Intraoperative assessment of regional myocardial perfusion using quantitative myocardial contrast echocardiography. J Am Coll Cardiol 16:1267–1279

Krieglstein CF, Granger DN (2001) Adhesion molecules and their role in vascular disease. Am J Hypertens 14:44S–54S

Kurose I, Anderson DC, Miyasaka M, Tamatani T, Paulson JC, Todd RF, Rusche JR, Granger DN (1994) Molecular determinants of reperfusion-induced leukocyte adhesion and vascular protein leakage. Circ Res 74:336–343

Lim YT, Skim S, Nakayama A, Stott NE, Bawendi MG, Grangioni JV (2003) Selection of quantum dot wavelengths for biomedical assays and imaging. Mol Imaging 2:50–64

Lin Y, Weissleder R, Tung CH (2002) Novel near-infrared cyanine fluorochromes: synthesis, properties, and bioconjugation. Bioconjug Chem 13:605–610

Lindner JR, Firschke C, Wei K, Goodman NC, Skyba DM, Kaul S (1998) Myocardial perfusion characteristics and hemodynamic profile of MRX-115, a venous echocardiographic contrast agent, during acute myocardial infarction. J Am Soc Echocardiogr 11:36–46

Lindner JR, Ismail S, Spotnitz WD, Skyba DM, Jayaweera AR, Kaul S (1998) Albumin microbubble persistence during myocardial contrast echocardiography is associated with microvascular endothelial glycocalyx damage. Circulation 98:2187–2194

Nakayama A, del Monte F, Hajjar RJ, et al. Functional near-infrared fluorescence imaging for cardiac surgery and targeted gene therapy. Molec Imaging 2002;1:365–377

Neppiras EA, Nyborg WL, Miller PL (1983) Nonlinear behavior and stability of trapped micron-sized cylindrical gas bubbles in an ultrasound field. Ultrasonics 21:109–115

Ntziachristos V, Bremer C, Weissleder R (2003) Fluorescence imaging with near-infrared fluorescence imaging for cardiac surgery and targeted gene therapy. Eur Radiol 13:195–208

Ophir J, Parker KJ (1990) Contrast agents in diagnostic ultrasound [published erratum] Ultrasound Med Biol 16(2):209

Porter TR, D'Sa A, Turner C, Jones LA, Minisi AJ, Mohantry PK, Vetrovec GW, Nixon JV (1993) Myocardial contrast echocardiography for the assessment of coronary blood flow reserve: validation in humans. J Am Coll Cardiol 21:349–355

Porter TR, Xie F (1995) Transient myocardial contrast following initial exposure to diagnostic ultrasound pressures with minute doses of intravenously injected microbubbles: demonstration and potential mechanisms. Circulation 92:2391–2395

Rangaraj AT, Ghanta RK, Umakanthan R, Soltesz EG, Laurence RG, Fox J, Cohn LH, Bolman RM 3rd, Frangioni JV, Chen FY (2008) Real-time visualization and quantification of retrograde cardioplegia delivery using near infrared fluorescent imaging. J Card Surg 23(6):701–708

Sheil ML, Kaul S, Spotnitz WD (1996) Myocardial contrast echocardiography: development, applications, and future directions. Acad Radiol 3:260–275

Simpson DH, Burns PN, Averkiou MA (2001) Techniques for perfusion imaging with microbubble contrast agents. IEEE Trans Ultrason Ferroelectr Freq Control 48:1483–1494

Soltesz EG, Laurence RG, DeGrand AM, Cohn LH, Mihaljevic T, Frangioni JV (2007) Image-guided quantification of cardioplegia delivery during cardiac surgery. Heart Surg Forum 10: E381–E385

Villarraga HR, Foley DA, Mulvagh SL (1996) Contrast echocardiography. Tex heart Inst J 23:90–97

Villanueva FS, Klibanov A, Wagner WR (2002) Microbubble-endothelial cell interactions as a basis for assessing endothelial function. Echocardiography 19:427–438

Villanueva FS, Lu E, Bowry S, Kilic S, Tom E, Wang J, Gretton J, Pacella JJ, Wagner WR (2007) Myocardial ischemic memory imaging with molecular echocardiography. Circulation 115:345–352

Villanueva FS, Spotnitz WD, Jayaweera AR, Gimple LW, Dent J, Kaul S (1992) On-line intraoperative quantitation of regional myocardial perfusion during coronary artery bypass graft operations with myocardial contrast two-dimensional echocardiography. J Thorac Cardiovasc Surg 104:1524–1531

We X, Liu H, Liu J, Haley KN, Treadway JA, Larson JP, Ge N, Peale F, Bruchez MP (2003) Immunofluorescent labeling of cancer marker Her2 and other cellular targets with semiconductor quantum dots. Nat Biotechnol 21:41–46

Zaroff J, Aronson S, Lee BK, Feinstein SB, Walker R, Wiencek JG (1994) The relationship between immediate outcome after cardiac surgery, homogeneous cardioplegia delivery, and ejection fraction. Chest 106:38–45

Author Index

A
Aliabadi, A., 249–262

B
Barker, A., 131–140
Burki, S., 221–242

C
Chambers, D.J., 41–52, 199–213
Chen, F.Y., 269–279

D
Dietl, W., 109–125

F
Fallouh, H.B., 199–213

G
Gunnes, S., 15–35

H
Hallström, S., 145–160

J
Jynge, P., 15–35

L
Large, S., 131–140
Lee, L.S., 269–279
Levitsky, S., 73–86

M
McCully, J.D., 73–86
Mehlhorn, U., 179–192
Milasinovic, D., 221–242
Mohl, W., 221–242

P
Parker, J.A.T.C., 179–192
Podesser, B.K., 3–10, 109–125, 145–160

R
Robich, M.P., 167–174

S
Seebacher, G., 249–262
Sellke, F.W., 167–174
Sodha, N.R., 167–174
Szabó, G., 93–105

T
Tchantchaleishvili, V., 269–279
Trescher, K., 109–125

W
Wojta, J., 57–65

Z
Zuckerman, A., 249–262

Subject Index

A
Age, 73–86
Ageing,
Aortic valve replacement, 111, 117, 118, 121
Apoptosis, 44–46, 49, 52

B
Brain stem death, 133, 134, 139

C
Calcium, 180, 181, 183, 191
 channel, 200, 201, 208–210, 212
 sensitiser, 103, 105
Cardiac surgery, 63–65
Cardioplegia, 15–35, 112, 120–123, 125, 269–279
Cardioprotection, 76, 80–86
Cardiopulmonary bypass, 167–174
Cell transplantation, 228–231, 234–237
Contrast echocardiography, 270
Coronary sinus, 222–228
Cyclooxygenase endothelial derived hyperpolarizing factor, 169, 174

D
Donor heart preservation, 249–262

E
Endothelial dysfunction, 57, 58, 61, 62, 64, 65
Endothelium, 57–65
Excitation-contraction coupling, 200, 201, 208, 213

F
Frailty, 9

G
Gender, 73–86
Gene therapy,

H
Heart failure, 109, 110, 113, 114, 117, 121, 124, 125
Heart transplantation, 131–140
Hypertrophy, 41, 46, 48, 49
Hypothermic perfusion, 253, 255, 257

I
Inflammation, 57, 59–61, 63, 65
Ischemia, 16, 18, 21, 23–29, 31–34, 41–52, 111, 113, 120–123
Ischemia/reperfusion, 74–76, 80, 83, 85

M
Metabolism, 16, 23, 25, 27, 31, 32, 34, 36
Microarray, 86
Mitochondria, 42–44, 46–50
Mitral valve replacement, 119
30d Mortality, 6
Myocardial infarction, 94
Myocardial protection, 110, 120, 121, 221–242

N
Near-infrared fluorescence imaging, 274, 277
Necrosis, 42, 44, 45, 52
Nitric oxide (NO), 57, 58, 61, 62, 64, 65, 168, 173, 174, 180, 182
 direct and indirect donors, 146, 148
 homeostasis, 146, 150–152, 154, 156, 159, 160
 ischemia/reperfusion, 146, 151, 160
 myocardial protection, 159, 160
 pathway, 146–148
Normothermic perfusion, 253, 258, 259

O
Organ preservation, 136
Outcome, 5–9

P

Pathophysiology, 94, 95, 99, 110, 111, 125
Perfluorocarbons, 270, 271
Polarized cardiac arrest, 204, 206, 208, 213
Pressure, 252–254, 257–259, 261

R

Reactive oxygen species (ROS), 179–185
Reperfusion, 16, 19, 21, 22, 26, 27, 29–35, 41–44, 47–49, 51
Resuscitation, 23
Retrograde cardioplegia, 222, 224, 225, 239–241

Right ventricle, 93–99
ROS. *See* Reactive oxygen species

S

Scavengers, 171–192
Sodium and potassium channel, 200–203, 212
Stunning, 75

V

Vascular dysfunction, 167, 170–172
Visualization, 269–279

About the Editors

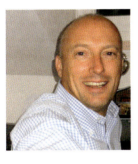

Dr. Bruno K. Podesser is Associate Professor of Surgery at the Department of Cardiac Surgery at the Landesklinikum St. Pölten, Austria. He is member of the Board of Directors of the Ludwig Boltzmann Cluster for Cardiovascular Research at the Medical University of Vienna, Austria. His research interests include myocardial protection, with particular emphasis on cardioplegic solutions. He has been at the Medical University of Vienna since 1991. In 1996 and 1997 he was working with Professor Carl S. Apstein at Boston University, Boston, USA. His current research interests focus on the preservation of endothelial function as an important aspect of myocardial protection. He enjoys golf and gardening.

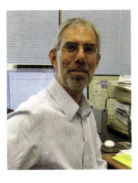

Dr. David Chambers is a Consultant Clinical Scientist and Director of Research for Cardiac Surgery at St. Thomas' Hospital (Guy's & St. Thomas' NHS Foundation Trust), London, UK. His research interests include myocardial protection, with particular emphasis on cardioplegic solutions. He has been at St. Thomas' since 1978, originally working with Mr Mark Braimbridge and Professor David Hearse, on the clinical and experimental development of the St. Thomas' Hospital cardioplegic solution. His current research interests focus on investigations into alternative cardioplegic solutions that induce a polarised, rather than depolarised, arrest. He enjoys golf and has recently started skiing.

Printing: Ten Brink, Meppel, The Netherlands
Binding: Stürtz, Würzburg, Germany